"Critical scholars approach com̲̲̲̲̲̲̲̲̲̲̲̲̲̲̲̲̲̲̲̲̲̲̲̲ as praxis—analytically and ethically interrogating the conditions that shape human suffering. This volume confronts the silences and inequalities that perpetuate systemic harm in health contexts, asking: Why do we accept such injustice? And how can we, as scholars and practitioners, demand and enact something better?"

Elaine Hsieh, *University of Minnesota, USA*

"*Critical Health Communication: Theory and Practice* explores how power, politics, and culture are entwined in all aspects of current health communication research, filling a much-needed gap in understanding current health issues. Bridging patients, professionals, and policy, it reveals the urgent need for conducting critical research to transform health communication—and ultimately, health outcomes—worldwide."

Kathryn Greene, *Rutgers University, USA*

CRITICAL HEALTH COMMUNICATION

This book offers strong rationales for adopting a critical view of health communication by demonstrating how theories and critical practices can be enriched by foregrounding issues of power, politics, and culture.

In health communication, critical approaches highlight the role of communication in constituting, reinforcing, and resisting inequitable power relations that underlie the sociocultural and structural barriers to well-being. This book highlights the theoretical and practical contributions of critical health communication to allow readers to gain in-depth understanding of the tools and methods required to conduct critical research. It includes a broad array of approaches to health communication scholarship such as rhetorical, feminist, anti-racist, and intersectional perspectives. Chapters present research from a variety of international and local contexts addressing medical and public health challenges and center issues of power, resistance, voice, and social change from marginalized perspectives.

Outlining the centrality of critical approaches to theorizing and practicing health communication in more equitable, ethical, and effective ways, this book will be of interest to scholars and graduate students in health communication, critical and cultural communication, as well as other health-related courses.

Shaunak Sastry is Professor of Communication in the School of Communication, Film, & Media Studies and Provost's Fellow at the University of Cincinnati, USA. Dr. Sastry is the second Vice-President of the National Communication Association (NCA). His award-winning health communication research has been funded by the National Institutes of Health, and he currently is Co-Principal Investigator and co-lead of the Community Engagement Core of the Cincinnati Center for Climate Change and Health. He is also a former Senior Editor of the journal *Health Communication* and sits on the editorial board of several leading academic journals.

Heather M. Zoller is a Professor in the School of Communication, Film, & Media Studies at the University of Cincinnati, USA. She is the Editor-in-Chief of the *Journal of Applied Communication Research* and former Senior Editor at *Health Communication*. She co-edited *Emerging Perspectives in Health Communication: Meaning, Culture, & Power* (Routledge, 2008) and serves on the National Academies of Sciences, Engineering, and Medicine Committee on PPE with NIOSH.

Ambar Basu is a Professor in the Department of Communication at the University of South Florida, USA. He is a co-editor of *Post-AIDS Discourse in Health Communication* (Routledge, 2021). He has served as Senior Editor for *Health Communication*, and he co-edits a Routledge book series titled *Critical Cultural Studies in Global Health Communication*.

CRITICAL HEALTH COMMUNICATION

Theory and Practice

Edited by
Shaunak Sastry, Heather M. Zoller,
and Ambar Basu

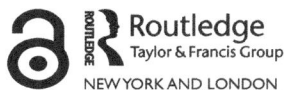
NEW YORK AND LONDON

Designed cover image: Irfan Ibrahim

First published 2026
by Routledge
605 Third Avenue, New York, NY 10158

and by Routledge
4 Park Square, Milton Park, Abingdon, Oxon, OX14 4RN

Routledge is an imprint of the Taylor & Francis Group, an informa business

© 2026 selection and editorial matter, Shaunak Sastry, Heather M. Zoller, and Ambar Basu; individual chapters, the contributors

The right of Shaunak Sastry, Heather M. Zoller, and Ambar Basu to be identified as the authors of the editorial material, and of the authors for their individual chapters, has been asserted in accordance with sections 77 and 78 of the Copyright, Designs and Patents Act 1988.

The Open Access version of this book, available at www.taylorfrancis.com, has been made available under a Creative Commons Attribution-NonCommercial-NoDerivatives (CC BY-NC-ND) 4.0 International license.

Any third party material in this book is not included in the OA Creative Commons license, unless indicated otherwise in a credit line to the material. Please direct any permissions enquiries to the original rightsholder.

For Product Safety Concerns and Information please contact our EU representative GPSR@taylorandfrancis.com. Taylor & Francis Verlag GmbH, Kaufingerstraße 24, 80331 München, Germany.

Trademark notice: Product or corporate names may be trademarks or registered trademarks, and are used only for identification and explanation without intent to infringe.

ISBN: 9781032730752 (hbk)
ISBN: 9781032725536 (pbk)
ISBN: 9781003426530 (ebk)

DOI: 10.4324/9781003426530

Typeset in Sabon
by codeMantra

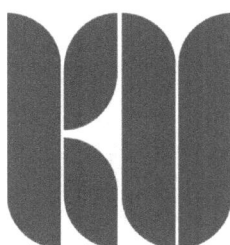

An electronic version of this book is freely available, thanks to the support of libraries working with Knowledge Unlatched (KU). KU is a collaborative initiative designed to make high quality books Open Access for the public good. The Open Access ISBN for this book is 9781003426530. More information about the initiative and links to the Open Access version can be found at www.knowledgeunlatched.org.

CONTENTS

List of Figures xi
List of Contributors xiii
Acknowledgments xxiii

1 Introduction 1
  Shaunak Sastry, Heather M. Zoller, and Ambar Basu

Critiquing Dominant Discourses **29**

2 From Symptoms to Transformation: Addressing the Root Causes of Hunger Through Critical Health Communication 31
  Rebecca de Souza

3 Reproductive Injustice, Feminicides, and the Intersections of Critical Health Communication and Journalism Praxis 56
  Leandra H. Hernández

4 God, Country, and Family: A Risk Orders Theory Approach to Deconstructing Health Messages About Family Planning in the Latine Community 75
  Kimberly Field-Springer and Julee Tate

5 Communicating Structural Violence: A Case Study of Entertainment Establishment Women Workers in Kathmandu, Nepal 96
Iccha Basnyat

Advocacy, Activism, and Social Change 113

6 Critical Pragmatism and the Politics of the Possible: Communicating for Critically Holistic Health in the Workplace and Beyond 115
Heather M. Zoller

7 HIV Interventions, Collectivization Efforts, and Citizenship on the Margins of the State in India 138
Shamshad Khan

8 Navigating the Terrain: Applying Critical Health Communication Methods to Participatory Action Praxis with Black Women Farmers 158
Andrew Carter

Critical Methods in Health Communication Research and Practice 183

9 Biocriticism in a Time of Precarity: Inventional Resources for Critical Health Communication 185
Lisa Keränen, Liliane Campos, and Jennifer Malkowski

10 Culture-Centered Approach as Critical Health Practice: The Body as Resistance 210
Mohan Dutta, Satveer Kaur-Gill, Pankaj Baskey, Selina Metuamate, Indranil Mandal, and Venessa Pokaia

11 Decolonizing Health Communication: Reflections on Critical Health Communication Research in Nigeria 231
C. T. Adebayo, O. O. Olusanya, and O. E. Ambrose

12 Journeys in Critical Health Communication:
   Meditations on Being/Becoming CCA Scholars   245
   Balkisa M. Sissy, Usman Bah,
   Yixuan Qi, and Shaunak Sastry

13 New Light: Critical Health Communication and
   Connections to Experiences from the Field   261
   Urmi Basu, Ambar Basu, Mavis Freeman Essel,
   and Roopam Mishra

   Index   277

FIGURES

9.1 *Masques virus* © Marie-Sarah Adenis, 2021
 (carbon fiber, beads and wire). Courtesy of the artist   199

CONTRIBUTORS

Comfort Tosin Adebayo is an Assistant Professor in the Department of Communication Studies at Towson University, Maryland. She takes a critical-interpretive approach to the study of health communication. Her journey into this field, using the method that she uses, began from her own lived experiences as an African immigrant woman accessing U.S. maternal healthcare services. She was not a "Black" woman" until she migrated to the U.S. It became apparent that her healthcare experiences were then nuanced by discourses of race and immigration. The works of Mohan Dutta and Collins Airhihenbuwa served as a launchpad in helping her navigate the critical approach to health communication scholarship and practice. Thus, her work, using a culture-centered approach, is focused on interrogating cultural codes that impact health behaviors and promotions, particularly in the African contexts—an often-understudied context.

Oluwaseyi Ambrose is currently a doctoral student in the Department of Communication, University of Wisconsin, Milwaukee, WI. She identifies as a health and intercultural communication scholar. Using the interpretive research paradigm, She seeks to understand cultural discourse surrounding maternal and child health, particularly for people of African descent. Her journey within the field of critical health communication is informed by the works of scholars like Tosin Adebayo and Megan McFarlane who study maternal healthcare experiences or marginalized groups from a critical lens.

Usman Bah is a PhD student at the University of Cincinnati, School of Communication, Film, and Media Studies. His research interests are in health and environmental (climate change) issues. He is at an early stage of his communication journey. For his master's thesis, he explored stories of climate change impact on the livelihoods, health, and wellbeing of Conakry Dee coastal community in Sierra Leone. His research in climate change is influenced by his work as project lead and head of programs for the Media Reform Coordinating Group in Sierra Leone where he led climate change awareness and resilience alternatives in six coastal communities in Sierra Leone for three years. His journey as a critical health communication scholar is ongoing. It sprung from his unforgettable experience with the Ebola crisis in Sierra Leone that claimed the lives of members of his family, friends, and fellow Sierra Leoneans. At that time, he was not satisfied with the response of the government and international partners in managing the Ebola outbreak. The country did not have health communication experts to account for factors such as cultural and religious beliefs, distrust of public officials, and ethnic diversity in their response to the epidemic. The country had to rely on external experts who arrived later and were not as informed about the local intricacies and often developed insufficient recommendations. That sense of loss and the desire to change health narratives in his country and underserved communities have shaped his journey so far.

Pankaj Baskey is a Santali community organizer and activist, leading the work of the Center for Culture-centered Approach to Research and Evaluation on Adivasi Education and Community-led Social Cohesion in West Bengal, India.

Iccha Basnyat is an Associate Professor of Global Health Communication in the Global Affairs Program with a joint appointment in the Department of Communication at George Mason University. For her Master's in Public Health project, she conducted fieldwork through an internship at an international non-profit organization with roots in a U.S.-based academic institution focused on implementing behavior change communication (BCC). More specifically, she investigated using entertainment education to change sexual and reproductive health behaviors such as family planning and contraceptive use among women in Nepal. While she gained a lot in doing fieldwork, assisting in program development, and interacting with the rural community members, this experience also left her with many critical questions about the intersections of culture, power, gender, health, and development. The search for answers resulted in her pursuing a degree in health communication and, soon after, her first critical health communication publication with her advisor. That juncture began her journey as a "critical health communication scholar."

Ambar Basu is a Professor in the Department of Communication at the University of South Florida, where he has spent his entire post-doctoral academic career—16 years now. His research explores how individuals and communities living at the margins of our societies communicate about health, illness, and well-being. With particular emphasis on theorizing culture as a site of change, his scholarship documents and analyzes narratives about health that emerge from dialogue between his SELF (as the researcher) and research participants. He remains interested in the stories of struggle, survival, and health inequities in the context of cultural and economic agendas in marginalized spaces. He is also intrigued by the methodological implications of knowledge production in collaboration with underprivileged communities. Self-reflexivity is an integral lens/method that shapes his thinking. He has served as Senior Editor for *Health Communication*, and he co-edits a Routledge book series titled *Critical Cultural Studies in Global Health Communication*.

Urmi Basu is the founder and leader of New Light. New Light is a not-for profit charitable organization that works with a community of poor women in sex work in Kalighat, Kolkata, India. Founded in 2000, New Light provides numerous services to the sex worker community in Kalighat, namely shelter, educational opportunities, healthcare, and legal aid to the children, girls, and women in the Kalighat community. This includes a crèche and night shelter, and three residential homes for young and teenaged children of sex workers working in Kalighat. A sociologist by academic training, Urmi Basu has received the Nari Shakti Puraskar, (literally translated to mean Woman Power Award), India's highest civilian award that recognizes the achievements and contributions of women. In 2009, she was honored by the Dalai Lama as one of the "Unsung Heroes of Compassion." The story of New Light and Urmi Basu's journey with the Kalighat sex worker community has been featured in the documentary series led by Nicholas Kristof and Sheryl WuDunn, called, "Half the Sky: Turning Oppression into Opportunity for Women Worldwide."

Liliane Campos is an Assistant Professor in English and Theatre Studies at the Sorbonne Nouvelle University in Paris, and a Research Fellow of the Institut Universitaire de France. After her doctoral research on the role of scientific discourse in contemporary performance, she broadened her field to contemporary literature and visual arts, and focused her research on artistic uses of biological and medical discourse. Her interest in health communication is primarily how artistic work engages with the rhetoric of health and medicine. Her critical orientation is inspired by post-Foucauldian philosophy, ecocriticism, medical humanities, and new materialism, but she works diagonally across those fields to question the political, ethical, and epistemological consequences of twenty-first-century representations of life. She directs the BioCriticism project, which fosters conversations between scholars, artists, and art-lovers.

Andrew Carter is an Assistant Professor in the Department of Public Health at San Jose State University. His orientation as a CHC scholar was first shaped by personal experience observing and helping his mother navigate a burdensome and confusing health care system in her lifelong journey with diabetes. When she ultimately passed away from the disease in 2011, he was enrolled at the time in a rhetoric MA program where he was studying persuasion and messaging in the context of intercultural and race communication. Applying what he was learning in the classroom to real-world contexts, he immediately connected the dots to her challenges navigating the health care system with the substandard quality of care and health communication practices by her doctors and care team. After graduating from his degree program, he was driven to apply his rhetoric and communication training to broader health contexts, which led him to pursue doctoral studies in health communication with an emphasis on critical methods.

Rebecca de Souza is an Associate Professor at the School of Communication at San Diego State University. Her critical perspective is deeply shaped by her upbringing in India, where the harsh realities of capitalism were inescapable. This awareness, along with her intellectual curiosity, flourished during her undergraduate years in the vibrant coffee shops of Bangalore, where she read and debated with friends the works of social thinkers such as Jean-Paul Sartre, Karl Marx, and B. R. Ambedkar. In graduate school, after a period of exploration, she found she was most interested in how the absence of basic needs—such as food, housing, and healthcare—shaped the health and well-being of communities. She came to understand that these deprivations, whether in the Global South or the Global North, are rarely due to individual choices, but shaped by the political distribution of resources. Her approach to health communication has been greatly influenced by the work of critical medical anthropologists like Paul Farmer and Richard Parker, as well as her engagements with Dr. Mohan Dutta's thinking on the culture-centered approach. Her critical lens was perhaps most sharply honed through her decades-long research and writing of *Feeding the Other*, which continues to guide her thinking today.

Mohan J. Dutta is Dean's Chair Professor of Communication and Director of the Center for Culture-Centered Approach to Research and Evaluation

(CARE) at Massey University in Aotearoa New Zealand, where they carry out various community-led projects of transformative social change across different countries and regions globally. The familial (he grew up in a joint family) and community environments of union organizing, lockouts, protest marches, and Left party organizing under the banner of the Communist Party of India (Marxist) shaped his learnings of critical theory, which he sees as at the core, Marxist theory. His father, through his gentle introductions to Lenin, was and is his first teacher of critical theory in its analysis of imperialism and anticolonialism (they used to have a large, human-size picture of Lenin hanging on the wall above our study table), with his uncles and aunts offering anchors for connecting the theory to praxis through Left party work. When he started performing in street theater and in productions of the Indian People's Theater Association (IPTA), he started learning about the roles of communication and performance in working class struggles for social change. These early lessons in community and amidst practice continue to guide his life journey as a scholar and practitioner of communication for social change.

Mavis Freeman Essel is a second-year doctoral student in the Department of Communication at the University of South Florida, studying health and interpersonal communication. Her research focuses on maternal and child health communication practices within Global South contexts. Through an African Feminist theoretical framework, she critically examines power dynamics, women's socio-cultural health challenges, and persistent health disparities pertaining to women and children in the Global South. She systematically documents and analyzes narratives concerning women's and children's health through dialogue between herself as a researcher and study participants. Self-reflexivity constitutes a fundamental framework that informs her scholarly inquiry and research methodology.

Kimberly Field-Springer is an Associate Professor of Communication at Berry College. Her research investigates how we negotiate meanings in health contexts, while also attending to the ways these interpretations inform identity, action, and transformative change. In exploring alternative potentialities of meaning, she strives to examine and unpack imagined possibilities from and in-between the sites of contested realities contingently informed by our lived experiences. She uses feminist theory, pragmatism, phenomenology, and critical approaches to examine communication phenomena. *Risk orders theory* (ROT) is a critical health communication framework that critiques bias, morality, and judgments embedded in messages about health risks.

Leandra H. Hernández is an Assistant Professor in the Department of Communication at the University of Utah. Her roots in critical health communication and media studies stem from her lived experiences as a queer Chicana feminist who witnessed gender violence and reproductive injustice in her community from an early age. Critical health communication spaces have served as a home for her in the Communication discipline because of her intersectional work and community-based social justice approaches. Early conversations with Dr. Jill Yamasaki, Dr. Tasha Dubriwny, and Dr. Richard Street, three of her graduate school mentors, helped her find her voice and footing in critical and feminist approaches to health communication.

Satveer Kaur-Gill is an Assistant Professor in the Department of Communication Studies at the University of Nebraska-Lincoln (UNL). Having always felt singled out by her peers, family, and friends for often being "unduly" concerned by the many injustices around her, she finally found her center in 2014, the CARE lab, housed at the National University of Singapore during her PhD program. Here, along with other like-minded scholars and her mentor, Mohan J. Dutta, she was allowed to be frustrated while finding her critical orientation, reading and learning from the works of Ambar Basu, Collins Airhihenbuwa, Barbara Sharf, Heather Zoller, Iccha Basnyat, Rebecca de Souza, and Shaunak Sastry. Her journey at CARE sowed her scholarly roots in critical health communication. Today, she continues to be enriched and inspired by the critical voices of her colleagues at UNL, Liahnna Stanley and Kate Siegfried, at their new academic home, The Center for Coalitional Praxis and Liberation.

Lisa Keränen is a Professor of Communication and Interim Associate Dean for Academic and Strategic Planning in the College of Liberal Arts and Sciences at the University of Colorado Denver. As a PhD student specializing in the rhetoric of science, she realized everything she was writing about had to do with medicine, the body, or surgery, so she decided to pursue a second MA in bioethics. Completing required clinical practica in intensive care units and in surgical clinics led her to an emerging scholarly community now known as the rhetoric of health and medicine. She came to critical health communication late in her career through its synergies with critical rhetoric and dialogues about the relations between RHM and CHC. Her critical voice emerged in a post-Foucauldian environment via bioethics, health humanities, and feminist care ethics. She also co-leads their health communication pathway and certificate program and is an affiliate of the Humanities in Healthcare Program of the Center for Bioethics & Humanities on the Anschutz Medical Campus.

Shamshad Khan is an Associate Professor in the Department of Communication at the University of Texas at San Antonio. He has an interdisciplinary background and has been immersed in public health and communication research for more than a decade. The groundwork for his critical health communication research was laid during his graduate studies in History and Social Sciences in Health, as well as during doctoral and post-doctoral training in communication studies and global public health that oriented him to the role that larger social and structural processes play in our everyday lives, including health and illness. His grant-funded research has focused on documenting the impact of large-scale global health interventions and building sustainable community-driven models, with a particular focus on HIV prevention among marginalized communities. In his research, he has drawn on a range of critical theoretical and methodological approaches, including political economy, structural violence and institutional ethnography, postcolonialism and subaltern studies, and cultural or culture-centered analyses of public health policies and media discourse.

Jennifer Malkowski is an Associate Professor of Communication Arts and Sciences at California State University, Chico. Early on in her academic career she was drawn to the intersections of public health and persuasive messaging as a source of constantly evolving current affairs. Regardless of training or disciplinary roots, she found that public health controversies invited opinions, conversations, and questions across diverse audiences and settings and, more often than not, showcased human capacities to work with and alongside one another in a common practical effort to take seriously the age-old question: *how ought we live?* And this emphasis on the we—the collective—continues to guide and characterize her work. Whether it be working directly with healthcare professionals to improve their communication with patients and colleagues, equipping students with theories to explain and challenge personal beliefs about health, or critiquing public messages for both their intentional and unanticipated influences, her scholarship foregrounds fissures in our well-crafted and choreographed symbolic realities, those moments wherein the natural world reminds us of our common humanity and demands a collective response.

Indranil Mandal is a community organizer and community researcher with Center for Culture-Centered Approach to Research and Evaluation (CARE). He has been working with CARE since 2012 in leading community led efforts of health organizing for justice.

Selina Metuamate is a Māori community researcher and organizer at the Center for Culture-Centered Approach to Research and Evaluation (CARE) at Massey University in Aotearoa New Zealand. Her research and activism engage with questions of land and food sovereignty.

Roopam Mishra is a PhD student in the Department of Communication at the University of South Florida, currently ending her second year. She identifies as a critical health and organizational communication researcher who examines the health narratives of marginalized individuals from the Global South. She focuses on documenting the role of culture, structure, and agency in shaping the health outcomes for these individuals and understanding how they navigate the structural barriers specific to their socio-cultural contexts. She is continually shaping and fine-tuning her current researcher identity as she embodies practices such as reflexivity, journaling, and field notes to be cognizant of her role as a researcher especially with the community in her interactions with them and to see them in totality, without being blinded by her own beliefs and ideologies. Beside this, she is also a bi-lingual poet and has been published in anthologies, magazines, and journals like *The Ekphrastic Review, Confluence Magazine, Setu, Loch raven Review, The Quiver Review, Borderless Journal, Hastaksher,* among others.

Oyewole. O. Olusanya, by training and practice, is a medical sociologist. His research centers on the sexual and reproductive health of females in Nigeria. His position as an academic informed his current research focus on health communication. Working with female students who experience enormous health information gaps about sexual and reproductive health sparked his interest in investigating barriers to sexual and reproductive health education for females in Nigeria. Through his ongoing collaboration with health communication scholars, he seeks to continue to unpack cultural barriers to the development and implementation of [sexual] health education in Nigeria. He is currently a Senior Lecturer in the Department of Sociology at Adekunle Ajasin University, Akungba-Akoko, Ondo State, Nigeria.

Venessa Pokaia is a Māori community leader and researcher, working with the Center for Culture-Centered Approach to Research and Evaluation (CARE) at Massey University in Aotearoa New Zealand in the work on developing migrant-Māori solidarities, refugee health, Māori food sovereignty, and Kaupapa Māori methods of healing.

List of Contributors xxi

Yixuan Qi is a PhD student at the University of Cincinnati in the School of Communication, Film, and Media Studies. Her research interest is in critical health communication, shaped by personal experiences. During the COVID-19 pandemic, she witnessed two close family members undergo cancer treatment under restrictive public health policies. This deeply influenced her understanding of health as not only medical, but also emotional, social, and cultural. While searching for a PhD program, she was especially drawn to the Cultural-Centered Approach (CCA), which led her to learn from Dr. Sastry. She approaches health as a socially constructed concept, shaped by cultural beliefs, power structures, and institutional barriers. Her work is grounded in the belief that everyone deserves to be heard, respected, and supported in their health journeys—especially those too often overlooked by dominant systems.

Shaunak Sastry is Professor of Communication and Provost Fellow at the University of Cincinnati. He is also the Co-Principal Investigator and Co-Director of the community engagement core of an NIH-funded center for climate change and health at the University of Cincinnati. From 2020–2025, he was senior editor of *Health Communication*. He did not define himself as a "critical health communication scholar" until late in his doctoral degree in Communication at Purdue, but the seeds were sown much earlier through introductions to Freud and the Indian psychoanalyst Sudhir Kakkar as an undergraduate Psychology major, and a specialization in cultural semiotics as a Master's student. His critical orientation was shaped through Marx, postcolonial and subaltern studies literature, and critical globalization studies, but he has honed his critical voice through leading two academic centers dedicated to community-engaged health communication, The Cincinnati Project, and the Cincinnati Center for Climate Change and Health (C4H).

Balkisa M. Sissy is a second-year MA student in Communication at the University of Cincinnati, transitioning into a PhD program at George Mason University. Her academic and personal journey has been anything but linear; it has been shaped by migration, motherhood, and an encounter with the often-overlooked spaces of women's well-being among marginalized communities. Her thesis, *"Voices Rising: The Untold Narratives of Maternal Mental Health in Ghana's Zango Communities,"* explores how cultural, religious, biomedical, and societal factors shape Zango women's understanding of perinatal depression. Passionate about gender, women, and infant health, She aims to build advocacy infrastructures and destigmatize mental health through co-creating knowledge and solutions, opening pathways for dialogue. Her journey reflects a commitment to co-creating solutions in being/becoming a critical health scholar grounded in both lived experience and academic rigor. She hopes to continue this work through her PhD and beyond, working alongside communities to reimagine what it means to be well, to be heard, and to be whole.

Julee Tate is a Professor of Spanish and Latin American Studies at Berry College. To date her research has focused primarily on applying gender and sexuality theories to Latin American texts, both written and visual. While she has dipped her toes into the field of health communication in her work that examines social messaging in telenovelas through the lens of entertainment-education theory, this project represents her first official foray into critical health communication. It has been intellectually stimulating and rewarding to work across disciplines with her colleague in the Communication Department.

Heather M. Zoller is a Professor in the University of Cincinnati's School of Communication, Film, and Media Studies. Her research focuses on the politics of public health, emphasizing participatory organizing for occupational, environmental, and economic health. Her journey as a health communication scholar altered course from studying provider-patient interaction at Texas A&M University when an architecture professor spoke to her public health class about organizing for illness prevention, highlighting how South American workers subsidize the cost of goods with their health. It was clear to her that you should not have to risk your life or your community's health to make a living. Her critical orientation grew out Howard Waitzkin's work (assigned by Rick Street) and was influenced by advisors and teachers including Tarla Rai Peterson (environmental communication), Charles Conrad and Kim Kline (rhetorical health issues management), Dennis Mumby (critical organizational communication), and Bill Rawlins (dialogue and communication theory). She is currently the Editor-in-Chief at the *Journal of Applied Communication Research*. She serves as the Director for the Communicating Health, Science, and Environment certificate and a member of the Committee on Personal and Protective Equipment with the National Academies of Sciences, Engineering, and Medicine.

ACKNOWLEDGMENTS

We (Shaunak, Heather, and Ambar) are grateful to work on this important project with our colleagues who contributed chapters. Thank you for your time and your solidarity.

At Routledge, we'd like to thank Zoya Gayle and Alexandra de Brauw for your patience and continued guidance.

We'd also like to acknowledge the anonymous reviewers of our book proposal. Your feedback was critical to our imagining this project.

Thank you, Irfan Ibrahim, for designing our book cover. Irfan's work was supported by a faculty excellence award that Shaunak received from the Office of Research and the Office of the Provost at the University of Cincinnati.

Finally, a big thank you to Yixuan Qi for the care you took to serve as our copy editor. Yixuan is a graduate student in the School of Communication, Film, & Media at the University of Cincinnati.

1
INTRODUCTION

Shaunak Sastry, Heather M. Zoller, and Ambar Basu

The overarching rationale of this book is to demonstrate how theories and practices of health communication can be enriched by foregrounding issues of power, politics, and culture. This book demonstrates the central role of critical research in the field of health communication. By critical, we refer to approaches that investigate how power and inequality shape communication contexts, messages, and processes. In the domain of health communication, critical approaches connect symbolic systems with questions of structural barriers to health, power and politics in healthcare, social and cultural determinants of health, and global health disparities. This edited collection offers a warrant for critical concepts in health communication to be centralized in the discipline going forward.

This edited collection demonstrates how sensitivity to the metatheoretical commitments of critical-cultural theories (in general, and critical health communication [CHC] in particular) benefits the discipline of health communication *in toto*. This book offers several strong rationales for adopting a critical view of health communication. First, a *timeliness* rationale: the differential global burden of disease during the COVID-19 pandemic along the lines of socioeconomic status, race/ethnicity, age, and gender is a reckoning for health communication practitioners. If epidemic disease outcomes are patterned through broad axes of social privilege, it follows that addressing social/structural determinants of health is of crucial importance to health communication theory and practice. Although health communication scholars have begun to address health disparities and social patterning of disease, critical research provides tools for moving beyond simply

DOI: 10.4324/9781003426530-1
This chapter has been made available under a CC BY-NC-ND license.

acknowledging or finding ways to adapt to disparities in order to promote communicative efforts that redress and prevent structural disparities.

A critical orientation to health also fulfills a *social justice* rationale. The ethical imperative to practice and theorize health communication from a justice orientation meets its fullest expression through a critical lens, which recognizes that communication processes can often impede human health and well-being rather than enhance it. The task at hand is not just to employ communication processes to transform health practices and behaviors but also to transform asymmetric communication practices themselves. Through its global scope and examples from across the field of communication, this book envisages a "critical turn" in health communication, wherein the unquestioned beneficence of communication interventions is challenged, and a reflexive orientation to theory and practice is encouraged.

A unique feature of this book is its emphasis on how critical approaches invigorate practitioner perspectives, or what we refer to as the *praxis* rationale. One of the prominent discontents of CHC—and of critical approaches writ large—is its purported disconnect to how "real" health communication is done by practitioners "out there." This line of critique creates a bifurcated version of health communication—one that is practiced in the "real world" and another that is discussed in graduate classrooms. By focusing on conversations with practitioners and their own reports on how critical concepts guide the practice of health communication, this book establishes critical sensibility as an inherently practice-oriented skill in health communication.

As health communication continues to grow, we are seeing a shift away from the dominance of more functionalist and quantitative research with much more interest in critical theories related to power, conflict, and social change. In part, this growing interest in critical research results from the fact that the communication discipline has begun to grapple seriously with questions related to diversifying and decolonizing our research. The field has also recognized the need for critical theories to engage with major social problems that influence health status, including growing economic inequities, racism and discrimination, social destabilization, and sustainability challenges.

Heather Zoller and Mohan Dutta published an edited volume in 2008 that highlighted both interpretive and critical approaches to health communication. Despite growing interest in critical perspectives, no book since that time has focused solely on critical research nor featured a broad array of critical scholarship. Therefore, this volume represents an important touchstone for the health communication discipline as well as related areas.

We begin this introductory chapter by defining "critical" in CHC and explaining how we conceptualize the field of CHC. We do this by offering a brief survey of the historical origins and foundational influences on the field. Following this, we survey the current state of CHC research. This is followed by a preview of the following twelve contributing chapters that comprise the collection.

How Do We Conceptualize CHC?

Let us start with a shared understanding of what the critical research paradigm in CHC means. Critical paradigms question the taken-for-granted notions of what is presented to us as a reality (Deetz, 1992; Lupton, 1994; Zoller & Dutta, 2008). Critical research asks us to interrogate the taken-for-granted notion that knowledge is neutral and to examine how power and ideology work in consort with the communicative production and circulation of knowledge to create and reinforce social and material structures of domination. We understand critical theory/research as a political calling to build knowledge practices that are committed to the struggle for a society that enables emancipatory change.

As a point of emphasis, we recognize that critical theory and critical research are not a monolith but rather a continuum (Dutta & Pal, 2020). This approach offers the latitude to include a variety of foci, methods, and theoretical perspectives into its domain. At the same time, taking a critical standpoint necessitates a scrutiny of research perspectives that (attempt to) co-opt its foundational premise—that of challenging existing modalities of power and knowledge that create and sustain material and communicative infrastructures of violence, death, and dispossession across the world. Critical theorizing thus contrasts with research that employs markers of inequality as discrete variables (in a quantitative and qualitative sense) without connecting intersecting inequalities with micro, meso, and macro structures of oppression. Critical theory challenges researchers to interrogate dominant frameworks of knowledge, considering how communicative constructions (e.g., identity and difference, culture, policy) create and reinforce multiple relations of power. This work goes beyond the superficial adaptation of concepts such as culture in ways that reinforce the status quo. As such, this edited volume centers issues of power, resistance, voice, and social change from marginalized perspectives. These insights can thus inform new approaches to postpositivist and interpretive theorizing as well as encourage more explicit critical theorizing in health communication.

As co-editors, we start from the view that both health and communication are sociocultural-political phenomena. As CHC scholars, our scholarship is focused on the ways that relations of power and inequality influence how individuals and communities make/share/negotiate meanings about health. The political commitments of CHC invite us and others to carefully examine how communicative constructions and interpretations of health influence lived experiences and colonize our identities and imagined futures. Critical perspectives encourage us to ask whose agendas are served through dominant articulations of how good health and well-being should be achieved, how these dominant articulations create and sustain the margins, and how the margins engage with and resist networks of oppression. Critical lenses connect these questions to local-global forces of life, dispossession, and death.

The three of us are often approached by junior scholars in the discipline who wonder whether they should "become critical scholars." When we have these discussions, we highlight the ways that "critical theories" encompassing neo-Marxist, feminist, poststructural, and decolonial perspectives provide tools to reclaim hidden conflict and highlight the role of communication in constructing and deconstructing relationships of dominance. The chapters in this book demonstrate the value of these approaches. At the same time, we recognize the value of multiple perspectives and methods in the field. What is important in our minds is not whether scholars identify as critical scholars, but that they consider how insights from critical scholarship influence their own research. Being "critically minded" involves de-centering dominant hierarchies and questioning foundational assumptions about the values embedded in conceptions of "objectivity" in postpositivist research and "intersubjectivity" in interpretive research. Critical perspectives can aid scholars from across the discipline in interrogating whose interests are served by the ways researchers define major concepts (e.g., what is health?, what counts as illness?, and what is culture?), pose research questions, and form interventions. This level of reflexivity is needed to spur the discipline to greater engagement with the realities of power and difference that suffuse health communication practices. In the next section, we offer a brief survey of the sources and influences of CHC.

CHC: Origins and Traditions

As we mentioned above, the aim of this edited collection is to demonstrate how theories and practices of health communication can be enriched by foregrounding issues of power, politics, and culture. In constituting CHC as a discernible field, we recognize that the area draws from a plethora of scholarly traditions. Having defined in the previous section what we mean by "critical" in CHC, here, we explore the early development of this critical tradition. We outline some of the key foundational texts, authors, and movements, out of which the field of CHC has emerged. In offering this genealogical survey, we recognize that any such telling is inevitably laden with our own telling of our "origin story" as scholars. We proceed with the proviso that this is not a historically "objective" or exhaustive genealogy. It is entirely likely that a different historical trajectory of this field (or any other field, for that matter) may be written by a different set of actors. For now, this is our version.

The received view is that CHC is a "new" or "recent" intervention into a field that was dominated by, initially, postpositivist, transmission-oriented models of communication, and then subsequently, by interpretivist and narrative-based modes of inquiry (Sharf, 1999; Sharf & Vanderford, 2003). This is a broadly accurate yet highly simplified telling of the evolution of critical approaches in the field. It is undeniable that there is more interest in critically oriented health communication in the last two decades, a shift first observed by Zoller and Kline (2008) and Zoller and Dutta (2008). However, invitations to think critically about health communication have always circulated in the field, albeit sporadically and at its margins. For example, writing a year before the first issue of the journal *Health Communication* was published, John McKnight (1988) already was making a case for distinguishing between the more instrumental needs of "medical communication" and the more social-structural bases of "health communication" (p. 40) and calling for a central focus on relations of power.

A major touchpoint for CHC was the publication of Deborah Lupton's essay "Towards the Development of Critical Health Communication Praxis," in the journal *Health Communication* (Lupton, 1994). Lupton offered three masterful critiques: First, that health communication remained rooted in social psychology; second, that its relationship with state-sponsored health promotion limited its potential, and finally, that it had a merely instrumental view of culture. Lupton urged the field to develop a critical-cultural stance, taking a broader view of medical discourse that drew from the increasing popularity of social constructionism in fields like sociology, anthropology, history, philosophy, and feminist studies. Finally, Lupton argued for health communication interventions that target the social and political environment around health behaviors rather than focus on behavior alone. The "critical-cultural theory" that Lupton articulated for the field was a response to broader tectonic shifts in social scientific terrain. Her work built on Foucauldian and feminist scholarship as well as an essay by Baer et al. (1986), who argued for a more critical version of medical anthropology nearly a decade earlier. Lupton's sociological view of biomedical power and its constitutive role in shaping social dynamics around health has had an indelible impact on the field (Lupton, 2012, 2022).

Yet another wellspring for CHC is Howard Waitzkin's scholarship on public health, medicine and the politics of healthcare (Waitzkin, 1991, 2000; Waitzkin & Waterman, 1974). As a Marxist physician interested in the reproduction of class ideology through public health and clinical encounters, Waitzkin provided a theoretical framework for CHC to critique the formative role of capitalism in the degradation of personal and social health. In a 1984 article in the *Journal of the American Medical Association* (JAMA), Waitzkin critiqued the asymmetrical and de-politicizing nature of doctor-patient communication training, warning about "social structural barriers to effective communication in medical encounters" (Waitzkin, 1984, p. 2441). Writing concurrently to the development of doctor-patient communication models in our field, Waitzkin elucidated how the clinic becomes a site for class politics; how doctors reproduce elite ideologies through their interactions with patients, and how clinical encounters can become an instrument for granular (conversation) analysis of class politics (Waitzkin, 1991). Waitzkin's writing provides a template for connecting capitalism, ideology, and biomedical dominance through the "everyday encounters" of the clinic, thereby offering a communicative window to view how broad institutional and discursive processes affect the experience of health. Writing from a squarely anti-capitalist position on the role of healthcare in society (Waitzkin & Working Group for Health Beyond Capitalism, 2018), this work provides an anchor for the broad structural critiques about health that CHC scholars have taken up.

The organizing principle that institutional structures condition individual and social well-being runs through the heart of CHC. The writing and activism of Paul Farmer, based on his pioneering work with Partners in Health, is another major influence on CHC scholarship. Methodologically, he demonstrated the value of ethnographic analysis (e.g., of the HIV epidemic in Haiti) (Farmer, 1996a), integrating the historical, cultural, and global aspects of health (Farmer, 1999; Farmer et al., 2013) and interweaving qualitative insights with epidemiological data (Farmer, 1996b). Farmer's insistence on an anthropological understanding of culture, vested in Geertzian "thick description" of everyday life rather than a psychological distilling of cultural variables, has been central to the development of not just the culture-centered approach (CCA), but an entire mode of thinking about health that is geographically broad and historically deep, to paraphrase an oft-use phrase that Farmer uses. Farmer's writings on structural violence expand on Galtung's (1969) definition of the term, connecting health experiences to the histories of colonial extraction (Farmer, 1996b). This structuralist notion of violence is a major source of theorizing within CCA and other "structurally oriented" models of health and development, such as the social-ecological model (SEM) (Bronfenbrenner, 1977;

Kilanowski, 2017). More importantly, Farmer's work in Haiti also leaves an imprint for health activism and advocacy as crucial aspects of CHC praxis (Basnyat & Dutta, 2012; Zoller, 2005, 2017).

A preponderance of CHC scholarship today emerges in the wake of the CCA, which is the subject of three individual contributing chapters in this collection. CCA offers a non-interventionist view of culture and a heuristic critical framework from which to regard the health experiences of marginalized communities. While the theoretical sources of the CCA have been discussed in detail elsewhere (see, for instance, Dutta, 2008; Sastry et al., 2021), we want to highlight the work of Collins Airhihenbuwa and colleagues' work on the PEN-3 model of health promotion (Airhihenbuwa et al., 2000, 2014; Airhihenbuwa & Obregon, 2000) as a major foundation of CCA research. PEN-3 is a health promotion model that theorized culture as non-pathological, challenging health social science research that equated "culture" with non-Western ways of knowing that were often described as "unscientific." Airhihenbuwa's work draws from pan-African traditions and customs to show how culture is more than just a barrier to health promotion; instead, it is existential, that is, formative of health beliefs and can be a positive force in shaping effective and humane health interventions. Writing against the "culture as difference" grain popular in Western social science at the time, where "culture existed elsewhere," Airhihenbuwa's PEN-3 model and other works demonstrated the importance of theorizing health promotion from non-Western contexts (Airhihenbuwa, 1995, 2007; Airhihenbuwa et al., 2000, 2024).

Although the PEN-3 model alludes to them in passing, it does not really delve into histories of colonial medicine and imperial public health governance that shaped the contours of global health today. Critiques of the colonizing impulse in global health, informed by postcolonial and subaltern studies, cultural studies, queer theory, and neo-Gramscian critiques of hegemony, represent yet another theoretical source for CHC scholarship (Anderson, 2002; Brown & Bell, 2008; Greene et al., 2013; King, 2002; Melkote et al., 2007, 2008; Yep et al., 2003).

Finally, we note that in addition to roots in health theorizing from other disciplines, CHC is indebted to the histories of critical theorizing in communication writ large. Rhetorical traditions including ideological and feminist criticism influenced the development of critical scholarship that now coheres around the rhetoric of health and medicine (RHM) (Bennett, 2022; Jensen, 2016; Lynch & Dubriwny, 2005; Meloncon & Scott, 2017; Segal, 2005a, 2005b) as well as health policymaking and corporate issues management (Conrad & McIntush, 2003; Conrad & Millay, 2001; Conrad & Barker, 2010). Cultural studies and media research laid the groundwork for investigating the politics of representation and inclusion in mediated and everyday discourse (Grossberg, 1993a, 1993b, 1997; Hall, 1985; Kline, 2011; Tulloch & Lupton, 2003). Critical organizational communication research (Deetz, 1992; Mumby, 1997; Parker, 2016) has influenced our understanding of the role of power in mediating the mutual influences among communication, health, and organizing. Chapters in this volume incorporate these perspectives and many others to theorize CHC.

Functionalist and interpretive approaches continue to be the norm in the discipline, reflected in the notable absence of a chapter on critical approaches to power and politics in the *Handbook of Health Communication*, and in the limited discussion of such approaches in leading textbooks (du Pre & Overton, 2021) Yet, this oversight misses significant growth in CHC scholarship. This edited volume represents just a sampling of the CHC scholarship being published. Researchers draw from multiple critical theories, perspectives, and methods to highlight the centrality of power to our understanding of health communication in a variety of domains.

Current State of Critical Research

As mentioned in the previous section, CCA has had a significant influence over the development of CHC over the last two decades (Basnyat & Dutta, 2012; Dutta, 2007, 2008; Dutta & Basu, 2008), and continues to be a driving force in producing critically informed research (Cao & Wang, 2021; Chandanabhumma et al., 2020; Jamil & Kumar, 2021; Kaur-Gill, 2022; Mukherjee & Ivancic, 2024; Pringle et al., 2022). CCA research draws attention to the politics of voice and the need to promote agency and participation in changing the structures that influence health. However, as the approach becomes more popular and is applied to varying health contexts, we also notice that not all of the research adopting a CCA lens is necessarily critical in its orientation. Many researchers invoke CCA when investigating how cultural values can aid in adapting communication interventions to local norms without attending to the theory's emancipatory elements of structure and agency. Sastry et al. (2021) point out that the "critical edge" of CCA scholarship emerges through reflexive practices about power, problem definition, and problem interpretation, which are commonly evidenced in long-term or at least medium-term engagements with marginalized communities' struggles for health. Many scholars today use CCA as a heuristic framework to provide a "thick description" of health experiences. While we do not claim orthodoxy in how a theory is to be taken up, it is useful to demarcate what precisely is "critical" about such theories.

There is now a palpable influence of postcolonial perspectives on health communication scholarship (Asante et al., 2025; Sastry, 2014; Sastry &

Dutta, 2011). Postcolonial research highlights epistemic politics of knowledge construction around health. Moreover, this line of research often highlights the communicative constitution of not just relations of consent but also coercion, and the necropolitics involved in organizing state-sanctioned death (Ban, 2016; Basu, 2011; Basu et al., 2022; de Souza, 2022; Dempsey et al., 2022; Sastry et al., 2023).

CHC scholars also draw from neo-Marxist and Gramscian theorizing, which sheds light on the communicative negotiation of consent and resistance to the relations of power embedded in the status quo (Khan, 2014; Zoller, 2003. Drawing from Lupton's early work in CHC and demonstrating the influences of cultural studies in communication, these approaches engage with questions of medicalization and demedicalization, biomedical hegemony, and relations of consent and resistance linked to health practices. Heather Zoller's chapter in this volume offers a summary of such approaches.

Health communication scholars also adopt poststructural perspectives that emphasize the communicative, power-laden constitution of truth, knowledge, and identity. Discourse frameworks examine the interrelationships among constructions of health, control, and identity (James et al., 2022). For example, scholars draw from Foucault to elucidate how power relations are embedded in disciplinary discourses we use to judge and evaluate the body (Dempsey & Gibson, 2017; Nadesan, 2008; Zoller, 2003). Ivancic (2018) used a Foucauldian biopower framework to examine discourses surrounding U.S. soda bans, finding that advocates challenged neoliberal "choice" narratives but could not overcome anti-government sentiments.

A small but growing number of health communication scholars employ critical race theory to highlight racial inequalities in health discourses and health outcomes. Vardeman-Winter (2017) looked at how grassroots community-based health workers manage whiteness frames that marginalize the experiences of women of color and perpetuate systemic biases. In a recent special issue of *Health Communication* focused on research by and for BIPOC communities, Adebayo et al. (2022) drew from critical race theory to discuss the structural causes of African American women's maternal health experiences, including racially insensitive biomedical approaches, cultural dismissal of Black women's pain, lack of insurance access, and other issues. Hawkins (2022) elucidated the impact of police violence as a threat to Black Americans' physical and mental health, demonstrating how foregrounding racial issues reshapes how the health communication discipline defines and attends to health risks.

Feminist researchers examine how gender inequalities influence health experiences and health outcomes. Feminist commitments to integrating the personal and political highlight the connections between embodied, lived experience and institutional health practices (Bute et al., 2010; Jensen 2016). For example, feminist scholars highlight public policy discourses, including the gendered implications of body mass index reporting in U.S. schools (Gerbensky-Kerber, 2011) and patriarchal assumptions embedded in U.S. Gardasil vaccine debates (Thompson, 2010). Scholars connect gender constructions with medical diagnoses and experiences of endometriosis (Krebs & Schoenbauer, 2020) and birth control practices (Zou & Liu, 2024). Feminist researchers also highlight structural violence that threatens women's health, particularly in low-income countries (Basnyat, 2017).

Queer theorizing investigates the mutual influences of sexuality and health discourses. For example, Eger (2024) et al. created and evaluated a peer advocate model for addressing structural causes of sexual and substance abuse risks among LGBTQ+ students. Research in this area demonstrates how greater understanding of intersectional identity, including the full LGBTQ+ spectrum, can produce more ethical and effective health communication interventions. An emerging line of health communication research integrates gender, queer, and "crip" theorizing of the body (Ellingson, 2009). As Yep (2013) articulated in discussions of body normativity, " …queering/quaring/ kauering/crippin'/transing can serve as useful analytical tools to unpack and deconstruct dominant discursive constructions of the body*and their embodied translation*in relationship to gender, sexuality, race, class, ability, nation, and culture" (p. 120). Consistent with this approach, Spieldenner (2016) drew from queer and quare theorizing to assess how the labeling of "Truvada whores" constructs and reinforces dirty/clean binaries and stigmatizes the use of HIV prophylaxis medicine.

This intersectional work builds on critical theorizing of dis/ability as a health communication issue (Alper et al., 2023; Coopman, 2016). Contributing to our understanding of creative forms of praxis, recent scholarship on ability status emphasizes the role of art, including a museum installation promoting agency and well-being among blind and visually impaired audiences (Makkawy & Moreman, 2025) as well as storytelling and cancer survivorship (Billingslea & Ellingson, 2015).

While this is by no means an exhaustive survey of the major theoretical perspectives fueling the developments in CHC today, we hope to have provided the interested reader a broad sense of the diverse, cross-pollinating, and dynamic nature of this emergent field. A consequence of this theoretical plurality is a widening of the conceptual scope of what "counts" as health communication. In the next section, we discuss some new and emergent ways in which CHC scholars are expanding and developing the scope of health communication.

Conceptual Developments in CHC

In addition to presenting an overview of major theoretical perspectives, we also want to briefly discuss the conceptual evolution of CHC. We do so by highlighting some key areas of research.

The interconnections between power, identity, and stigma have opened the door to a plethora of scholarship in the field. Linked to the theoretical focus on the communicative construction and negotiation of identity, a significant body of critical scholarship considers how stigma is linked with dominant and resistant power relations. For example, Davis and Quinlan (2017) described how both popular and health promotion discourses about body size construct and reinforce cultural biases that reinforce false and misleading depictions of the relationship between weight and illness (see also Lupton, 2018; Shugart, 2011). Given critical commitments to praxis, CHC research investigates communicative pathways toward countering stigma (Basnyat, 2020; Basu, 2010; Zou & Liu, 2024). In this volume, Khan et al. (Chapter 6) describe grassroots organizing to counter stigma among sex workers. Also in this volume, de Souza (2022) (Chapter 1) broadens stigma research to theorize the relationships among political ideologies, policy, and marginalization in constructing "neoliberal stigmas" around not only identities but also public benefits that support health and well-being.

Another major contribution of CHC research is extending our understanding of health disparities and their linkages to economic and sociopolitical power. Unlike more functionalistic research that often treats disparities as a group-level phenomenon, CHC situates these disparities within communicatively constructed power relations (see Chapter 5 for Zoller's discussion). Sastry et al. (2017) chronicled how community health workers transformed a prevention-oriented patient navigation initiative by listening to low-income community members and addressing structural barriers to cancer prevention.

National and global health disparities became highly visible during the COVID-19 pandemic. Critical scholars have lent insights into the management of global disease outbreaks, elucidating how we can reduce the spread of illness and mitigate social impacts by addressing the cultural and political organization of inequality (Sastry et al., 2021). For example, Dove et al. (2024) investigated how multiple and intersecting layers of marginalities led to unique vulnerabilities in San Antonio and South-Central Texas in the U.S., many of which were not addressed in the "one-size-fits-all official response at the national or state level on the other" (n.p.).

COVID-19 also made visible the central role of work and employment in relation to health disparities (Fujishiro et al., 2022; Kaur-Gill, 2020). Critical research highlighted tensions between the need for quarantine/

distancing to prevent illness and making a living for low-wage and precarious workers (Villamil & D'Enbeau, 2021). Dempsey et al. (2022) theorized necropolitics in the meatpacking industry's rhetoric, which used security discourses surrounding a supposed "meat shortage" to undermine health protections when the low-wage, often minoritized, and immigrant laborers experienced significant outbreaks. Dutta (2021) highlighted the intersections between structural barriers, agency, and voice in the everyday negotiations of COVID-19 among low-wage male Bangladeshi migrant workers in Singapore.

CHC scholars have investigated how global economic organizing and migration drives health disparities (de Souza et al. 2008; Sastry & Dutta, 2012; Zoller, 2008). In addition, CHC work has interrogated international development discourses that aim to remediate the health effects of economic disparities (Olufowote, 2017). Recently, Asante et al. (2025) detailed an alternative framework for NGO engagement with marginalized groups based on their community-based action research project among LGBTS groups in Ghana.

Linked to development discourses, a growing number of scholars connect health disparities to the communicative construction of food policies and agricultural practices. As de Souza (Chapter 1) and Carter (Chapter 7) describe, critical researchers highlight inequities in the production and distribution of food at the local, national, and international levels. Researchers examine the neoliberal foundation of Western food policy and address the role of community organizing in reinforcing and resisting those ideologies to promote equitable food production and access (Carter & Alexander; de Souza et al., 2008; Ivancic, 2020; Okamoto, 2017; Thomson, 2009; Zoller, 2021, 2023).

In addition to public health, CHC builds on early work by scholars such as Howard Waitzkin, Patricia Geist-Martin, and Barbara Sharf to investigate communication in medical contexts. Patient-centered and cultural competence theorizing incorporates the social, cultural, and economic contexts of patients into medical interactions (Dean & Street, 2014; Teal & Street, 2009) and technological access (Merrill Jr, 2024). Theorizing "communicative disenfranchisement" considers how interactions create or suppress opportunities for voice (Hintz & Tucker, 2023). Researchers also consider how issues of economic and social difference influence access to medical providers (Hudak & Bates, 2019). More explicitly *critical* theorizing extends this research by highlighting the connections between micro-level interactions and larger cultural and political inequities, including race, country of origin, language, class, gender and sexuality, ability, migration status, and other issues (see Robb, 2023). For example, Babu et al. (2025) draw from critical theorizing to look at how women "critique, resist, and transform the contexts of their dismissal" (p. 1090) in the U.S. health system. Tucker et al. (2024) used a quantitative approach to address intersectional differences based on gender, race, and socioeconomic status in the experiences of chronic pain patients.

In addition to public health and medicine, critical research is concerned with cultural discourses about health and their link to knowledge production. For example, critical research highlights the role of media in shaping public perceptions of health issues among marginalized groups (Khan, 2014). LaPoe et al. (2022) consider how mainstream media blame Indigenous people for health disparities rather than systemic deprivation by the U.S. Hernandez et al. (Chapter 3) and Field-Springer & Tate (Chapter 4) address linkages among media and women's bodily autonomy, reproductive rights, and violence.

Finally, another major contribution of critical research has been to reformulate what counts as a communication campaign or intervention, moving from top-down media interventions toward participatory, community, and activist organizing (Basu & Dutta, 2009; Dutta & Pal, 2010; Zoller, 2005). Critical researchers demonstrate how community organizing improves health by increasing access to education, public health resources, and countering environmental racism (De Los Santos Upton et al., 2022). Critical research highlights the role of activism in contesting elite-dominated policies influencing health. Digital activism has become a key technique for resisting dominant approaches to disease funding and management (Parsloe & Holton, 2018; Vicari & Cappai, 2016). Bennett (2022) examined disability activists' efforts to resist healthcare indexing and its influence on access to services. Critical research also highlights activism aimed at cultural and institutional practices that undermine worker health (Zoller, 2021; Zoller et al., 2023). Critical scholarship also examines how activists contest corporate power and the health effects of neoliberal capitalism (Zoller, 2017), including soda bans (Ivancic, 2018), gun safety (Zoller & Casteel, 2021), pharmaceutical influence (Thomson, 2009), addiction and incarceration (Stanley & Basu, 2023), and agricultural policies (Dutta & Thaker, 2019). Critical scholars also engage in activism directly (Hernández & De Los Santos Upton, 2019).

These are just some examples of critical health communication research. The chapters in this book build on this intellectual foundation and chart new directions for developing health communication theory and practice.

Preview of Chapters

The first section of the book highlights work that draws from an array of critical concepts to identify and critique dominant relations of power that influence health experiences. In Chapter 2, titled "From Symptoms to Transformation: Addressing the Root Causes of Hunger through Critical Health Communication," Rebecca de Souza explores the role of CHC in addressing structural inequalities and systemic failures contributing to hunger and poverty. De Souza adopts a critical modernism framework to understand the root causes of hunger and poverty and provides examples of how CHC can engage with real-world health issues to uncover systemic inequalities and offer potential solutions through community organizing and collective action.

Gendered violence finds a sharp voice in Chapter 3, by Leandra Hernandez, titled "Reproductive Injustice, Feminicides, and the Intersections of Critical Health Communication and Journalism Praxis." This chapter discusses health communication and journalism practices regarding reproductive feminicides. It emphasizes the need for ethical coverage and framing of gender-based violence in media, particularly in Latin American contexts. The chapter advocates for trauma-informed journalism and ethical witnessing to improve news coverage and public health responses to gender-based violence. It also provides examples of how news framing can perpetuate harmful stereotypes and stigmatize victims of gender-based violence. In addition, Hernandez explores the role of journalists in shaping public perceptions of gender-basedviolence and the importance of using feminist news framing practices to promote more equitable and sensitive coverage. The author calls for collaboration between journalists, public health practitioners, and health communication scholars to develop best practices for framing health messages that center gender-based violence

Chapter 4, authored by Kimberly Field-Springer and Julee Tate, is titled "God, Country, and Family: A Risk Orders Theory Approach to Deconstructing Health Messages about Family Planning in the Latine Community." The chapter examines the spread of misinformation and disinformation about abortion within the Latine community following the U.S. Supreme Court's decision to overturn Roe v. Wade on June 24, 2022. Using risk orders theory, a framework that calls into question the dominant techno-scientific and cognitive approaches that aim to measure and control risks, the authors analyze anti-abortion messages on Eduardo Verástegui's Spanish-language social media platform. This analysis reveals how medically inaccurate information is used to propagate ideological patterns and the political constructions concealed within Verástegui's motto: "God, country, and family." Further, the chapter highlights the impact of these messages on public health discourse, exposing the power dynamics and moral, social, and identity risks embedded in anti-abortion rhetoric. The findings underscore the importance of combating misinformation with accurate, evidence-based information to protect women's health and reproductive rights.

The following chapter by Iccha Basnyat, "Communicating Structural Violence: A Case Study of Entertainment Establishment Women Workers in Kathmandu, Nepal," also delves into gendered violence, this time in the workplace. Basnyat explores the lived experiences of women workers in entertainment establishments in Kathmandu. This chapter highlights how structural violence and societal stigma impact their mental and physical health. Basnyat shares how everyday communicative acts perpetuate structural violence, such as verbal threats, belittling, and denigration, that lead to negative health outcomes. This chapter connects communication about health with work-related vulnerabilities faced by women in entertainment establishments in Asia due to migration patterns, income disparities, and societal norms. Finally, the chapter calls for a shift in health communication research to prioritize interventions in structural forms of violence faced by women in marginalized contexts and to consider broader structural conditions that frame policies and interventions to address health inequalities, particularly in the global South

The next section of the book highlights the centrality of advocacy, activism, and social change to health communication theorizing and practice. In Chapter 5, Heather Zoller highlights relationships between critical health and organizational communication. Drawing from Gramscian and poststructural theorizing, Zoller elucidates how illness attributions and constructions of health and wellness construct, reinforce, or resist the organization of dominant social hierarchies (and vice versa). The chapter describes the ideological implications of major illness attributions in health communication research and practice, including four different ways of addressing health disparities. Zoller argues that the discipline should give more attention to transformative and collective organizing aimed at the "fundamental causes" of illness. Integrating a critical pragmatist perspective, she highlights improvisational and experimental forms of activism that promote healthy and safe work in sustainable and equitable economies. The chapter promotes a Critically Holistic framework that (1) broadens the focus of wellness movements (physical, mental, social, and spiritual health) to address fundamental causes, (2) promotes substantive worker participation, and (3) creates accountability to ensure that programs equitably address workers' social, economic, and political needs. Zoller highlights an agricultural certification program, the Equitable Food Initiative (EFI), and the worker-owned union cooperative movement 1worker1vote, to demonstrate both the benefits and the feasibility of a Critically Holistic approach for reconfiguring workplace health promotion and health communication practices more broadly.

Shamshad Khan's chapter, titled "HIV Interventions, Collectivization Efforts, and Citizenship on the Margins of the State in India," calls attention to the role of health activism in not only resisting dominant relations of power that undermine health, but also in promoting grassroots social change. The chapter explores the impact of the community-led structural intervention (CLSI) program by Ashodaya Samithi, a sex worker collective in South India that addresses HIV prevention through mutual empowerment. This chapter further investigates the intersections among power, working conditions, and health status. The chapter connects with CHC theorizing that highlights the centrality of work to public health. Khan's CHC perspective challenges sexual health promotion models that target individual behavior change among sex workers as a way to prevent the spread of HIV and STIs among the public (and, possibly, the workers themselves). The study demonstrates how Ashodaya Samithi's comprehensive approach, including health education, financial stability, and civil rights awareness, transformed members' lives, enabling them to assert their rights and identities. The collective's work highlights the need for marginalized workers to advocate for larger sociopolitical changes, including resisting stigma and discrimination, in order to advance their own physical, mental, social, and economic health and safety. The chapter also underscores the importance of participatory, community-driven interventions in CHC for marginalized populations.

In Chapter 8, Andrew Carter describes his engagement in critical participatory action research with the National Women in Agriculture Association (NWIAA), a major non-profit that represents Black women in agriculture and advocates for food system justice. This chapter reflects the centrality of food and agricultural policies to public health. Carter's approach to research reflects his commitments to understanding how Black women farmers can communicatively challenge structural inequalities, advocate for themselves and their cultural heritage, and reduce health disparities by promoting food access. The author also discusses how CHC insights guide his academic-community partnership with NWIAA. He gives us an insider view of his role as a researcher and advocate with the group. He elucidates how four conceptual anchors of CCA (participation, communication infrastructures, partnerships, and reflexivity) guide these efforts. To highlight these anchors, Carter describes how he navigates power dynamics, drawing from his positionality as an academic researcher to advocate for the group while simultaneously centering the experiences and voices of group members themselves. Insights from this chapter are crucial for scholars interested in ethical and effective forms of engaged research that promote democratic forms of social change as a way to transform the health of the public.

The third section of book addresses critical health communication methods, considering both academic research and practitioner perspectives. Chapter 9, by Mohan Dutta et al., titled "Culture-centered Approach as Critical Health Practice: The Body as Resistance" outlines CCA as a transformative meta-theory in health communication. The chapter describes how CCA emerged from community struggles for justice and aims to dismantle the whiteness embedded in health communication. By centering the voices of marginalized communities, the CCA redefines health through the lens of cultural, structural, and agency interplays. It charts the complex critique of postcolonial theory that is often produced by privileged upper-caste academics and addresses epistemic violence linked to health disparities. The CCA employs voice infrastructures to amplify marginalized voices, exemplified by projects like Listening 1965, which co-created narratives with Indonesian genocide survivors. The approach emphasizes critical reflexivity, urging researchers to interrogate their positionality and power dynamics. This chapter advocates for embodied activism, where researchers engage deeply with communities, which can involve risking personal well-being to challenge oppressive structures, or what the authors refer to as "body on the line."

Chapter 10, titled "Biocriticism in a Time of Precarity: Inventional Resources for Critical Health Communication" brings together an interdisciplinary team of scholars invested in the rhetoric of health, cultural studies, and health communication. Lisa Keränen, Liliane Campos, and Jennifer Malkowski discuss biocriticism as a critical framework for analyzing the intersections of biology, culture, and politics. Earmarking the current moment as the "age of biology," the authors offer biocriticism as an important way to apprehend the power dynamics and implications of biological discourses in health. The authors provide examples of biocriticism in practice, focusing on how scholars use biocriticism to unpack the dynamics and implications of biological discourses, contexts, artifacts, symbols, images, and assemblages. They discuss the theoretical underpinnings of biocriticism, drawing on Foucauldian biopolitics. This chapter emphasizes the need for CHC scholars to engage with broader conversations in the humanities and describes how biocritical approaches can foster collaborations with diverse academic audiences.

Adebayo, Olusanya and Ambrose's Chapter 11, titled "Decolonizing Health Communication: Reflections on Critical Health Communication Research in Nigeria," explores the evolution of their scholarly journey. This journey was spurred by the dissonance between Western theorizing of health communication and the African contexts where they have lived and worked. The authors' reflexive approach foregrounds the need to interrogate the connections among researchers' social location, epistemological frameworks, and research goals. In addition to challenging the dominance of Western ideologies, the chapter makes a strong case for Africa-centered theories and methodologies that prioritize local voices and give attention to the cultural and structural factors that influence health care practices.

In Chapter 12, Balkisa Sissy, Usman Bah, Yixuan Qi, and Shaunak Sastry also offer a discussion that highlights their academic trajectories as CHC researchers. Titled "Journeys in Critical Health Communication: Meditations on Being/becoming CCA Scholars," the piece is crafted as a conversation on CCA (and critical approaches to health in general) from the unique co-points of scholars at very different parts of their academic journey, including a Master's student, two doctoral students, and a senior scholar. The essay weaves between defining what CCA means at these various stages and thinking through the activist and emancipatory aims of CHC by politicizing the nature of health and defining/destabilizing the Global South. The chapter is written expressly to invite early career scholars and students in a journey toward understanding the often jargon-heavy world of CHC.

Finally, in Chapter 13, "New Light: Critical Health Communication and Connections to Experiences from the Field," Ambar Basu, Mavis Essel Freeman, and Roopam Mishra engage in a discussion with Urmi Basu, the founder of New Light, an NGO in Kolkata, India, that is dedicated to health and safety of women in sex work and their children. This chapter highlights relationships among local cultural and communicative systems, power, politics, and health inequities, showing how such inequities play out on the ground in the lives of those who bear the brunt of these inequities. In other words, this chapter presents a CHC praxis that explores how local and global knowledge and communicative systems come into play in a marginalized community as an NGO facilitates pathways for the transformation of the health and lives of members of the community. Lessons learned from New Light's and Urmi Basu's journey with a community of sex workers in Kalighat, Kolkata are illustrative and instructive in this context. Hopefully, the readers will see how critical health initiatives that aim to transform the lives of the marginalized in meaningful ways came to fruition.

Conclusion

As editors, we want to thank the authors of these chapters. Their work provides valuable insights that can be taken up in a number of different ways to center critical questions in health communication. At the same time, as critical health scholars, we recognize that in curating our book, there are several scholars-thinkers-practitioners engaged in stellar transformative health work whose stories we have missed. We hope this edited volume serves as a call to center such stories from every corner of the world. We write at a time when health is imperiled by economic inequality, violence, war and human rights violations, environmental degradation and climate change, the dismantling of medical and public health infrastructures, rising online disinformation and political radicalization, and other major crises. This means that foregrounding the role of communication in establishing, reinforcing, resisting, and reformulating relationships of power is more crucial than ever. Health communication as a discipline can play a more central role in promoting public health based on insights from this book, incorporating the voices of the marginalized as central to understanding linkages between health and culture, connecting with deeper structures of power as we theorize what counts as "empowerment," and acknowledging and working closely with activists to address sociopolitical conditions and policy change.

References

Adebayo, C. T., Parcell, E. S., Mkandawire-Valhmu, L., & Olukotun, O. (2022). African American women's maternal healthcare experiences: A critical race theory perspective. *Health Communication*, *37*(9), 1135–1146. https://doi.org/10.1080/10410236.2021.1888453

Airhihenbuwa, C. O. (1995). *Health and culture: Beyond the Western paradigm*. Sage.

Airhihenbuwa, C. O. (2007). *Healing our differences: The crisis of global health and the politics of identity*. Rowman & Littlefield Publishers. https://www.loc.gov/catdir/toc/ecip0614/2006017494.html

Airhihenbuwa, C. O., Ford, C., Iwelunmor, J., Griffith, D. M., Ameen, K., Murray, T., & Nwaozuru, U. (2024). Decolonization and antiracism: Intersecting pathways to global health equity. *Ethnicity & Health*, *29*(7), 846–860. https://doi.org/10.1080/13557858.2024.2371429

Airhihenbuwa, C. O., Ford, C. L., & Iwelunmor, J. I. (2014). Why culture matters in health interventions: Lessons from HIV/AIDS stigma and NCDs. *Health Education & Behavior*, *41*(1), 78–84. https://doi.org/10.1177/1090198113487199

Airhihenbuwa, C. O., Makinwa, B., & Obregon, R. (2000). Toward a new communications framework for HIV/AIDS. *Journal of Health Communication: International Perspectives*, *5*(1 supp 1), 101–111. https://www.informaworld.com/10.1080/108107300406820

Airhihenbuwa, C. O., & Obregon, R. (2000). A critical assessment of theories/models used in health communication for HIV/AIDS. *Journal of Health Communication*, *5 (Supplement)*, 5–15. https://doi.org/10.1080/10810730050019528

Alper, M., Rauchberg, J. S., Simpson, E., Guberman, J., & Feinberg, S. (2023). TikTok as algorithmically mediated biographical illumination: Autism, self-discovery, and platformed diagnosis on #autisktok. *New Media & Society*, *27*(3), 1378–1396. https://doi.org/10.1177/14614448231193091

Anderson, W. (2002). Going through the motions: American public health and colonial "Mimicry". *American Literary History, 14*(4), 686–719. https://doi.org/10.2307/3568021

Asante, G., Adjaka, G., & Nartey, I. (2025). Rethinking (LGBT) Empowerment: Exploring the potential of community-based participatory research project among human rights NGOs in Ghana. *Journal of Applied Communication Research, 53*(2), 91–112. https://doi.org/https://doi.org/10.1080/00909882.2025.2470232

Babu, S., Koven, M., Thompson, C., & Makos, S. (2025). (Re)making scales: Communicative enfranchisement in women's narrative discourses about health dismissal. *Health Communication, 40*(6), 1–11. https://doi.org/10.1080/10410236.2024.2386716

Baer, H. A., Singer, M., & Johnsen, J. H. (1986). Toward a critical medical anthropology. *Social Science & Medicine, 23*(2), 95–98. https://doi.org/10.1016/0277-9536(86)90358-8

Ban, Z. (2016). Delineating responsibility, decisions and compromises: a frame analysis of the fast food industry's online CSR communication. *Journal of Applied Communication Research, 44*(3), 1–20. https://doi.org/10.1080/00909882.2016.1192290

Basnyat, I. (2017). Structural violence in health care: Lived experience of street-based female commercial sex workers in Kathmandu. *Qualitative Health Research, 27*(2), 191–203. https://doi.org/10.1177/1049732315601665

Basnyat, I. (2020). Stigma, agency, and motherhood: Exploring the performativity of dual mother–female sex workers identities in Kathmandu, Nepal. *Journal of International and Intercultural Communication, 13*(2), 98–113. https://doi.org/10.1080/17513057.2020.1735486

Basnyat, I., & Dutta, M. J. (2012). Reframing motherhood through the culture-centered approach: articulations of agency among young Nepalese women. *Health Communication, 27*(3), 273–283. https://doi.org/10.1080/10410236.2011.585444

Basu, A. (2010). Communicating health as an impossibility: Sex work, HIV/AIDS, and the dance of hope and hopelessness. *Southern Communication Journal, 75*(4), 413–432. https://doi.org/10.1080/1041794x.2010.504452

Basu, A. (2011). HIV/AIDS and subaltern autonomous rationality: A call to re-center health communication in marginalized sex worker spaces. *Communication Monographs, 78*(3), 391–408. https://doi.org/10.1080/03637751.2011.589457

Basu, A., & Dutta, M. J. (2009). Sex workers and HIV/AIDS: Analyzing participatory culture-centered health communication strategies. *Human Communication Research, 35*(1), 86–114. https://doi.org/10.1111/j.1468-2958.2008.01339.x

Basu, A., Spieldenner, A. R., & Dillon, P. J. (Eds.). (2022). *Post-AIDS discourse in health communication: sociocultural interpretations*. Routledge.

Bennett, J. A. (2022). Resisting the rhetoric of indexing: Disability, access, and the 2005 Tennessee State Capitol sit-in. *Communication and Critical/Cultural Studies, 19*, 1–19. https://doi.org/10.1080/14791420.2022.2086280

Billingslea, R., & Ellingson, L. (2015). Voicing late effects: Stories of long-term cancer survivorship [Art installation]. Santa Clara, CA: Special Collections Gallery, Santa Clara University, 8.

Bronfenbrenner, U. (1977). Toward an experimental ecology of human development. *American Psychologist*, *32*(7), 513–531. https://doi.org/10.1037/0003-066x.32.7.513

Brown, T., & Bell, M. (2008). Imperial or postcolonial governance? Dissecting the genealogy of a global public health strategy. *Social Science & Medicine*, *67*, 1571–1579.

Bute, J., Harter, L., Kirby, E., & Thompson, M. (2010). Politicizing personal choices? The storying of age-related infertility in public discourses. In S. Hayden & D. L. O'Brien Hallstein (Eds.), *Contemplating maternity in an era of choice: Explorations into discourse of reproduction* (pp. 49–72). Rowman & Littlefield Publishing Group, Inc.

Cao, A., & Wang, M. (2021). Exploring the health narratives of Chinese female migrant workers through culture-centered and gender perspectives. *Health Communication*, *36*(2), 158–167. https://doi.org/10.1080/10410236.2019.1669269

Carter, A. L., & Alexander, A. (2020). Soul food: [Re]framing the African-American farming crisis using the culture-centered approach [Original Research]. *Frontiers in Health Communication*, *5*(5). https://doi.org/10.3389/fcomm.2020.00005

Chandanabhumma, P. P., Duran, B. M., Peterson, J. C., Pearson, C. R., Oetzel, J. G., Dutta, M. J., & Wallerstein, N. B. (2020). Space within the scientific discourse for the voice of the other? Expressions of community voice in the scientific discourse of community-based participatory research. *Health Communication*, *35*(5), 616–627. https://doi.org/10.1080/10410236.2019.1581409

Conrad, C., & McIntush, H. G. (2003). Organizational rhetoric and healthcare policymaking. In *The Routledge handbook of health communication* (pp. 417–436). Routledge.

Conrad, C., & Millay, B. (2001). Confronting free market romanticism: Health care reform in the least likely place [Article]. *Journal of Applied Communication Research*, *29*(2), 153.

Conrad, P., & Barker, K. K. (2010). The social construction of illness: Key insights and policy implications. *Journal of Health and Social Behavior*, *51 Suppl*, S67–S79. https://doi.org/10.1177/0022146510383495

Coopman, S. J. (2016). Communicating disability: Metaphors of oppression, metaphors of empowerment. *Communication Yearbook*, *27*(1), 337–394. https://doi.org/10.1080/23808985.2003.11679030

Davis, C. S., & Quinlan, M. M. (2017). Communicating stigma and acceptance. In J. Yamasaki, P. Geist Martin, & B. Sharf (Eds.), *Storied health and illness* (pp. 191–220). Waveland Press.

De Los Santos Upton, S., Tarin, C. A., & Hernández, L. H. (2022). Construyendo conexiones para los niños: Environmental justice, reproductive feminicidio, and coalitional possibility in the borderlands. *Health Communication*, *37*(9), 1242–1252. https://doi.org/10.1080/10410236.2021.1911386

de Souza, R. (2022). Communication, carcerality, and neoliberal stigma: The case of hunger and food assistance in the United States. *Journal of Applied Communication Research*, *51*, 1–18. https://doi.org/10.1080/00909882.2022.2079954

de Souza, R., Basu, A., Kim, I., Basnyat, I., & Dutta, M. J. (2008). The paradox of "fair trade:" The influence of neoliberal trade agreements on food security and health. In H. M. Zoller & M. J. Dutta (Eds.), *Emerging perspectives in health communication* (pp. 411–430). Routledge.

Dean, M., & Street, R. L. (2014). A 3-stage model of patient-centered communication for addressing cancer patients' emotional distress. *Patient Education and Counseling*, *94*(2), 143–148. https://doi.org/https://doi.org/10.1016/j.pec.2013.09.025

Deetz, S. (1992). *Democracy in an age of corporate colonization: Developments in communication and the politics of everyday life*. State University of New York.

Dempsey, S., & Gibson, K. E. (2017). Food, biopower, and the child's body as a scale of intervention. In P. Marcell & F. Bosco (Eds.), *Food and place: A critical introduction* (pp. 253–269). Rowman & Littlefield.

Dempsey, S. E., Zoller, H. M., & Hunt, K. P. (2022). The meatpacking industry's corporate exceptionalism: racialized logics of food chain worker disposability during the COVID-19 crisis. *Food, Culture & Society*, *26*(3), 571–590. https://doi.org/10.1080/15528014.2021.2022916

Dove, S. A., Khan, S., & Kline, K. N. (2024). Structural violence, social suffering, and the COVID-19 syndemic: Discourses and narratives on the margins of the state in Texas. *Frontiers in Communication*, *9*. https://doi.org/10.3389/fcomm.2024.1369796

DuPré, A., & Overton, B. C. (2021). *Communicating about health: Current issues and perspectives* (6th ed.). Oxford University Press.

Dutta, M. J. (2007). Communicating about culture and health: Theorizing culture-centered and cultural-sensitivity approaches. *Communication Theory*, *17*, 304–328. https://doi.org/10.1111/j.1468-2885.2007.00297.x

Dutta, M. J. (2008). *Communicating Health: A culture-centered approach*. Polity.

Dutta, M. J. (2021). Singapore's extreme neoliberalism and the COVID outbreak: Culturally centering voices of low-wage migrant workers. *American Behavioral Scientist*, *65*(10), 1302–1322.

Dutta, M. J., & Basu, A. (2008). Meanings of health: Interrogating structure and culture. *Health Communication*, *23*(6), 560–572.

Dutta, M. J., & Pal, M. (2010). Dialog theory in marginalized settings: A Subaltern studies approach. *Communication Theory*, *20*(4), 363–386. https://doi.org/10.1111/j.1468-2885.2010.01367.x

Dutta, M. J., & Pal, M. (2020). Theorizing from the global south: Dismantling, resisting, and transforming communication theory. *Communication Theory*, *30*(4), 349–369.

Dutta, M. J., & Thaker, J. (2019). 'Communication sovereignty' as resistance: Strategies adopted by women farmers amid the agrarian crisis in India. *Journal of Applied Communication Research*, *47*(1), 24–46. https://doi.org/10.1080/00909882.2018.1547917

Ellingson, L. L. (2009). "Do we need to make it look good?" Form, function, and femininity for women with disabilities. In E. Kirby & C. McBride (Eds.), *Gender actualized: Cases in communicatively constructing realities* (pp. 69–70). Kendall/Hunt.

Farmer, P. (1996a). *AIDS and accusation: Haiti and the geography of blame*. University of California Press.

Farmer, P. (1996b). On suffering and structural violence: A view from below. *Daedalus*, *125*(1), 261–283. https://www.mitpressjournals.org/toc/daed/125/1/

Farmer, P. (1999). *Infections and inequalities: The modern plagues*. University of California Press.

Farmer, P., Kleinman, A., Kim, J., & Basilico, M. (Eds.). (2013). *Reimagining global health: An introduction*. University of California Press.

Fujishiro, K., Ahonen, E. Q., & Winkler, M. (2022). Investigating employment quality for population health and health equity: A perspective of power. *International Journal of Environmental Research and Public Health*, *19*(16), 9991. https://www.mdpi.com/1660-4601/19/16/9991

Galtung, J. (1969). Violence, peace, and peace research. *Journal of Peace Research*, *6*(3), 167–191. https://doi.org/10.1177/002234336900600301

Gerbensky-Kerber, A. (2011). Grading the "good" body: A poststructural feminist analysis of body mass index initiatives. *Health Communication*, *26*(4), 354–365. https://doi.org/10.1080/10410236.2010.551581

Greene, J., Basilico, M. T., Kim, H., & Farmer, P. (2013). Colonial medicine and its legacies. In P. Farmer, J. Y. Kim, A. Kleinman, & M. Basilico (Eds.), *Reimagining global health: An introduction* (pp. 33–73). University of California Press.

Grossberg, L. (1993a). Can cultural studies find true happiness in communication? *Journal of Communication*, *43*(4), 89–97. https://doi.org/10.1111/j.1460-2466.1993.tb01308.x

Grossberg, L. (1993b). Cultural studies and/in new worlds. *Critical Studies in Mass Communication*, *10*(1), 1–22. https://doi.org/10.1080/15295039309366846

Grossberg, L. (1997). *Bringing it all back home: Essays on cultural studies*. Duke University Press.

Hall, S. (1985). Signification, representation, ideology: Althusser and the poststructuralist debates. *Critical Studies in Media Communication*, *2*(2), 91–114. https://doi.org/10.1080/15295038509360070

Hawkins, D. S. (2022). "After Philando, I had to take a sick day to recover": Psychological distress, trauma and police brutality in the black community. *Health Communication*, *37*(9), 1113–1122. https://doi.org/10.1080/10410236.2021.1913838

Hernández, L. H., & De Los Santos Upton, S. (2019). Critical health communication methods at the U.S.-Mexico border: Violence against migrant women and the role of health activism [conceptual analysis]. *Frontiers in Communication*, *4*. https://doi.org/10.3389/fcomm.2019.00034

Hintz, E. A., & Tucker, R. V. (2023). Contesting illness: Communicative (dis)enfranchisement in patient–provider conversations about chronic overlapping pain conditions. *Human Communication Research*, *49*(2), 170–181. https://doi.org/10.1093/hcr/hqad004

Hudak, N., & Bates, B. R. (2019). In pursuit of "queer-friendly" healthcare: An interview study of How queer individuals select care providers. *Health Communication*, *34*(8), 818–824. https://doi.org/10.1080/10410236.2018.1437525

Ivancic, S. R. (2018). Body sovereignty and body liability in the wake of an "obesity epidemic": A poststructural analysis of the soda ban. *Health Communication*, *33*(10), 1243–1256. https://doi.org/10.1080/10410236.2017.1351266

Ivancic, S. R. (2020). "No one's coming to save us": Centering lived experiences in rural food insecurity organizing. *Health Communication*, *36*, 1–5. https://doi.org/10.1080/10410236.2020.1724644

James, E. P., Zanin, A. C., & Damon, Z. (2022). Blue-collar and healthy worker identities: How parallel ideal worker identities sustain unobtrusive control on

the shop-floor. *Management Communication Quarterly, 37*(3), 542–571. https://doi.org/10.1177/08933189221134116
Jamil, R., & Kumar, R. (2021). Culture, structure, and health: Narratives of low-income Bangladeshi migrant workers from the United Arab Emirates. *Health Communication, 36*(11), 1297–1308. https://doi.org/10.1080/10410236.2020.1750773
Jensen, R. (2016). *Infertility: Tracing the History of a Transformative Term*. The Penn State University Press.
Kaur-Gill, S. (2020). The COVID-19 pandemic and outbreak inequality: Mainstream reporting of Singapore's migrant workers in the margins. *Frontiers in Communication, 5*, 65.
Kaur-Gill, S. (2022). The meanings of heart health among low-income Malay women in Singapore: Narratives of food insecurity, caregiving stressors, and shame [Article]. *Journal of Applied Communication Research, 50*(2), 111–128. https://doi.org/10.1080/00909882.2022.2033298
Khan, S. (2014). Manufacturing consent?: Media messages in the mobilization against HIV/AIDS in India and lessons for health communication. *Health Communication, 29*, 288–298. https://doi.org/10.1080/10410236.2012.753139
Kilanowski, J. F. (2017). Breadth of the socio-ecological model. *Journal of Agromedicine, 22*(4), 295–297. https://doi.org/10.1080/1059924X.2017.1358971
King, N. B. (2002). Security, disease, commerce: Ideologies of postcolonial global health. *Social Studies of Science, 32*(5-6), 763–789. http://www.jstor.org/stable/3183054
Kline, K. N. (2011). Popular media and health: Images, effects, and institutions. In T. L. Thompson, R. Parrott, & J. F. Nussbaum (Eds.), *Handbook of health communication* (2nd ed., pp. 252–267). Routledge.
Krebs, E., & Schoenbauer, K. V. (2020). Hysterics and heresy: Using dialogism to explore the problematics of endometriosis diagnosis. *Health Communication, 35*(8), 1013–1022.
LaPoe, V. L., Carter Olson, C. S., Azocar, C. L., LaPoe, B. R., Hazarika, B., & Jain, P. (2022). A comparative analysis of health news in indigenous and mainstream media. *Health Communication, 37*(9), 1192–1203. https://doi.org/10.1080/10410236.2021.1945179
Lupton, D. (1994). Toward the development of critical health communication praxis. *Health Communication, 6*, 55–67. https://doi.org/10.1207/s15327027hc0601_4
Lupton, D. (2012). *Medicine as culture: Illness, disease, and the body* (3rd ed.). SAGE.
Lupton, D. (2018). *Fat* (2nd ed.). Routledge.
Lupton, D. (2022). *COVID societies: Theorising the coronavirus crisis*. Routledge.
Lynch, J., & Dubriwny, T. (2005). Drugs and double binds: Racial identification and pharmacogenomics in a system of binary race logic. *Health Communication, 19*(1), 61–73.
Makkawy, A., & Moreman, S. T. (2025). Wellbeing for the blind and visually impaired: An arts-based cripistemological ethnography of Alexandria, Egypt's Taha Hussein Library. *Health Communication*, 1–13. https://doi.org/10.1080/10410236.2025.2458247
McKnight, J. (1988). Where can health communication be found? *Journal of Applied Communication Research, 16*(1), 39–43. https://doi.org/10.1080/00909888809365270.

Meloncon, L., & Scott, J. B. (Eds.). (2017). *Methodologies for the rhetoric of health and medicine*. Routledge.

Melkote, S. R., Krishnatray, P., & Krishnatray, S. (2007). Destigmatizing leprosy: Implications for communication theory and practice. In Zoller, H.M. & Dutta, M. (eds.), *Emerging perspectives in health communication: Meaning, culture, and power*. Routledge.

Merrill Jr., K. (2024). Using artificial intelligence to address health disparities: Challenges and solutions. in Srividya, R., & Banjo, O. O. (eds.), *The Oxford handbook of media and social justice*, 234. Oxford Academic. https://doi.org/10.1093/oxfordhb/9780197744345.013.25

Mukherjee, P., & Ivancic, S. (2024). Safe water as empowerment, structural dilemma, and savior: Conflicting discourses about arsenic groundwater contamination in West Bengal. *Journal of Applied Communication Research*, 52(4), 435–454. https://doi.org/10.1080/00909882.2024.2345211

Mumby, D. K. (1997). The problem of hegemony: Rereading Gramsci for organizational communication studies. *Western Journal of Communication*, 61(4), 343–375. https://doi.org/10.1080/10570319709374585

Nadesan, M. (2008). *Governmentality, biopower, and everyday life*. Routledge.

Okamoto, K. E. (2017). "It's like moving the titanic:" Community organizing to address food (in)security. *Health Communication*, 32(8), 1047–1050. https://doi.org/10.1080/10410236.2016.1196517

Olufowote, J. O. (2017). An Institutional field of people living with HIV/AIDS organizations in Tanzania: Agency, culture, dialogue, and structure. *Frontiers in Communication*, 2. https://doi.org/10.3389/fcomm.2017.00001

Parker, P. S. (2016). Control, resistance, and empowerment in raced, gendered, and classed work contexts: The case of African American women. *Annals of the International Communication Association*, 27(1), 257–291. https://doi.org/10.1080/23808985.2003.11679028

Parsloe, S. M., & Holton, A. E. (2018). #Boycottautismspeaks: Communicating a counternarrative through cyberactivism and connective action. *Information, Communication & Society*, 21(8), 1116–1133. https://doi.org/10.1080/1369118X.2017.1301514

Pringle, W., Sachal, S. S., Dhutt, G. S., Kestler, M., Dube, E., & Bettinger, J. A. (2022). Public health community engagement with Asian populations in British Columbia during COVID-19: Towards a culture-centered approach. *Can J Public Health*, 113, 1–10. https://doi.org/10.17269/s41997-022-00699-5

Robb, J. S. (2023). A clash of culture and structure: Considering barriers to access for people without papers. *Health Communication*, 38(13), 3003–3011.

Sastry, S. (2014). Postcolonial studies of health. In T. L. Thompson (Ed.), *Encyclopedia of health communication* (pp. 1081–1084). Thousand Oaks, CA: SAGE Publications, Inc.

Sastry, S., & Dutta, M. J. (2011). Postcolonial constructions of HIV/AIDS: Meaning, culture, and structure. *Health Communication*, 26(5), 437–449. https://doi.org/10.1080/10410236.2011.554166

Sastry, S., & Dutta, M. J. (2012). Public health, global surveillance, and the "emerging disease" worldview: A postcolonial appraisal of PEPFAR. *Health Communication*, 27(6), 519–532. https://doi.org/10.1080/10410236.2011.616626

Sastry, S., Siegenthaler, B., Mukherjee, P., Abdul Raheem, S., & Basu, A. (2023). The (mis)uses of community: A critical analysis of public health communication for COVID-19 vaccination in the United States. *Human Communication Research*, *49*(4), 396–407. https://doi.org/10.1093/hcr/hqad018

Sastry, S., Stephenson, M., Dillon, P., & Carter, A. (2021). A meta-theoretical systematic review of the culture-centered approach to health communication: Toward a refined, "nested" model. *Communication Theory*, *31*(3), 380–421. https://doi.org/10.1093/ct/qtz024

Sastry, S., Zoller, H. M., Walker, T., & Sunderland, S. (2017). From patient navigation to cancer justice: Toward a culture-centered, community-owned intervention addressing disparities in cancer prevention. *Frontiers in Communication*, *2*. https://doi.org/10.3389/fcomm.2017.00019

Segal, J. (2005a). *Health and the rhetoric of medicine*. Southern Illinois University Press.

Segal, J. (2005b). Interdisciplinarity and bibliography in rhetoric of health and medicine. *Technical Communication Quarterly*, *14*(3), 311–318.

Sharf, B. F. (1999). The present and future of health communication scholarship: Overlooked opportunities. *Health Communication*, *11*, 195–199. https://doi.org/10.1207/s15327027hc1102_5

Sharf, B. F., & Vanderford, M., L. (2003). Illness narratives and the social construction of health. In T. L. Thompson, A. Dorsey, M., K. Miller, I., & R. Parrott (Eds.), *Handbook of health communication* (1st ed., pp. 9–34). Routledge.

Shugart, H. A. (2011). Shifting the balance: The contemporary narrative of obesity. *Health Communication*, *26*(1), 37–47. https://doi.org/10.1080/10410236.2011.527620

Spieldenner, A. (2016). PrEP whores and HIV prevention: The queer communication of HIV Pre-Exposure Prophylaxis (PrEP). *Journal of Homosexuality*, *63*(12), 1685–1697. https://doi.org/10.1080/00918369.2016.1158012

Stanley, B. L., & Basu, A. (2023). 'Chemical jail': Culture-centered theorizing of carcerality in methadone maintenance treatment and addiction recovery in the United States. *Journal of Applied Communication Research*, *51*(5), 463–480.

Teal, C. R., & Street, R. L. (2009). Critical elements of culturally competent communication in the medical encounter: A review and model. *Social Science & Medicine (1982)*, *68*(3), 533–543. https://doi.org/10.1016/j.socscimed.2008.10.015

Thompson, M. (2010). Who's guarding what? A poststructural feminist analysis of Gardasil discourses [Article]. *Health Communication*, *25*(2), 119–130. https://doi.org/10.1080/10410230903544910

Thomson, D. M. (2009). Big food and the body politics of personal responsibility. *Southern Communication Journal*, *74*, 2–17. https://doi.org/10.1080/10417940802360829

Tucker, R. V., Gunning, J. N., Hintz, E. A., & Denes, A. (2024). A critical quantitative approach to intersectionality: Interrogating race and class in the context of female chronic pain. *Communication Studies*, *75*(4), 425–444. https://doi.org/10.1080/10510974.2024.2344404

Tulloch, J., & Lupton, D. (2003). *Risk and everyday life*. Sage Publications. https://www.loc.gov/catdir/enhancements/fy0657/2002113233-t.html; https://www.loc.gov/catdir/enhancements/fy0657/2002113233-d.html

Vardeman-Winter, J. (2017). The framing of women and health disparities: A critical look at race, gender, and class from the perspectives of grassroots health communicators. *Health Communication*, *32*(5), 629–638. https://doi.org/10.1080/10410236.2016.1160318

Vicari, S., & Cappai, F. (2016). Health activism and the logic of connective action. A case study of rare disease patient organisations. *Information, Communication & Society*, *19*(11), 1653–1671.

Villamil, A. M., & D'Enbeau, S. (2021). Essential work in the U.S. during COVID-19: Navigating vulnerability–sustainability tensions. *Sustainability*, *13*(19), 10665. https://www.mdpi.com/2071-1050/13/19/10665

Waitzkin, H. (1984). Doctor-patient communication. *JAMA*, *252*(17), 2441–2446. https://doi.org/10.1001/jama.1984.03350170043017

Waitzkin, H. (1991). *The politics of medical encounters: How patients and doctors deal with social problems*. Yale University Press.

Waitzkin, H. (2000). *The second sickness: Contradictions of capitalist health care* (Rev. and updated ed.). Rowman & Littlefield. Table of contents https://www.loc.gov/catdir/toc/fy022/99046590.html

Waitzkin, H., & Waterman, B. (1974). *The exploitation of illness in capitalist society*. Bobbs-Merrill.

Waitzkin, H., & Working Group for Health Beyond Capitalism. (2018). *Health care under the knife: Moving beyond capitalism for our health*. Monthly Review Press.

Yep, G. A. (2013). Queering/Quaring/Kauering/Crippin'/Transing "Other Bodies" in intercultural communication. *Journal of International and Intercultural Communication*, *6*(2), 118–126. https://doi.org/10.1080/17513057.2013.777087

Yep, G. A., Reece, S., & Negron, E. (2003). Culture and stigma in a bona fide group: Boundaries and contexxt in a 'closed' support group for Asian Americans living with HIV infection. In L. R. Frey (Ed.), *Group Communication in context: Studies of bona-fide groups* (pp. 157–180). Lawrence Erlbaum Associates.

Zoller, H. M. (2003). Health on the line: Identity and disciplinary control in employee occupational health and safety discourse. *Journal of Applied Communication Research*, *31*(2), 118–139.

Zoller, H. M. (2005). Health activism: Communication theory and action for social change. *Communication Theory*, *15*(4), 341–364. https://doi.org/10.1111/j.1468-2885.2005.tb00339.x

Zoller, H. M. (2008). Technologies of neoliberal governmentality: The discursive influence of global economic policies on public health. In H. M. Zoller & M. J. Dutta (Eds.), *Emerging perspectives in health communication: Meaning, culture and power* (pp. 390–410). Routledge.

Zoller, H. M. (2017). Health activism targeting corporations: A critical health communication perspective. *Health Communication*, *32*(2), 219–229. https://doi.org/10.1080/10410236.2015.1118735

Zoller, H. M. (2021). Re-Imagining localism and food justice: Co-Op Cincy and the union cooperative movement [Community Case Study]. *Frontiers in Communication*, *6*(118). https://doi.org/10.3389/fcomm.2021.686400

Zoller, H. M. (2023). Addressing health inequalities through worker and consumer cooperatives: Co-op Cincy's organizing for food justice. In S. Dempsey (Ed.),

Organizing eating: Communicating for equity across U.S. food systems (pp. 139–165). Routledge.

Zoller, H. M., & Casteel, D. (2021). #March for our lives: Health activism, diagnostic framing, gun control, and the gun industry. *Health Communication, 37*(7), 813–823. https://doi.org/10.1080/10410236.2020.1871167

Zoller, H. M., & Dutta, M. J. (2008). *Emerging perspectives in health communication: Meaning, culture, and power*. Routledge, Taylor & Francis Group.

Zoller, H. M., & Kline, K. N. (2008). Theoretical contributions of interpretive and critical research in health communication. *Annals of the International Communication Association, 32*(1), 89–135. https://doi.org/10.1080/23808985.2008.11679076

Zoller, H. M., Strochlic, R., & Getz, C. (2023). An employee-centered framework for healthy workplaces: Implementing a critically holistic, participative, and structural model through the Equitable Food Initiative. *Journal of Applied Communication Research, 51*(2), 164–184. https://doi.org/10.1080/00909882.2022.2106579

Zou, W., & Liu, Z. (2024). Body politics, reproductive rights, and digital media advocacy within stigmatized contexts: A critical discourse analysis of Weibo discussions on IUDs in modern-day China. *Journal of Applied Communication Research, 52*(1), 27–46. https://doi.org/10.1080/00909882.2023.2282514

Critiquing Dominant Discourses

2
FROM SYMPTOMS TO TRANSFORMATION

Addressing the Root Causes of Hunger Through Critical Health Communication

Rebecca de Souza

Even as scientists figure out how to micro-edit genes, we have not solved the most fundamental problems of our times: poverty and hunger. In an era of neoliberal expansionist agendas and technological advancement, poverty is not just unprofitable to solve, but it is the calculated collateral damage of a "capitalism-on-speed" agenda. The corporate capture of the food system globally has meant a concentration of wealth for a few and growing hunger and health disparities worldwide (Spring et al., 2024). With regard to hunger, approximately 15% of the U.S. population suffers from hunger and food insecurity (Coleman-Jensen et al., 2019), and over the last five decades, there has been little change to this number despite advances in agricultural production (Carolan, 2011). Indeed, scholars point out that the U.S. government is more invested in "counting" the hunger problem than finding long term solutions (Chilton & Rose, 2009). Women, parents, and communities of color face the brunt of hunger often experiencing devastating physical, social, and mental outcomes (de Souza, 2023). The failure of the state to ensure good food for all through progressive and regulatory policies reflects the strategic politics of "care and abandonment" in a neoliberal regime (Dickinson, 2020; Pine & de Souza, 2023).

Historically, much health communication scholarship has focused on individual factors that affect health such as attitudes, values, and beliefs, while structural, systemic, and environmental conditions within which health behaviors arise have been ignored (see Dutta, 2008; Dutta & de Souza, 2008). For example, there is a plethora of research examining the role of "self-efficacy" or "perceived behavioral control" on an individual's motivation and ability to engage in healthy behaviors (e.g., Denison et al., 2023). These cognitive-behavioral approaches are appealing because they offer avenues for health interventions and can have short-term results (e.g., changes in knowledge). However, without attending to the root causes of hunger and poverty, these interventions are mere blips in the landscape that do little to bring about large-scale transformation. In his groundbreaking treatise, Dutta (2008) observed that dominant theories and approaches to health communication are rooted in Eurocentric middle-class ideologies that myopically offer cognitive-behavioral approaches for preventing illness while leaving structural inequities unchecked.

Critical health communication (CHC) scholarship sits at the key juncture of health and structural transformation. CHC intervenes in the dominant health paradigm by recognizing that health is not just about individual choices, but about systems, structures, cultures, and environments that facilitate or inhibit those choices. Sometimes referred to as the "social determinants of health," these factors include food, housing, employment, education, and healthcare to name a few (World Health Organization, n.d.). CHC makes an important move by shifting the conversation from "outcomes" to root causes pointing out that the distribution of health and life opportunities are heavily influenced by the interaction of social, economic, communicative, and political factors. Several decades ago, medical anthropologist Farmer (2005) used the phrase "structural violence" to refer to the large-scale forces of poverty and political violence that shape the distribution of disease. Going beyond the more neutral phrase social determinants of health (SDH), Farmer emphasized the role of power in creating health inequities: he noted that politics determined who had access to HIV anti-retroviral therapy and who did not, and this was the result of systematic political-economic oppression. Within the paradigm of social determinants research, CHC plays a crucial role in illuminating how power is intricately woven into the fabric of discourse, knowledge, and institutional structures, ultimately affecting the health and well-being of individuals, communities, and environments.

This chapter will offer a brief overview of critical modernism, outlining the fundamental assumptions that underpin the critical modernist perspective on hunger. It will also explore four primary areas of CHC scholarship: (a) hunger discourse, identity, and materiality; (b) organizing hunger and hunger solutions; (c) hunger policy and political action; and (d) culture-centered approaches (CCAs) to hunger. The chapter concludes by presenting two case studies that serve as examples of specific pathways for CHC scholarship; these case studies illustrate how CHC can engage with tangible, real-world issues to uncover systemic inequalities and offer insights into potential solutions.

Critical Modernism and Communication

The term "critical" is rooted in Marxist political economy, signifying an intensified focus on the power structures that perpetuate inequity alongside a desire to address these imbalances in the pursuit of justice (Cohen & Arato, 1994; Held, 1980; Macey, 2009). While scholars may conceptualize power in myriad ways, in the field of communication, critical theory tends to focus on political and economic structures, discourse, ideology, language, and the social/political construction of knowledge (e.g., Fairclough & Wodak, 1997; Lupton, 1994, 1996, 2003; Mumby, 1997; van Dijk, 1989, 2004). Some health communication researchers focus on power linked to economic, racial, and gender-based exploitation (e.g., Adebayo et al., 2022; De Los Santos Upton et al., 2022), while others explore cultural, linguistic, and symbolic forms of power, including the authority to present, represent, and produce knowledge (e.g., Lupton, 2003).

In my own scholarship, I adopt a "critical modernist" approach, which serves as a bridge between the intellectual traditions of modernism and postmodernism (Mumby, 1997; Pal & Dutta, 2008). Critical modernism and postmodernism diverge in significant ways (Berube, 2001); critical modernism maintains a belief in a realist, objective world, whereas postmodernism expresses skepticism toward the notion of objective reality, viewing the world as socially constructed. Critical modernists embrace grand narratives, particularly those focused on emancipation and justice, while postmodernists reject overarching narratives, contending that truth is fragmented and ultimately unattainable. Critical modernists view the subject as a rational agent, capable of critique, and resistant to oppression; postmodernism, in contrast, questions the existence of a coherent and stable subject, perceiving identity as fragmented, fluid, performative, discursively produced and perpetually in flux. Critical modernism negotiates the tensions between modernism and postmodernism, engaging with how power operates within structures and institutions as well as knowledge, language, and discourse (Pal & Dutta, 2008). Critical modernism provides an entry point for theorizing and praxis in CHC by elucidating how power resides within structures and discourse.

The critical modernist approach I employ to study hunger does not adhere to a single set of tenets; rather, it draws from a diverse array of principles that align with similar epistemological and ontological truths. I incorporate insights from various social theorists to examine the hunger problem, aiming to reveal the power dynamics embedded in hunger discourses, practices, and policies while opening pathways for food system transformation. For instance, by drawing on critical theorists and poststructuralists such as Foucault (1975, 2003), Gramsci (1992), and

Bourdieu (1984), I utilize concepts of power, hegemony, ideology, materiality, discourse, and governmentality to analyze issues of food justice. I also engage with the more applied work of communication scholars (e.g., Dutta, 2015; Ivancic, 2018; van Dijk, 1989, 2004) to gain insights on the application of critical theory to health concerns. Given my focus on equity and marginality, I lean on critical race theory (e.g., Crenshaw et al., 1991), whiteness studies (e.g., Frankenberg, 1993), critical feminism (Harding & Hintikka, 1983; hooks, 2004), and cultural and postcolonial theorizing (Appadurai, 1996; Talpade Mohanty, 1984) to provide more nuanced understandings of power and to address common critiques of critical theory. For example, scholars point out that it is possible to engage in critical theory while only addressing the experiences of white people. This evaluation has led me to the work of Black and Third World feminists (e.g., Collins, 2009), who offer incisive critiques of how women, and women of color, are symbolically and materially marginalized through masculinist structures of knowledge and power. In my research on hunger for instance, I integrate abstract Foucauldian concepts with feminist theorizing to illustrate how governance functions to construct some populations as full citizens with rights of belonging, while rendering others (e.g., women) outside the folds of citizenship (see de Souza, 2022).

An important facet of critical modernism is its engagement with knowledge construction. While dominant health communication research prioritizes results, outcomes, and findings, CHC recognizes that researchers—and the institutions that support them—are deeply implicated in any reported findings. The process of "discovery," from Christopher Columbus to contemporary grant-funded research, is frequently marred by exploitation, colonization, and the subjugation of "subjects." Critical ethnographic methods (e.g., Conquergood, 1991; Huffman & Tracy, 2018; Madison, 2020) emerge as pathways to restore power to participants, emphasizing dialogue as a central component. The next section will delve into fundamental assumptions about hunger from a critical modernist perspective, challenging the prevailing scientific, economic, and political rationalities surrounding hunger.

Key Assumptions of the Critical (Modernist) Approach to Hunger

A critical approach to hunger challenges the fundamental belief that hunger arises solely from food shortages. Instead, it posits that hunger is caused by a lack of access to political and legal power and that governments are responsible for ensuring food security through "good governance" and political action (de Souza, 2022; Pine & de Souza, 2023). A second key assumption involves recognizing that historical factors shape food disparities and injustices (Pine & de Souza, 2023). In the United States, as in many developing nations, hunger is linked to historical systems of patriarchy, racism, colonization, and imperialism, which contribute to disproportionate levels of hunger and poverty among certain populations. Black and Brown communities, burdened by a legacy of systemic discrimination, experience higher rates of hunger (Spring et al., 2024), and women face the disproportionate burden of food insecurity due to factors such as gender-based violence and reproductive caring labors (de Souza, 2023). A third assumption of the critical approach involves scrutinizing mainstream solutions, such as charitable food distribution. In my work, for example, I examine how charity does not truly "solve" or "end" hunger but instead manages the issue, treating hunger as a symptom rather than addressing its structural roots in the deregulation of labor and capitalist markets under neoliberalism (de Souza, 2019; Dickinson, 2020; Poppendieck, 1999). The relationship between food banks, agribusiness, and anti-hunger organizations—often referred to as the "hunger industrial complex" (Fisher, 2017)—is deeply problematic. This system channels inadequate and unhealthy food to low-income communities through charitable food programs, ultimately reinforcing stigma and marginalization (de Souza, 2019). Lastly, the critical approach to hunger challenges the notion that change is impossible or that "there will always be hungry people." Instead, it advocates for social transformation by questioning and dismantling accepted norms and structures. Critical scholars focus on envisioning new possibilities to replace the profit-driven capitalist food system grounded in human rights and moral principles surrounding justice and equity. For example, Zoller's (2024) study examines how 1worker1vote.org leaders practice "pragmatic utopianism" by advancing a counter-narrative to extractive capitalism through worker ownership, sustainability, and solidarity. The movement cultivates "realistic hope" by turning systemic challenges into opportunities for innovation while adapting strategically to obstacles. It underscores the power of grassroots organizing in shaping alternative economies and driving meaningful social change. Another piece by Zoller (2021) examines the Co-Op Cincy's food sector organizing as a form of resistance to the industrial, corporate food system. Rooted in a commitment to social justice, Co-Op Cincy raises awareness of the deep connections between food systems, racial and class-based inequities, and the imperative for sustainability. By embedding these values into its daily operations and embodying these commitments, the cooperative offers valuable insights into creating a more equitable food system and a just economy. Next, we turn our attention to how CHC contributes to the literature on hunger.

Key Contributions of the Critical Communication Approach to Hunger

While hunger is a well-studied phenomenon in public health and nutritional sciences, critical approaches to hunger are only now gaining traction in the field of communication, with a notable increase in research on hunger, food, and food systems emerging over the past decade. Overall, critical communication research tends to view food, both its presence and absence, as an entry point to understanding power, privilege, identity, and culture (Dempsey, 2023; Frye & Bruner, 2012). Food is a material reality that "organizes" social, economic, and civic life in important ways as witnessed by how communities come together around food for both celebration and in mundane acts of social reproduction. The materiality of food and its discursive practices are inextricably linked to each other influencing identities, environments, policies, and structures (Dempsey, 2023). Furthermore, food and eating offer key sites of power, resistance, and activism that challenge hegemonic ideologies and systems (e.g., Dempsey, 2023; Dutta & Thaker, 2019). Indeed, a fundamental contribution of CHC has been to offer counter-cultural and counter-hegemonic interpretations and analyses of health-related concerns by examining structural and linguistic vectors of power. Scholars have made unique contributions to CHC through four overlapping lines of inquiry: (a) hunger discourses, identity, and materiality, (b) organizing hunger and hunger solutions, (c) hunger policy and politics, and (d) the CCA to hunger. This body of work spans diverse communication subdisciplines of health, rhetoric, organizational, and environmental communication, but taken together offer new and poignant ways of understanding hunger's root causes, impacts, and solutions. This section reviews some key studies that offer counter-hegemonic assessments of the hunger problem through a communication lens. Although some studies may appear "outdated," I present them as exemplars of transformative scholarship that have shaped my own academic trajectory and the discipline itself.

Discourse, Identity, and Materiality

CHC scholarship within this domain aims to unravel the layers of meaning inscribed upon the condition of hunger and hungry people illuminating how food is not only a biological necessity but also deeply implicated with issues of identity, discourse/ideology, and materiality. From the quality of food we eat to where we get our food, food shapes our sense of self and perceptions of others with implications for health and well-being. One entry point for communication scholars has been to study how hungry and "obese" people are represented in media and cultural discourses. Ratzinger

(2012) for example examined verbal and visual imagery of hunger and obesity on international and domestic hunger relief websites. Her analysis revealed that hunger is often approached through numbers and statistics, enumerating both the hungry population and the amount of food needed to meet their needs. This focus on quantification reinforces public health scholars Chilton and Rose's (2009) critique of hunger as an overly counted phenomenon, reflecting a preoccupation with "counting" rather than addressing the deeper causes of the problem. While hunger discourses focused on quantification and victimhood, obesity discourses focus on the objectification of the body; overweight individuals were dehumanized, portrayed in terms of their body parts, and portrayed as lacking in personal responsibility. The study reveals how mainstream hunger discourses shape inaccuracies about who suffers from hunger and obesity (and why) while at the same time concealing the root causes of hunger—the role of the food industry and corporate "irresponsibility." Theorizing the medicalization of weight, Lupton's (2018) book, *Fat* examines how fat bodies are central to social stigma, medical discourse, and public health interventions; fatness is often framed as a pathological condition within the so-called "obesity epidemic" and efforts to regulate and contain fat bodies are deeply rooted in societal and medical anxieties.

Communication scholars have done important work linking food with social class and identity. For example, Dougherty et al. (2018) used a discursive-material framework to explore how food security and economic insecurity were experienced and articulated by unemployed people across social classes. In the first category comprising low-income individuals, participants focused on the materiality of food and what it was like to experience a shortage of food. In the second category, participants who were most threatened by class slippage had developed a middle-class form of communication that concealed their food (in)security. In the third category, resource-secure participants relegated the materiality of food to the background; unemployment for this group meant that they did not have to worry about their next meal, so they talked about food more broadly as a means to build community and maintain classed relationships (e.g., going to a coffee shop to network with other professionals). The study illuminates how food, identity, and social class are intimately linked, produced, and performed through discourse.

Rhetorical studies, though not always directly focused on human health and well-being, cogently articulate how language, symbols, and discourse indirectly affect politics and policies concerning human health. Cooks' (2015) analysis of foodie discourses and food recovery/ rescue discourses found disjunctures between dominant cultural discourses and lived experiences of hunger. She found that while foodie discourses almost universally recognized taste as a primary marker of culture and identity, food insecurity discourses almost universally left out matters of taste and desirability. She writes: "Once again, we can see the separation of those for whom the taste of food should be important from those for whom 'wasted' food would be welcomed" (p. 131).

This body of scholarship linking class and identity has provoked me to think more deeply about the mundane processes through which stigma is produced through food and how it influences our health and well-being especially for those on the receiving end of food assistance—themes which I have taken up in my own work on hunger (de Souza, 2023, 2024). For example, in interviews with women experiencing hunger (de Souza, 2024), I found that even though food insecure women sometimes consumed whatever food was available to them through charitable programs, taste, healthfulness, and desirability of food were important factors in their decision-making. In a neoliberal era, where personal responsibility and discipline are valued, women worked hard to make good food choices but were unable to choose the foods they wanted to eat because of a lack of resources and inadequate social safety net protections.

Overall, this line of communication research highlights the complex relationship between food, identity, and material reality, demonstrating that food is not merely a biological need but a site for symbolic and material conflict. Hunger challenges individuals' ability to survive and uphold their class and social identity. Moreover, prevailing hunger discourses often obscure its true causes and perpetuate class-based stereotypes about who experiences hunger and why. The gap between dominant narratives of hunger and people's actual experiences reveals how the root causes of hunger are often overlooked or concealed, preventing the development of comprehensive solutions to hunger and poverty.

Organizing Hunger and Hunger Solutions

Communication studies within the "organizing hunger" domain demonstrate how the presence and absence of food organizes, structures, and orders society in important ways (Dempsey, 2023). Anthropologists have long argued that food operates similarly to language to the extent that it has a structure and code that expresses patterns about social relationships (Julier, 2013; Van Esterik, 1999). The role of volunteer labor and faith-based organizing around hunger has been an important site of exploration in communication research illuminating patterns of hierarchical social and racial structures. For example, a pioneering study by Papa et al. (2006) examined a participatory soup kitchen in rural Appalachia, where food was served family style and the responsibility for cooking and cleaning was shared by staff and clients. However, even with restructuring the soup kitchen and encouraging staff/volunteers to mingle with clients, staff ending up sitting with each other while clients sat on their own. In this instance, despite well-intentioned efforts, the soup kitchen was unable to disrupt class and social boundaries even as it distributed free food to hungry people. More recently, Ivancic and Dooling (2023) offered the concept of "entangled shame" to describe how discourses about poverty, materiality, and marginality cohere to produce shame among clients of food assistance programs, while also cautioning that drawing clean distinctions between "givers and receivers" can sidestep the labor, complexity, and generosity that emerges in spaces of oppression (Ivancic, 2020).

In charitable food settings, scholars have illuminated contentions surrounding "good" and "bad food" and demonstrated potential health and safety implications on clients' health (de Souza, 2023). On the one hand, communities come together volunteering time and labor to distribute food to those in need, but on the other hand, the quality of food handed out is less than adequate and therefore exacerbates health vulnerabilities of already marginalized populations. Schuwerk (2011) explored contradictions in nutrition messages in food pantries; she found that while food safety was an important part of the organization's discursive practices, food safety guidelines were not always followed, because staff and volunteers saw no reason to throw out food they thought was "perfectly fine food" (p. 395). Schuwerk writes that despite good intentions, "...nutrition takes a proverbial back seat to making the donors feel like they are being generous and helpful" (p. 397). More recently, Okamoto (2017) explored how community members in a small public school district in Appalachian Ohio formed the Appalachian Nutrition Advisory Council (ANAC) to address the nutritional needs of low-income students. Despite constraints, ANAC was able to join together to create a salad bar and institute "healthy celebration campaigns" with plans to open a food pantry. In the end however the food pantry ANAC set up offered extremely restricted food choices illuminating class-based disparities in food access. The disjuncture calls into question food banking as a safe and adequate solution to hunger, which while designed to help may instead contribute to health disparities.

Communication scholarship has played an important role illuminating how neoliberal solutions to hunger do not always serve clients' needs and in many cases reinforce racial and class-based discrimination. For example, in my research monograph *Feeding the Other: Whiteness, Privilege, and Neoliberal Stigma in Food Pantries* (de Souza, 2019), I examined how clients and volunteers in two food pantries in Minnesota articulated varying constructions of health, food, and racial privilege. The book offers a powerful critique of food pantries as a solution to hunger centered on the notion of "neoliberal stigma" defined as "…a particular kind of Western and American narrative that focuses on individualism, hard work, and personal responsibility as defining attributes of human dignity and citizenship" (p. 17). Through ethnographic accounts, I show how neoliberal stigma is perpetuated within food pantries reinforcing the material and symbolic marginalization of food insecure people while simultaneously glorifying white volunteers for their good works. I demonstrate how clients constructed health meanings around "good food" based on the types of food accessible to them. Clients' attempts to maintain a healthy diet were consistently undermined by inadequate resources and the poor quality of foods offered at food pantries. Overall, this body of work questions the capacity of food banks to genuinely "end hunger" and resonates with Dutta's (2015) assertion that modernist solutions can become vectors of neoliberalism that reproduce health disparities.

The relationship between the state, the labor market, and citizens has become a key area of study for organizational communication scholars. Dempsey's (2023) edited volume, *Organizing Eating: Communicating for Equity Across US Food Systems*, highlights how communication and power dynamics shape eating, working, and organizing within U.S. food systems. The collection covers various issues such as community responses to water injustice in Detroit, Michigan (Mitra et al., 2023), collective organizing by marginalized food workers to challenge corporate power (Zoller, 2023), intersectional food organizing in Denver, Colorado in the context of gentrification (Gordon, 2023), and "place-based organizing" in Appalachia (Ivancic & Okamoto, 2023). From food producers to farmworkers and warehouse workers, each case study illuminates the powerful interplay among institutions, discourses, practices, and policies that serve to undermine or advance social equity. The book illuminates and calls for a deeper exploration of "how socially constructed meanings—such as neoliberal stigma—become sedimented into hierarchies, policies, organizations, and institutions" (Dempsey, 2023, p. 3), a key focus of my own work over the last decade.

A novel contribution to the communication literature featured within this collection (Dempsey, 2023) is in the realm of place-based narratives linked to organizing around poverty, hunger, and housing. The field of communication has typically conceptualized stigma as a "spoiled identity" (e.g., Goffman, 1963), and while race, poverty, and gender have been studied as sources of devalued identities, "place" has rarely been linked to stigma and as such remains undertheorized in the CHC literature. In their chapter, Ivancic and Okamoto (2023) draw attention to the importance of histories, cultures, and contexts in theorizing communication. Specifically, they elaborate on how nonprofit organizations use "place-based" food organizing to build their movements. While dominant narratives about Appalachian identity construct people and place "as close-minded, undesirable, or inadequate," these organizations offer transformative narratives shifting local imaginaries around people and place. The research thus illuminates the role of discursive constructions of space and place in informing identity, stigma, and community organizing. In an earlier chapter, Ivancic (2022) shows how the local community food security movement in rural Appalachia engaged in "place based narrative labor" not only to change local food systems but also to challenge dominant (negative) perceptions of the region. The book *Everybody Eats: Communication and the Paths to Food Justice* (LeGreco & Douglas, 2021) deals with similar themes of community organizing around food, place, and divergent interests. LeGreco and Douglas used eight case studies of food justice activism in Greensboro, North Carolina (e.g., urban farms, mobile farmers markets, and food policy councils) to show how residents came together to participate in political action for sustainable solutions to hunger. The book underscores the crucial role communication plays not only in fostering values and commitments necessary for movement building but also the infrastructure needed to create a just food system—the key foundation for health and well-being.

All in all, this avenue of CHC illustrates the fundamental role food plays in organizing and ordering health and social well-being. The research clarifies the limitations and opportunities associated with charitable food organizing; on the one hand, local movements can use discursive strategies to challenge negative stereotypes and positively impact identity, but on the other hand, charitable food organizing can reinforce "neoliberal stigma," white saviorism, and health disparities. As Dempsey (2023) poignantly writes: "A focus on organizing provides a way to understand how meanings get accomplished and how these meanings come to matter" (p. 3). If we are to adopt a broader lens on health, shifting our focus from direct effects to root causes, then organizational communication offers important points of entry for understanding the broader social and institutional determinants of health.

Policy and Political Action in the Hunger Context

Communication scholarship within this domain has been crucial to revealing power dynamics intertwined within food systems and food policy. While closely linked to organizational perspectives in the previous section, I differentiate this body of scholarship by its focus on health and food-related policy texts and enactments—how people come together for the direct purpose of influencing policy and political action and how policy itself is enacted and put into practice in hunger contexts.

Communication scholars have clarified how communication is critical to policymaking and coordinating the interests of multiple stakeholders (LeGreco, 2012; LeGreco & Douglas, 2021). For example, LeGreco (2012) analyzed how multiple stakeholders participated in the enactment of two policy texts aimed at restructuring healthy eating practices in Arizona schools: the Arizona Nutrition Standards (AZNS) and the Child Nutrition Act policy. LeGreco's analysis highlights the importance of attending to policy as text and policy as talk; in other words, policy is not only what is written down but also how it is talked about and enacted on the ground.

An important line of critical communication research draws on Foucauldian biopolitical theory (Foucault, 2003) to illuminate how policy serves as a technology of governance intervening in the health of citizens. For example, using a Foucauldian lens, Ivancic (2018) showed how complex neoliberal political formations emerged in reaction to Mayor Bloomberg's proposed soda ban in New York City aimed at preventing obesity. This critical analysis made visible the market logics and cultural fears that shaped conversations and understandings about the causes of obesity, what produces good health, and who is responsible for maintaining public health.

My article on communication and carcerality (de Souza, 2022) develops, theorizes, and refines the concept of "neoliberal stigma," offering a critical framework for unraveling symbolic violence perpetuated through U.S. hunger policy. I argue that U.S. hunger policy functions as a form of racial biopolitics and structural racism, disproportionately impacting the health of communities of color. Instead of comprehensive solutions, the United States has constructed a patchwork of government and charitable hunger programs that are intertwined with racist and carceral logics structured around the discursive practices of "shame, suspicion, and surveillance"; these practices are implemented by millions of ordinary people in everyday spaces like schools, food pantries, and hospitals, so even when we claim to "help" poor people, the welfare system is designed to reinforce hurt poor and racialized communities physiologically, materially, and symbolically. This is central to how racism operates in an era of colorblind racism.

There have been a few analyses of policy texts directly related to hunger, agriculture, and/or nutrition. Hunt's (2023) analysis of the U.S. Farm Bill and how it impacts food system inequities is a case in point. The Farm Bill is a comprehensive piece of legislation renewed every five years; Hunt critically examines the policy's impact on agricultural practices, food production, and nutrition. Drawing on Giddens structuration theory, Hunt observes that the "recursive dynamics" of the Farm Bill's agriculture and nutrition subsidies reproduce capitalist food politics. Hunt highlights how agricultural subsidies benefit large agribusinesses at the expense of small farmers as well as how nutritional subsidies (i.e., food assistance programs for hungry and food insecure individuals) undermine equity.

Using a similar approach, in a previously published chapter, my colleagues and I (de Souza et al., 2008) analyzed three major global trade policies, including the General Agreement on Trade and Tariffs (GATT), and their effects in Asia, Latin America, and the African-Caribbean region. This policy analysis revealed how unjust agricultural and trade policies contributed to hunger in the Global South. For instance, GATT facilitated the establishment of banana plantations across Latin America, where local workers earned as little as 1% of the banana's market price—wages far too low to meet their basic needs. Moreover, the rise of industrial plantations led to, land colonization, river contamination, and the displacement of indigenous communities. This analysis exposed the stark contradiction between modernist development narratives and reality; rather than progress, neoliberal trade liberalization resulted in higher food prices, lower wages, and the erosion of food sovereignty. What is important to point out is that the critiques of the U.S. Farm Bill and the GATT are identical! These policies prioritize corporate agriculture and the commodification of the food system at the expense of individuals and communities in the Global North and Global South. These "free trade" legislations are tied to each other through the consolidation of power, lobbying efforts, and the unchecked influence of Big Agriculture, wreaking havoc on the health of communities around the world (Dutta, 2015).

Overall, critical communication scholarship has been crucial for understanding the power dynamics that operate at the policy level in the Global North and South. The research illuminates how discursive practices around food and hunger policy hinder food justice ultimately impacting the health and livelihoods of individuals and communities.

A Culture-Centered Approach to Hunger

The CCA is an important critical theoretical lens used to study hunger in Global North and South contexts. Developed by CHC scholar Mohan Dutta (Dutta, 2008, 2015), the CCA argues that communicative marginalization works alongside material deprivation and that poverty is sustained through the erasure of subaltern voices from mainstream policy platforms. Given these erasures, the CCA stresses decolonizing knowledge structures through the co-construction of community narratives as entry points for social transformation (Dutta-Bergman, 2004). The CCA utilizes the tripartite framework of "culture, structure, and agency" to unpack the communicative aspects of hunger and poverty, where "culture" refers to the web of meaning making that individuals are embedded within, "structures" refer to institutions and systems which influence the distribution of resources including access to food, healthcare, and employment, and "agency" highlights people's ability to understand, negotiate, and participate in social transformation (Sastry et al., 2021).

Over the last two decades, a robust body of CCA scholarship on hunger and poverty has emerged in local and global contexts illuminating the corporatization of food and agriculture as root causes of hunger and health disparities. These studies articulate people's lived experiences of hunger and health in the backdrop of neoliberal systems of oppression. For example, drawing connections between global and local manifestations of poverty, the Voices of Hunger project analyzed hunger experiences in two economically disenfranchised communities—West Bengal, India and Tippecanoe County, Indiana (Dutta et al., 2013). At both sites, participants showed heightened awareness of the neoliberal logics that operated within the context of food insecurity. A CCA study in Singapore similarly found oppressive neoliberal forces in play (Tan et al., 2017). The Singaporean neoliberal political framework titled "Many Helping Hands" conceptualized welfare as a shared responsibility between families, self-help organizations, and government. In the absence of state food assistance, people turned to their families and welfare organizations but were still not able to make ends meet. Low-skilled contractual labor left communities vulnerable to the vicissitudes of unemployment and market failures. Participants discussed skipping meals and eating bread, biscuits, and instant noodles to survive resonating with experiences of food insecurity in the global North where food insecure people are also forced to eat unhealthy foods in order to survive (de Souza, 2019).

Another set of CCA studies in the Global South focuses on food sovereignty concerns brought about by the corporatization of agriculture and neocolonial landgrabs (Dutta & Thaker, 2019). Several of these studies have taken place in India, where neoliberal policies have resulted in an agrarian crisis and compounded hunger and food insecurity. In one study, researchers talked to farmers in the rural Uttar Pradesh to understand their conceptions of agriculture, land, and development (Rastogi & Dutta, 2015). For these farmers, agriculture *was* culture; something passed down from generation to generation. Farmers worked the land even as they struggled with limited access to resources (including food), and they questioned the narrative of development articulated by the state, noting that because of corruption, development does not "trickle down" to rural areas. Another study centered the voices of farmer widows from Maharashtra highlighting patriarchal structures that unfold amid neoliberal agrarian reform (Falnikar & Dutta, 2019). In this study, the widows discussed how new agrarian structures such as high-investment BT cotton cost their husbands their lives and how gendered division of labor and patriarchal attitudes meant that women were excluded from decision-making. Agrarian communities around the world are connected in their experiences of colonization, racism, and capitalism, a theme which is highlighted in the CCA study of the African American farming crisis in the United States (Carter & Alexander, 2020), which identified land loss and the erasure of the African-American farming tradition as central to ongoing hunger and health challenges.

CCA studies further illuminate most profoundly how communication is central to community resistance. While multinational agrochemical corporation spin positive narratives around profitability and growth, local communities come together to tell their own truths around hunger and food. For example, Dutta and Thaker (2019) narrate how rural women farmers were able to interrupt neoliberal hegemonic narratives of agricultural reform. To raise awareness about local agricultural practices, the women held an annual biodiversity festival traveling to different villages with carts full of seeds and singing songs of food sovereignty. Owning communication infrastructures or "communication sovereignty" allowed these women farmers to resist the large advertising and PR budgets of the agro-corporations selling neoliberal narratives of profit. In another examination of people's resistance, Pal and Dutta (2013) explored farmer protests against the state and a multinational corporation in West Bengal who were trying to acquire their lands. The company withdrew from the project a year after fieldwork had begun because of this resistance movement. Conversations with farmers revealed alternate ways of being, where they expressed an intricate and intimate relationship with their land linked to customary right and economic self-sufficiency. Farming was seen as a way of life and even though farmers were offered money for the land, they rejected this money stating that money was not an adequate replacement for land loss and health. In so doing, the farmer narratives illuminate etiologies of health and development that defy neoliberal logics grounded in western capitalism.

All in all, research using the CCA highlights both the adverse effects of neoliberalism on food security and health and the ways in which local communities resist and challenge these injustices through collective action. By attending to the voices of local communities, CCA research offers critiques of dominant modernist development narratives while highlighting alternative rationalities as entry points for structural transformation.

Bridging the Gaps: Critical Health Communication and Social Change

In terms of moving forward, there are still several pieces of the food, hunger, and health puzzle that CHC scholars can address. My most urgent call is for health communication scholars to enter the arena of social and political change. If we recognize that health is deeply entangled with intricate webs of power, capital, and a range of political, communicative, historical, and cultural forces, then creating lasting improvements in health means not only studying the impacts, outcomes, and health effects but also the root causes of health and health disparities such as poverty, hunger, and food insecurity. We must notice and call attention to the communicative operation of injustice (and its inevitable impacts on health) across contexts and scales. Our theories, frameworks, and methods offer much needed clarity and illumination in a world of chaotic "wicked problems." In the last few years, critical communication scholars have proposed important agendas for food justice and "food systems" approaches to communication (Gordon & Hunt, 2019; LeGreco & Douglas, 2021) that call into focus the interplay between individuals, organizations, discourses, and policy. These approaches recognize the fundamental, constitutive functions of communication in enabling and constraining possibilities for organizing around food, health, and social and political well-being. This shift offers powerful openings and directions for future research often working across traditional subdisciplines of communication to thread important connections.

In this section, rather than offering a set of future research directions, I invite readers to join me in thinking through complex intersections between food, health, and social justice, and how CHC might enter into these stories to offer an illuminating and clarifying perspective. Specifically, I offer two anecdotes from my own academic journey rife with possibilities for more research and theorizing. These examples deal with the central dilemma of how socially and politically constructed truths become sedimented and inscribed in structures, systems, and policies impacting the health and everyday lives of people. I hope these stories serve to elucidate the critical mindset required to draw linkages between food, health, and communication.

There's No Such Thing as a Free Lunch

The first example is that of "lunch shaming" and "lunch debt"—issues that became apparent to me while working on my book *Feeding the Other*. During my fieldwork, I encountered a Legal Aid lawyer in Minneapolis involved in lawsuits against school districts who used lunch shaming tactics to discourage students from accessing school lunches. "Lunch debt" refers to when parents or caregivers are unable to pay even the subsidized amount for school meals provided by the National School Lunch Program (NSLP) leading to students accumulating a debt, while "lunch shaming" involves various practices used by public schools to embarrass students and their families into paying off overdue meal bills (McConkie et al., 2020). These practices can include disposing of students' lunches, serving alternative meals, stamping students' hands, or publishing lists of students with outstanding meal debts. The aim is to shame families into paying what they owe, thus recovering funds for the school district. The NSLP, established by President Harry Truman in 1946, is the second largest food assistance program in the United States, operating in 100,000 public and nonprofit private schools. In 2019, it provided low-cost or free lunches to 29.6 million children each school day, at a cost of $14.2 billion (Suarez-Sousa & Bradbury, 2017). Given the program's crucial role in alleviating childhood hunger, the practice of lunch shaming exacerbates the very issue that school meal programs aim to solve—ensuring that every child has access to nutritious food.

From a research perspective, this bizarre and egregious phenomenon provides several compelling lines of inquiry for CHC scholars. Given the health and political dimensions of these issues, researchers who study the interpersonal dimensions of health communication could explore how children and families internalize "political" shame, how they communicate with each other about it, and the ways in which lunch shaming impacts the physical, mental, and social health and well-being of individuals and communities. Scholars focused on the rhetorical dimensions of health could investigate how lunch shaming discourses reinforce social and political attitudes surrounding welfare, racial neoliberalism, and discourses of personal responsibility, reinforcing age-old tropes and stereotypes in new ways. Health and organizational communication scholars could examine how school staff enforce or resist lunch shaming practices, the embodied health impacts of discipline and punishment on marginalized communities, and how shame is deployed as a political weapon with children's bodies as collateral damage. Overall, this body of work can contribute to a larger communicative theoretical intervention that shame is not only a psychological construct but a technology for political oppression. "Shame is produced through a complex assemblage of social and institutional discursive practices that erase the structural causes of poverty and hunger, reducing them to individual problems" (de Souza, 2022, p. 6). In all, these brief examples show how the single phenomenon of lunch shaming offers myriad opportunities for health communication scholars to engage in significant work that spans both the health and political domains, offering entry points to comment on health disparities and use scholarship to activate policy change.

Alfalfa Sprouts in a (Food) Desert

The second example I want to share deals with the complexity of a simultaneously local and global food system. When I moved to San Diego a few years ago, I entered a new political and cultural environment with its own unique history and geography. While driving to give a talk on hunger and food justice at the San Diego State University-Imperial Valley (SDSU-IV) campus located south of San Diego County near the US-Mexico border, I was struck by the sight of vast fields of green alfalfa sprouts growing in what is essentially a desert. I soon discovered that these sprouts were being cultivated in the Imperial Valley to be shipped to South Korea, where they would be used as cattle feed. This feed would eventually contribute to beef exports worldwide. The irony of growing alfalfa in a natural desert, with irrigation dependent on advanced technology and affected by climate change, was striking. Learning that much of the water supply and irrigation system has been owned intergenerationally by a few white farmers was also startling. This level of agriculture was not possible in the Imperial Valley until the construction of the Alamo Canal, also known as the Imperial Canal, in 1901, which diverted water from the Colorado River.

Against this historical backdrop of racial and environmental injustice, it was not surprising to learn that Imperial County is listed by the United States Department of Agriculture (USDA) as a food desert. Furthermore, students studying at SDSU-IV—many of whom cross the border daily—have limited access to food while on campus. To address the immediate hunger concern, campus stakeholders started, you guessed it, a food pantry to provide packaged snacks to students. Although I have criticized food pantries as an inadequate and unsustainable solution to hunger, the SDSU-IV food pantry is the only support available for students.

From a CHC perspective, the food pantry is just the tip of the iceberg that obscures the hunger problem. The root causes of hunger in this region are in fact linked to the alfalfa crops, racist agricultural policy, and imperialist U.S. policies in Latin America. A burning question that I am left with is how does racial neoliberalism shape global food policy and local institutional practices around "solving" hunger? Furthermore, how does US immigration policy and politics impact hunger and food insecurity for communities living in border regions? The issue of sustainability and environmental justice, particularly in relation to racial and Indigenous sovereignty, is raised. While government programs offer financial incentives to irrigate deserts –essentially driving agriculture into deserts –the broader impacts of climate change are overlooked, impacting the health and livelihoods of communities. This complex case study offers multiple avenues of inquiry for health communication researchers, activists, and advocates approaching the topic from diverse perspectives. For scholars focusing on the interpersonal dimensions of health communication, they might explore how living in border communities impacts the health, identity, culture, pride, and resilience of students and the broader community. Questions such as, "How do communities make sense of who they are and 'where' they come from in a deeply place-based context?" or "How do healthcare and food systems intersect in these environments?" can guide this exploration. Scholar-activists examining the rhetorical dimensions of health could investigate how border-related discourses shape political attitudes toward immigrants, the fentanyl crisis, and agricultural workers reinforcing age-old racist stereotypes. Ultimately, this case study—which started with the witnessing of alfalfa sprouts—raises broader questions spanning both health and political domains. In this border setting, agricultural, trade, criminal justice, and immigration policies intersect daily, profoundly affecting student and community health and upward mobility in embodied ways. Here, hunger is not merely a biological issue but one deeply connected to the environment, migration, and trade policy offering rich opportunities for CHC scholarship and activism.

These two examples have complicated and clarified my own thinking around food, health, and social justice issues. The critical modernist is always interested in seeing something old in a new and startling light; this was certainly true of lunch shaming as "political strategy" or the juxtaposition of alfalfa sprouts with food insecurity in the Imperial Valley. Critical modernism asserts that surface level meanings and behaviors obscure deep structural conflicts that systematically disrupt the potential of a genuinely democratic society (Pal & Dutta, 2008). Although rooted in poststructuralism, I reflect on how Foucault, decades ago, unified prisons, schools, and mental health institutions within a single conceptual frame. He saw these institutions as apparatuses of the modern world, designed to discipline, control, and punish individuals who deviated from established norms. I also think about the chilling insight that Crenshaw (1991) had when she noticed that the discrimination Black women faced was not the same as white women or Black men, but a combination of both that was not yet addressed by the legal system. There is nothing "armchair" about this kind of counter-hegemonic theorizing; these analyses have genuinely transformed the world—not just our thinking, but our environments and our policies. Indeed, the best critical modernist theorizing is accomplished through touch with life and lived realities, in conversation with people, and vigilant about noticing and bearing witness to the invisible and concealed contradictions in the modern world. I therefore encourage CHC scholars, and all health communication scholars to look with renewed enthusiasm at the entangled structures, cultures, and discourses that enable and constrain our health in consequential ways. This witnessing will inevitably lead you into the arena of health and politics where transformative change can take root.

Conclusion

To conclude, this chapter has shown how critical scholars have contributed to the CHC literature in four primary arenas: (a) discourse, identity, and materiality; demonstrating how food is not just a biological necessity but also a site of symbolic and material struggle; (b) organizing hunger and hunger solutions; illuminating opportunities and limitations of charitable food organizing, (c) hunger policy and politics showcasing the discursive and interactive dimensions of policy and political action, and (d) the CCA to hunger, which offers critiques of dominant modernist narratives while highlighting entry points for structural change. Consistent with critical modernist leanings, this body of work shows how dominant narratives and practices around hunger obscure its root causes and advocates for the transformation of the food system, moving away from profit-driven models toward systems that ensure equitable access to food, dignity, and human rights. This body of work disrupts dominant hunger narratives around root causes, impacts, and solutions to hunger. As critical modernists, there are several opportunities and encounters in our daily lives calling for attention. We must respond, through scholarship, advocacy, and activism, in a way that contributes to critical and counter-hegemonic readings of the world in the interests of a more genuinely democratic and just society.

References

Adebayo, C. T., Parcell, E. S., Mkandawire-Valhmu, L., & Olukotun, O. (2022). African American women's maternal healthcare experiences: A critical race theory perspective. *Health Communication*, *37*(9), 1135–1146. https://doi.org/10.1080/10410236.2021.1888453

Appadurai, A. (1996). *Modernity at large: Cultural dimensions of globalization*. University of Minnesota.

Berube, M. R. (2001). *Beyond modernism and postmodernism: Essays on the politics of culture*. Bloomsbury Publishing USA.

Bourdieu, P. (1984). *Distinction: A social critique of the judgement of taste*. Harvard University Press.

Carolan, M. (2011). *The real cost of cheap food*. Earthscan.

Carter, A., & Alexander, A. (2020). Soul food: [Re]framing the African-American farming crisis using the culture-centered approach. *Frontiers in Communication*, *5*(5). https://doi.org/10.3389/fcomm.2020.00005

Chilton, M., & Rose, D. (2009). A rights-based approach to food insecurity in the United States. *American Journal of Public Health*, *99*(7), 1203–1211.

Cohen, J. L., & Arato, A. (1994). *Civil society and political theory*. MIT Press.

Coleman-Jensen, A., Rabbitt, M., Gregory, C., & Singh, A. (2019). *Household food security in the United States in 2019, ERR-275*. United States Department of Agriculture, Economic Research Service. Retrieved from https://www.ers.usda.gov/publications/pub-details?pubid=99281

Collins, P. H. (2009). *Black feminist thought: Knowledge, consciousness, and the politics of empowerment*. Routledge..

Conquergood, D. (1991). Rethinking ethnography towards a critical cultural politics. *Communication Monographs, 58*, 179–194.

Cooks, L. (2015). Constructing taste and waste as habitus. In S. Boerboom (Ed.), *The political language of food* (pp. 123–140). Rowman and Littlefield.

Crenshaw, K. (1991). Mapping the margins: Intersectionality, identity politics, and violence against women of color. *Stanford Law Review, 43*(6), 1241–1299. https://doi.org/10.2307/1229039

De Los Santos Upton, S., Tarin, C. A., & Hernández, L. H. (2022). Construyendo conexiones para los niños: Environmental justice, reproductive feminicidio, and coalitional possibility in the borderlands. *Health Communication, 37*(9), 1242–1252. https://doi.org/10.1080/10410236.2021.1911386

Dempsey, S. E. (2023). *Organizing eating: Communicating for equity across U.S. food systems*. Routledge.

Denison, B., Dahlen, H., Kim, J. E. C., Williams, C., Kranzler, E., Luchman, J. N., Trigger, S., Bennett, M., Nighbor, T., Vines, M., Petrun Sayers, E. L., Kurti, A., Weinberg, J., Hoffman, L., & Peck, J. (2023). Evaluation of the "We Can Do This" campaign paid media and COVID-19 vaccination uptake, United States, December 2020–January 2022. *Journal of Health Communication, 28*(9), 573–584. https://doi.org/10.1080/10810730.2023.2236976

de Souza, R. (2019). *Feeding the other: Whiteness, privilege, and neoliberal stigma in food pantries*. MIT Press.

de Souza, R. (2022). Communication, carcerality, and neoliberal stigma: The case of hunger and food assistance in the United States. *Journal of Applied Communication Research, 51*, 1–18. https://doi.org/10.1080/00909882.2022.2079954

de Souza, R. (2023). "Motherwork" and communicative labor: A gendered analysis of hunger in marginalized US women [Original Research]. *Frontiers in Communication, 8*. https://doi.org/10.3389/fcomm.2023.1057472

de Souza, R. (2024). Women in the margins: A culture-centered interrogation of hunger and "food apartheid" in the United States. *Health Communication, 39*, 1–11. https://doi.org/10.1080/10410236.2023.2245206

de Souza, R., Basu, A., Kim, I., Basnyat, I., & Dutta, M. (2008). Who agreed to the neoliberal trade agreements? A discussion of the impact of "fair trade" on the health of marginalized communities. In H. Zoller & M. Dutta (Eds.), *Emerging perspectives in health communication: Interpretive, critical, and cultural approaches* (pp. 411–430). Lawrence Erlbaum.

Dickinson, M. (2020). *Feeding the crisis: Care and abandonment in America's growing food safety net*. University of California Press.

Dougherty, D., Schraedley, M., Gist-Mackey, A., & Wickert, J. (2018). A photovoice study of food (in)security, unemployment, and the discursive-material dialectic. *Communication Monographs, 85*(4), 443–466. https://doi.org/10.1080/03637751.2018.1500700

Dutta, M. (2008). *Communicating health: A culture-centered approach*. Wiley.

Dutta, M. (2015). *Neoliberal health organizing: Communication, meaning, and politics*. Left Coast Press.

Dutta, M., Agaptus, A., & Jones, C. (2013). Voices of hunger: Addressing health disparities through the culture-centered approach. *Journal of Communication*, *63*, 159+.

Dutta, M., & de Souza, R. (2008). The past, present, and future of health development campaigns: reflexivity and the critical-cultural approach. *Health Communication*, *23*(4), 326–339. https://doi.org/10.1080/10410230802229704

Dutta, M., & Thaker, J. (2019). 'Communication sovereignty' as resistance: Strategies adopted by women farmers amid the agrarian crisis in India. *Journal of Applied Communication Research*, *47*(1), 24–46. https://doi.org/10.1080/00909882.2018.1547917

Dutta-Bergman, M. (2004). The unheard voices of Santalis: Communicating about health from the margins of India. *Communication Theory*, *14*(3), 237–263.

Fairclough, N., & Wodak, R. (1997). Critical discourse analysis. In T. van Dijk (Ed.), *Discourse studies: A multidisciplinary introduction, Vol 2, Discouse as social interaction* (pp. 258–284). Routledge.

Falnikar, A., & Dutta, M. (2019). Voices of farmer-widows amid the agrarian crisis in India. *Women's Studies in Communication*, *42*(4), 432–451. https://doi.org/10.1080/07491409.2019.1669756

Farmer, P. (2005). *Pathologies of power: Health, human rights, and the new war on the poor*. University of California Press.

Fisher, A. (2017). *Big hunger: The unholy alliance between corporate America and anti-hunger groups*. MIT Press.

Foucault, M. (1975). *The birth of the clinic: An archeology of medical perception* (A. M. S. Smith, Trans.). Vintage Books.

Foucault, M. (2003). *'Society must be defended': Lectures at the Collège de France, 1975–76*. Picador

Frankenberg, R. (1993). *White women, race matters: The social construction of whiteness*. University of Minnesota Press.

Frye, J., & Bruner, M. (Eds.). (2012). *The rhetoric of food: Discourse, materiality, and power*. Routledge.

Goffman, E. (1963). *Stigma: Notes on the management of spoiled identity*. Simon and Schuster.

Gordon, C. (2023). Communicative considerations for urban food governance: Toward food privilege or food justice in Denver, Colorado. In S. Dempsey (Ed.), *Organizing eating: Communicating for equity across U.S. food systems.* (pp. 114–138). Routledge.

Gordon, C., & Hunt, K. P. (2019). Reform, justice, and sovereignty: A food systems agenda for environmental communication. *Environmental Communication*, *13*(1), 22–29.

Gramsci, A. (1992). *Prison notebooks* (J. Buttigieg & A. Callari, Trans.; J. Buttigieg, Ed.). Columbia University Press.

Harding, S., & Hintikka, M. (Eds.). (1983). *Discovering reality: Feminist perspectives on epistemology, metaphysics, methodology, and philosophy of science*. Kluwer.

Held, D. (1980). *Introduction to critical theory: Horkheimer to Habermas*. University of California Press.

hooks, b. (2004). Choosing the margin as a space of radical openness. In S. Harding (Ed.), *The feminist standpoint theory reader: Intellectual and political controversies* (pp.153–160). Routledge.

Huffman, T., & Tracy, S. J. (2018). Making claims that matter: Heuristics for theoretical and social impact in qualitative research. *Qualitative Inquiry, 24*(8), 558–570. https://doi.org/10.1177/1077800417742411

Hunt, K. (2023). "The rules for the food system we all eat by": How the U.S. Farm Bill (re)structures capitalist food politics. In S. Dempsey (Ed.), *Organizing eating: Communicating for equity across U.S. food systems.* (pp. 48–68). Routledge.

Ivancic, S. (2018). Body sovereignty and body liability in the wake of an "obesity epidemic": A poststructural analysis of the soda ban. *Health Communication, 33*(10), 1243–1256. https://doi.org/10.1080/10410236.2017.1351266

Ivancic, S. (2020). "No one's coming to save us": Centering lived experiences in rural food insecurity organizing. *Health Communication, 36*, 1–5. https://doi.org/10.1080/10410236.2020.1724644

Ivancic, S. (2022). (Re)storying Appalachia: Navigating the tensions of place-based narrative labor. In B. Peterson & L. Harter (Eds.), *Brave space-making: The poetics and politics of storytelling* (pp. 555–580). Kendall Hunt.

Ivancic, S., & Dooling, D. (2023). Navigating entangled shame: Examining the sociomaterialities of food assistance programs. *Communication Monographs, 90*(3), 293–316. https://doi.org/10.1080/03637751.2023.2202710

Ivancic, S. R., & Okamoto, K. E. (2023). Building collaborative empowerment through regionally attentive organizing: A comparative case study of place-making within two Appalachia food nonprofits. In S. Dempsey (Ed.), *Organizing eating: Communicating for equity across U.S. food systems* (pp. 214–235). Routledge.

Julier, A. (2013). *Eating together: Food, friendship, and inequality*. University of Illinois Press.

LeGreco, M. (2012). Working with policy: Restructuring healthy eating practices and the circuit of policy communication. *Journal of Applied Communication Research, 40*, 44–64.

LeGreco, M., & Douglas, N. (2021). *Everybody eats: Communication and the paths to food justice*. University of California Press.

Lupton, D. (1994). Toward the development of critical health communication praxis. *Health Communication, 6*(1), 55–67.

Lupton, D. (1996). *Food, the body and the self*. Sage.

Lupton, D. (2003). *Medicine as culture: Illness, disease and the body in western societies* (2nd ed.). Sage Publications.

Lupton, D. (2018). *Fat*. Routledge.

Macey, D. (2009). Rethinking biopolitics, race, and power in the wake of Foucault. *Theory, Culture & Society, 26*(6), 186–205. https://doi.org/10.1177/0263276409349278

Madison, D. S. (2020). *Critical ethnography: Method, ethics, and performance* (3rd ed.). https://doi.org/10.4135/9781071878965

McConkie, M., Andersen Spruance, L., Goates, M., & Vaterlaus Patten, E. (2020). P111 A content and thematic analysis of lunch shaming in the news media.

Journal of Nutrition Education and Behavior, 52(7), S68–S69. https://doi.org/10.1016/j.jneb.2020.04.158

Mitra, R., Gaber, N., Bouier, R., & Howell, S. (2023). Contesting institutional narratives and core assumptions about Detroit's mass water shutoffs: Collaborative writing for water justice. In S. Dempsey (Ed.), *Organizing eating: Communicating for equity across U.S. food systems*. (pp. 69–94). Routledge.

Mohanty, C. T. (1984). Under Western eyes: Feminist scholarship and colonial discourses. *Boundary 2, 12/13*, 333–358. https://doi.org/10.2307/302821

Mumby, D. K. (1997). Modernism, postmodernism, and communication studies: A rereading of an ongoing debate. *Communication Theory, 7*(1), 1–28.

Okamoto, K. E. (2017). "It's Like Moving the Titanic:" Community organizing to address food (in)security [Article]. *Health Communication, 32*(8), 1047–1050. https://doi.org/10.1080/10410236.2016.1196517

Pal, M., & Dutta, M. J. (2008). Public relations in a global context: The relevance of critical modernism as a theoretical lens. *Journal of Public Relations Research, 20*(2), 159–179. https://doi.org/10.1080/10627260801894280

Pal, M., & Dutta, M. J. (2013). "Land is our mother": Alternative meanings of development in subaltern organizing. *Journal of International and Intercultural Communication, 6*(3), 203–220. https://doi.org/10.1080/17513057.2013.765954

Papa, M., Singhal, A., & Papa, W. (Eds.) (2006). Dialectic of fragmentation and unity in rural Appalachia. In *Organizing for social change: A dialectic journey of theory and praxis* (pp. 196–230). Sage Publications.

Pine, A., & de Souza, R. (2023). Hunger, survivance, and imaginative futures: A racial analysis of the "right to food". In S. E. Dempsey (Ed.), *Organizing eating: Communicating for equity across U.S. food systems* (pp. 17–47). Routledge.

Poppendieck, J. (1999). *Sweet charity?: Emergency food and the end of entitlement*. Penguin Putnam Books.

Rastogi, R., & Dutta, M. (2015). Neoliberalism, agriculture and farmer stories: Voices of farmers from the margins of India. *Journal of Creative Communications, 10*(2), 128–140. https://doi.org/10.1177/0973258615597380

Ratzinger, J. (2012). Empty bellies/empty calories: Representing hunger and obesity. In J. Frye & M. Bruner (Eds.), *The Rhetoric of Food: Discourse, Materiality, and Power* (pp. 22–41). Routledge.

Sastry, S., Stephenson, M., Dillon, P., & Carter, A. (2021). A meta-theoretical systematic review of the culture-centered approach to health communication: Toward a refined, "nested" model. *Communication Theory, 31*(3), 380–421. https://doi.org/10.1093/ct/qtz024

Schuwerk, K. (2011). Food bank culture: Food and nutrition communication in a hunger relief organization. In J. M. Cramer, C. P. Greene, & L. M. Walters (Eds.), *Food as communication/Communication as food* (pp. 381–403). Peter Lang.

Spring, C., de Souza, R., & Garthwaite, K. (2024). Surplus food and the rise of charitable food provision. In *Oxford research encyclopedia of food studies*. Oxford University Press. https://doi.org/10.1093/acrefore/9780197762530.013.97

Suarez-Sousa, X. P., & Bradbury, B. L. (2017). *National school lunch program as proxy for socioeconomic status and its impact on academic performance: A mixed-methods study*. Sage.

Tan, N., Kaur-Gill, S., Dutta, M. J., & Venkataraman, N. (2017). Food insecurity in Singapore: The communicative (dis)value of the lived experiences of the poor. *Health Communication, 32*(8), 954–962. https://doi.org/10.1080/10410236.2016.1196416

van Dijk, T. A. (1989). Structures of discourse and structures of power. *Communication Yearbook, 12*, 18–59.

van Dijk, T. A. (2004). Discourse, knowledge and ideology: Reformulating old questions and proposing some new solutions. In M. Pütz, N. Neff, & T. van Dijk (Eds.), *Communicating ideologies: Multidisciplinary perspectives on language, discourse and social practice* (pp. 5–38). Peter Lang.

Van Esterik, P. (1999). Gender and sustainable food systems: A feminist critique. In M. Koc, R. MacRae, L. J. A. Mougeot, & J. Welsh (Eds.), *For hunger-proof cities: Sustainable urban food systems* (pp. 103–109). International Development Research Centre.

World Health Organization. (n.d.). Social determinants of health. Retrieved from https://www.who.int/health-topics/social-determinants-of-health#tab=tab_1.

Zoller HM (2021) Re-imagining localism and food justice: Co-Op Cincy and the union cooperative movement. *Frontiers in Communication* 6. doi: 10.3389/fcomm.2021.686400

Zoller, H. (2023). Addressing health inequalities through worker and consumer cooperatives: Co-op Cincy's organizing for food justice. In S. Dempsey (Ed.), *Organizing eating: Communicating for equity across U.S. food systems.* (pp. 166–189). Routledge.

3
REPRODUCTIVE INJUSTICE, FEMINICIDES, AND THE INTERSECTIONS OF CRITICAL HEALTH COMMUNICATION AND JOURNALISM PRAXIS

Leandra H. Hernández

Gender violence is a significant public health concern, impacting at least 1 in 3 women worldwide (World Health Organization, 2024). Recently, news reports in the United States and throughout Latin America have lamented one particular type of gender violence: violence against pregnant women. In early 2018, three pregnant women were murdered in Mexico, leading Mexico's independent presidential candidate to call for a moment of silence to remember the slain women. The murder of pregnant women—reproductive feminicides, as I will discuss later in this chapter—is a gruesome developing trend in the larger gender-based system of feminicidal violence in Mexico and across Latin America. In March 2018, 20-year-old Jessica Gabriela was found dead in Tamaulipas after having gone missing for a few days. She was eight months pregnant. News reports stated that a woman and her husband murdered Jessica Gabriela and extracted her fetus (Stevenson, 2018). Similarly, 23-year-old Jenny Judith Seba Velasco, one of the three aforementioned victims, was murdered in April 2018 by Brianda Padrón Cano. She allegedly lured Seba Velasco on the pretext of giving her free baby clothes and later murdered her and extracted her fetus (Macfarlan, 2018). News reports of the murders utilized spectacle-based frames to illustrate the reproductive nature of the gender violence, referring to the murder as "an 'outbreak of womb raiders' in Mexico" and utilizing terms such as "cutting her baby out" and "brutal murder" (Hernández & De Los Santos Upton, 2018b; Macfarlan, 2018). Such framing is one example of many that highlights the precarious implications of news framing of reproductive violence against women, with concerns surrounding journalistic practice, ethical practice, and public health framing of violence.

DOI: 10.4324/9781003426530-4
This chapter has been made available under a CC BY-NC-ND license.

This chapter situates itself within scholarship that explores the role of news framing in public health contexts. It seeks to assist journalists and practitioners in developing more equitable and sensitive news coverage, particularly with positive impacts for criminal justice interventions and policy debates (Morgan & Simons, 2017; Palazzolo & Roberto, 2011; Savage et al., 2017; Simons & Morgan, 2017). This chapter is also part of my decade-long advocacy for health communication journals, divisions, and research spaces to recognize feminicides as a global public health concern and legitimate area of research inquiry and to welcome Latin American feminist scholarship as a legitimate frame for critical health communication scholarship. Thus, I explore news framing of reproductive feminicides through the lens of critical, intersectional health communication and journalism praxis. This methodological case study will illustrate how feminist news framing practices and principles (Hardin & Whiteside, 2009) elucidate how gendered violence is represented in contemporary news outlets in Latin American contexts. Further, it will provide a set of best practices for public health practitioners, journalists, and health communication practitioners regarding framing health messages in the mass media, particularly health messages that focus on gender-based violence.

Case Study: Gender Violence and Feminist News Framing

Feminicidios: Definitions and Trends

Building upon other Latin American feminist scholars of gender violence, I assert that feminicidios—and the violence-based ideologies undergirding them—are weapons of terror that both operate within and function as acts of structural and systemic violence (Fregoso & Bejarano, 2010; Fregoso, 2023). The systemic web of feminicidal violence is "the extreme, the culmination of many forms of gender violence against women that represent an attack on their human rights and that lead them to various forms of violent death" (Lagarde y de los Ríos, 2010, p. xxi). Further, feminicidal violence is created "by the patriarchal, hierarchical, and social organization of gender, based on supremacy and inferiority, that creates gender inequality between women and men" (Lagarde y de los Ríos, 2010, p. xxi). It is perpetuated by the exclusion of women from power structures, the exclusion of women's voices and agency in broader contexts, and the tolerance of machismo, patriarchy, and misogyny (Lagarde y de los Ríos, 2010).

Before progressing further, however, I contextualize my use of the terms femicide and feminicide. As other scholars have noted (Finnegan, 2018), there is a long and rich debate on the terms and their origins. Femicide was first defined by Diana Russell in 1976. Radford and Russell (1992) defined femicide as the killing of women specifically because they are women, which highlights how patriarchy and misogyny serve as the impetus for violence. As Russell and Harmes (2001) state,

> Femicide is on the extreme end of a continuum of the sexist terrorization of women and girls. Rape, torture, mutilation, sexual slavery, incestuous and extrafamilial child sex abuse, physical and emotional battery, serious cases of sexual harassment are also on this continuum.
> *(p. 4)*

Feminicidio is a term that was later circulated in the mid-1990s when the kidnapping, mutilation, and murders of women around maquiladoras at the U.S.-Mexico border became known. The term feminicidio emphasizes the assassination and murder of women, as well as the cultural contexts that contribute to this violence, such as machismo, religious beliefs, and policing systems, to name a few (Lozano, 2019). Mexican and Latin American feminists assert that the term feminicidio is a more appropriate cultural transition because it follows linguistic conventions for compound nouns in Spanish and it allows for a more thorough inclusion and investigation of state-sanctioned violence in perpetrating cases of violence in multiple contexts (Finnegan, 2018; Hernández & De Los Santos Upton, 2018a). As Fregoso and Bejarano (2010) explain, electing to use the term feminicide in research contexts aligns scholars and activists in "mark[ing] our discursive and material contributions and perspectives as transborder feminist thinkers from the global South (the Americás) in its redefinition" (p. 4). The term feminicidio allows scholars to center critical transborder perspectives and theories originating in the global South (Fregoso & Bejarano, 2010). In Latin American contexts, dominant categories of feminicide include intimate partner feminicide, familial feminicide, and systematic sexual feminicide (Fregoso & Bejarano, 2010). Further, Hernández and De Los Santos Upton (2018a) proposed the term reproductive feminicide, which refers to feminicidal acts that women face in reproductive contexts. Ultimately, the differences between the terms femicide and feminicidio are both linguistic and contextual, given that feminicidio highlights the contributions of Latin American feminist scholars, as well as the Latin American cultural contours that contribute to such violence.

Taken together, feminicidios constitute a global public health crisis and significant violation of women's human rights. The World Health Organization (2024) estimates that 1 in 3 women worldwide have been subjected to at least one act of gender-based violence in their lifetime and that such violence has deleterious health outcomes, negatively impacting women's physical, mental, emotional, and sexual and reproductive health. Additionally, gender-based violence contributes to structural, social, and economic problems such as isolation, decreased or loss of wages, and limited ability to care for themselves and their children, among others (World Health Organization, 2024). A woman is a victim of feminicide across Latin America every two hours (Green, 2022). The COVID-19 pandemic spotlighted a parallel shadow pandemic across Latin America, as feminicidio rates doubled in various countries because of women's isolation, inability to escape violent home situations, and lack of access to support systems (Green, 2022; United Nations, 2021a). The United Nations (2021b) reported at least 4,000 women were victims of feminicide in Latin America and the Caribbean in 2020, despite more awareness and social condemnation thanks to feminist activism from groups such as Ni Una Menos and others. In 2020, Mexico reported 1.5 feminicides per every 100,000 women, Belize reported 3.5 feminicides per every 100,000 women, and Honduras reported 6 feminicides per every 100,000 women (Statista, 2022). Ultimately, in many countries across Latin America, rates of feminicides either remain stable or are increasing (Statista, 2024), highlighting continued concerns about gender-based murders as a global public health epidemic.

Journalists play an important role in this context, as they communicate about the origins, facts, and impacts of gender violence to communities that might not have previous knowledge of the topic. Further, journalists have the power to affect the public's perceptions of topics such as gender violence, its causes, and its attributions (Palazzolo & Roberto, 2011), which I discuss in more detail in the next section.

News Framing of Violence Against Women

In their most basic sense, news frames are "prepackaged social constructions that function as fully developed templates for understanding a given social phenomenon" (Gillespie et al., 2013, p. 225). Similar to the metaphor of a picture frame, news frames assist viewers and readers in categorizing and making sense of information. As Entman (1993) elaborated, "To frame is to select some aspects of a perceived reality and make them more salient in a communicating text in such a way as to promote a particular problem definition, causal interpretation, moral evaluation, and/or treatment recommendation" (p. 52). News frames significantly impact how readers recall information about news events and define strategies that individuals use to present information about certain news topics (Valkenburg et al., 1999). Brüggemann (2014) proposed that the news production continuum oscillates between frame setting and frame sending.

On the one hand, frame sending occurs when one passively passes on interpretations provided by others, and frame setting occurs when a journalist provides the audience with their interpretations of a particular event or topic (Brüggemann, 2014). Ultimately, such considerations shed light on how journalists engage in the frame building process, which explores how frames are transmitted into media content (Scheufele, 1999). Two frames that are relevant to this study are thematic frames, which focus on the isolated news event at hand, and episodic frames, which link the story and crime to larger social contexts (Iyengar, 1991).

Further, both news production and news reception are processes of sense-making wherein individuals make important interpretations and conclusions about the world (Brüggemann, 2014). In the larger ecosystem of gender-based violence, journalistic coverage of violence is significant because it shapes society's views of the causes of violence, the impacts of violence, and perceptions of perpetrators, victims, and survivors (Richards et al., 2011). Earlier feminist scholars asserted that representations of women in the mass media are indicative of women's status in society (Croteau & Hoynes, 1997), and concepts such as symbolic annihilation highlight how the mass media historically and contemporarily demonize, trivialize, and/or underrepresent women and other minoritized groups (Tuchman, 2000). Research that explores news coverage of feminicide in both domestic and international contexts raise concerns about culpability and blame, the overrepresentation of certain voices and stifling of others, and ethics regarding language use and visual depictions of violence.

As one of the first scholars to explore news coverage of violence against women, Meyers (1994) found that crime reporting largely ignored violence against women, representing a form of symbolic annihilation. She also found that journalists who did cover the issue framed violence episodically as an individual or pathologized issue rather than a case representative of larger structural and gendered patterns of control and domination. Another historically significant study conducted by Taylor (2009) empirically supported Meyer's findings that violence was treated as an individual or isolated even rather than a structural issue. In addition, Taylor found that coverage (1) most commonly cited police officials as sources in news coverage of violence against women, highlighting a disparity in how individuals are treated and framed as experts in articles, and (2) used victim-blaming language to refer to the women involved in the cases.

Recent research continues to find that victim-blaming frames persist in news coverage of various types of violence against women (Correia & Neves, 2024; Richards et al., 2011; Gillespie et al., 2013; Sutherland et al., 2016). Violence against women is often referred to as normal or commonplace, alongside other myths (Gillespie et al., 2013; Sutherland et al.,

2016). Violence is continuously referred to as an isolated event, not a structural event (i.e. an overuse of episodic frames versus thematic frames; Andelsman & Mitchelstein, 2019; Gillespie et al., 2013; Pröll & Magin, 2022; Sela-Shayovitz, 2018; Sutherland et al., 2016; Taccini & Mannarini, 2024). By utilizing language that blames victims and treats cases of violence as isolated incidents, larger journalism discourses contribute to the obfuscation of blame for perpetrators, the lack of accountability for the justice system, the detraction of violence as a larger structural issue, and the normalization of acts of violence (Bouzerdan & Whitten-Woodring, 2018; Correia & Neves, 2024). Moreover, women are erased as reports cite law enforcement and criminal justice voices more frequently than other voices, such as victim advocates, local organizers, community resources, and family members (Richards et al., 2011; Sutherland et al., 2016).

In Mexican and other Latin American contexts specifically, journalists continue to use victim-blaming frames that justify perpetrators' actions, refrain from discussing structural causes of feminicide (García & Villanueva, 2020; Herscovitz, 2023). Scholars have referred to news discourses about gendered violence at the U.S.-Mexico border as violence journalism, one that reproduces and exacerbates perceptions of the border as a violent entity (Corona, 2012; Dominguez-Ruvalcaba & Corona, 2012). Framing feminicidal violence as normal and inevitable leads to a weakening of public sympathy for the victims of feminicide and a lack of justice for victims and their families (Finnegan, 2018; Wright, 2011). In their edited volume on representations of gender violence at the U.S.-Mexico border, Domínguez-Ruvalcaba and Corona (2012) illustrate how the news media play a significant, instrumental role in shaping the dissemination of and reception of information about gender violence against women. News discourses can misinterpret news information and events, neutralize events, impact perceptions of blame and culpability, and serve to incite fear amongst community members and those detached from geopolitical locations of violence. In Latin American contexts, for example, Guatemalan news outlets have featured up to 15 articles about feminicidios daily, which feed the fear of residents with sensationalized, gory details about the murdering of women throughout the country (Godoy-Paiz, 2012). As Godoy-Paiz (2012) aptly notes, "How the media portrays stories of violence toward women, and the discussions and narratives these news stories feed, reveals a great deal about the routinization of violence and fear" (p. 99).

Violence journalism both "depicts (in both fact and opinion) and produces (in its discursive formalization) a more violent reality" of the violence that exists at the U.S.-Mexico border and beyond (Corona, 2012, p. 106). Other strategies utilized by violence journalism include the implementation of "not knowing" politics. Corona's analysis of feminicides news coverage in Ciudad Juarez that "not knowing" politics occurs when news transfers...

> ...the documented facts about particular events to the background and [replaces] them with "news" about social or intergroup conflicts, which may be related to or in some cases generated by the occurrence of the primary events. Such politics infuse media "noise" to fill the void created by the public relevance or impact of events for which there is not enough proven or sanctioned information."
>
> *(p. 106)*

In addition to producing violent journalism, Corona (2012) found that news coverage in Mexico offered surface level descriptions of violence without examining root causes:

> In their pursuit of objectivity and unambiguous causal relations, the reporter and the newspaper editors may reproduce a vision of social reality that refuses to examine the roots of the problem and the basic structures of patriarchal society and its relationship to the economy, the use of urban space, political power and class privilege, the role of the authorities, the professional preparation of the security forces — all of which are important in the string of unsolved femicides.
>
> *(p. 118)*

Even further, news coverage of feminicidios throughout Latin America utilizes voyeuristic themes and representations to depict feminicidios. Bodies are shown in print and television in ways that promote sensationalism and normalize the crisis of violence (Corona, 2012). By showing body parts and utilizing sensationalizing headlines like "Womb Raiders Strike Again," slain individuals' consent is not honored, and bodies are treated as proverbial "battlefields" for likes, metrics, and increased engagement (Hernández & De Los Santos Upton, 2018b).

Bodies are also depicted as *the unknown* or *las desconocidas*. By framing women as unknown victims, it is easier for journalists and community members to avoid calling for justice or accountability regarding their death and the violence they endured. Corona (2012) argues that this "journalistic treatment of the murders does not provide enough elements for rational discourse, for collective memory, or for avoiding a discourse of victimization" (Corona, 2012, p. 109). In the case of *la desconocida* referenced above, a Mexican woman was brutally dismembered and murdered by members of the Sinaloan Cartel, and pictures of her remains were circulated on social media and hardly blurred in news coverage of her death. Videos also circulated on various media outlets that included live footage of her death. This sensationalistic and voyeuristic framing of her death negatively impacted her postmortem legacy (Hernández, 2023). Her death—one feminicidio among many—highlights journalism ethics concerns associated with consent, privacy, and dignity (Hernández, 2023). From a health communication perspective, her death also highlights concerns about journalistic framing of the causes, impacts, and outcomes of her death. By highlighting the spectacle of her death, journalists framed the violence episodically, not thematically, and failed to link her murder to women's well-being and the larger structures of gender violence and cartel violence (Hernández, 2023).

Ultimately, victims of feminicidio across Latin America are overdetermined as subjects of violence. As Fregoso (2000) illustrates, the trope of sexual violence and dehumanization both dominates news coverage of feminicides and further reifies its functioning, particularly through the representation of discarded and brutalized female remains. Such "ultraviolence" (Agnew, 2015) is further detailed by Wright (2011) in a discussion of the framing of *desconocidas* (or public women):

> If a public woman is the source of violence, then her murder provides a means for ending it. Her removal performs a kind of urban cleansing. The public woman discourse, in short, was a key tool for positioning the dead women and girls in the political order; it was a pillar of the necropolitics demonstrating that the publicness of the victims, as evidenced by the corpses' location in public places and the mutilations of their raped bodies, caused the violence that was disrupting the social and political peace of northern Mexico.
>
> *(pp. 714–715)*

Building upon the lens of necropolitics, scholars such as Montiel Valle and Martin (2023) assert that Latin American media utilize news coverage of feminicidios as opportunities to reaffirm state power, depict women as empty vessels, and normalize the commodification of excess violence through the gore and spectacle used to frame cadavers.

Through the public woman discourse that vilifies victims of feminicidio and presents their death publicly, victims of feminicidio are ungrievable victims, never lost in the full sense because they never received full humanity at the outset (Butler, 2016; Hernández, 2023). An analysis of the reproductive femicides of Jenny Judith Seba Velasco and other victims mentioned in the introduction showed that violence journalism exacerbated the details of violence utilized in their deaths. Coverage framed reproductive feminicide as spectacle by overfocusing on images and linguistic descriptions of their deaths, with references to the murderers as "womb raiders." Coverage also gave attention to anti-violence activism, highlighting how local activists and organizations banded together to protest such violence (Hernández et al., 2020). Given the chapter's focus thus far on the politics of news framing, in the next section I transition to the politics of news reception, particularly through the lens of witnessing, and its impact on audience reception of gender violence as a public health concern.

Ethical Witnessing and News Coverage of Feminicidios

Given trends shaping news framing of feminicidios, it is perhaps no surprise that scholars, activists, and educators have called for more culturally sensitive and trauma-informed approaches to journalistic coverage of gender violence. Concerns about objectivity as a dominant journalistic value also surface, particularly in considering the role of objectivity when covering state-sanctioned violence. Which facts are important, which facts should dominate the framing of the case, what is the role of activists' and educators' voices, and what are the best ways to memorialize the victims (Hernández, 2023b)? As media historian David Mindich (1998) discusses, "if American journalism were a religion, as it has been called from time to time, its supreme deity would be 'objectivity'" (p. 1). Mindich (1998) further explains that objectivity occupies a complex space in legal, political, and academic contexts because, despite its moral supremacy and constant privileging, its definition and applications are often elusive. Reporters often seek to enact objectivity by demonstrating detachment or nonpartisanship, using the inverted pyramid model, privileging facts, and demonstrating "balance" (Hernández, 2023b; Sutherland et al., 2016). However, many journalists and communication scholars question whether impartiality is possible and investigate the effects of these choices. For example, Wallace (2023) provides the following guiding questions: "Is impartiality ever possible? Is detachment the same as nonpartisanship? What is the difference between attempting 'balance' and attempting to *appear* 'balanced'? When 'objectivity' responds to public perceptions, which public is it?" (p. 7). In news coverage of violence against women, one could ask similar questions about whether valuing objectivity privileges micro-level case facts as opposed to structural causes of violence and whether privileging "facts" of the case leads to victim-blaming, audience detachment, and desensitization.

Such questions are of utmost importance for health communication scholars, students, and practitioners alike. Given that gender violence is a global public health concern, it is imperative for scholars, students, and practitioners to explore the role of news coverage in reinforcing this pandemic of violence, as well as to theorize how news coverage could be harnessed as a tool to curb feminicide. This focus encourages health communication scholars to consider which—and whose—issues get framed as health problems and crises deserving of public intervention.

Health Communication and Grievability

In addition to the question of agenda setting and framing of public health crises, this case raises important concerns about how inequities linked with necropolitics are tied to the politics of emotion. News framing of feminicidios raises significant ethical and moral questions about the ways in which victims are memorialized and how that coverage is tied to calls for justice. Judith Butler's (2016) work on grievability, mourning, and justice asserts that specific lives cannot be "apprehended as injured or lost if they are not first apprehended as living" (p. 1). Further, Butler (2016) states, "If certain lives do not qualify as lives or are, from the start, not conceivable as lives within certain epistemological frames, then these lives are never lived nor lost in the full sense" (p. 1). While Butler (2016) considers the relationship between grievability and war, her reflections carry significant implications for non-war-related violence. As Butler (2004, 2016) reminds us, such framing is a political operation of power that renders specific conclusions about the precarity about certain lives over others and who has a right to live (or further, a right to living). In the case of feminicidios, for example, do women not deserve to live because of certain actions that may have impacted their deaths? Do they not have a right to life or a right to living, as is often questioned in certain news articles? These questions have implications for the strategies journalists utilize to communicate about gender violence, for the ability of advocates and politicians to enact change against gender violence, and for the ways in which news consumers make sense of gender violence as a public health concern.

Resisting Feminicide

One strategy that journalists and health communication practitioners can utilize to communicate about gender violence more effectively is ethical witnessing, which has been presented as one solution to problematic news coverage of feminicidios. Scholars such as Tait (2011), Bovee (1991), Durham Peters (2001), and others have debated the role of witnessing in media ethics, mass communication, and journalism contexts. The term witness involves three points of a communicative encounter: (1) the agent who bears witness, (2) the utterance or text itself, and (3) the audience who witnesses (Peters, 2001). It can be a sensory experience, such as locating the video of the aforementioned feminicidio of *la desconocida* and watching and listening with one's own senses. Witnessing can also be the "discursive act of stating one's experience for the benefit of an audience that was not present at the event and yet must make some kind of judgment about it" (Peters, 2001, p. 709). Ultimately, witnessing communicates about an evil or atrocity and then exposes the evil to a larger community. It has two components: the passive one of seeing and the active one of saying. One limitation of this conceptualization of witnessing is that it does not identify how it makes space for a story that is later told by someone in lieu of a person who no longer has the agency or ability to tell their own story, such as the victims of feminicidios.

Witnessing as a concept involves both the moral responsibility of the journalist and the reader, particularly concerning stories of violence, war, trauma, and murder. Journalists, for example, often serve as communicative witnesses to a story by first witnessing the story at hand (either through lived experience or through the stories of those interviewed and filmed) and by then transmitting the story to readers and community members. Readers and community members, on the other hand, can serve as witnesses in the construction of a journalism story or as the reception audience for the story. As Peters (2001) explicates, witnessing is an "intricately tangled process" that "raises questions of truth and experience, presence and absence, death and pain, seeing and saying, and the trustworthiness of perception—in short, fundamental questions of communication" (p. 707).

Taking witnessing one step further, scholars have interrogated the concept of bearing witness, which provides a rationale for journalistic practice and implies that certain events require being borne witness to because they require some form of public response (Tait, 2011). Ultimately, inciting public response is central to the concept of bearing witness (Tait, 2011; Zelizer, 1998). It invokes an ethos of response-ability that encourages readers, community members, and journalists alike to share responsibility for the suffering of others. Nicholas Kristof's coverage of violence in Darfur attempted to mobilize readers by including the affective, textual, and visual responses of horror, shame, and anger. In doing so, he created a visceral phenomenon of such violence to incite readers to action. As Tait (2011) explains, "Central to this appeal is the attempt to elicit affect, to move the body to participation" (p. 1232).

In the context of feminicidios, one must question whether the textual and visual incorporation of violent imagery can lead readers to some moral action (researching feminicidios further, donating to local organizations, etc.) or whether such violent journalism leads a reader to feel overwhelmed and hopeless. Again, the question remains: what purpose does such textual and visual imagery serve? Is a victim's life and right to live worthy of being grieved *because* of the violent imagery included in the article? While research suggests that images of atrocity could be utilized to make a call to conscience (Tait, 2008), are there better, more moral, just, and humane strategies that could be used to discuss the senseless feminicidio violence one endures? What is the moral position of both the circulation and reception of such imagery, particularly when considering the role of Internet spectatorship?

Ultimately, journalists—community journalists, local journalists, and large news organizations—must continue to investigate stories about gendered violence against women. Rodriguez (2015) poignantly describes how journalists must continue to strive to tell stories with honor, truth, and respect, particularly for those who are victims of violence. In discussing the work of Kent Patterson, an investigative journalist who has covered femicides extensively, Rodriguez (2015) ponders:

> This made me think about the bigger picture of journalism: the practice of consciously investigating and revisiting these important issues that society must address. The issues may be local, but they have national, or even global implications. The issues are not just a headline for one day, they are not simply print and paper – they convey the stories of humans and their realities. Their lives are constantly evolving and developing over time, and therefore their stories must, as well. Those stories must speculate on our morals as humans and as a community. They deal with life and death, just like we all do.

Rodriguez's (2015) statement conveys the passion underlying her journalistic efforts. Conveying the human aspects of the narratives of victims in feminicidal justice contexts can radically enhance the impact of this news coverage. Further, Connie Walker, an award-winning investigative reporter, podcast producer, and podcast host, has written several stories on missing and murdered Indigenous women. She is a tireless advocate for trauma-informed journalism approaches that focus on transparency, context, consent, victim and family agency, and relationship-building with individuals, family members, and community members. She also stresses that when journalists are telling stories about those subjected to violence, such as Indigenous women, journalists should remember that women are more than just the violence inflicted upon them. In other words, journalists have both a moral responsibility and a moral obligation to "be mindful of the incredible strength and resilience that exists within Indigenous women and girls and within our communities" (McCue, 2023, p. 139). Journalism about violence against women should focus on both the violent act *and* the larger conversation, change, and anti-violence efforts comprising the larger storytelling context. In news coverage of feminicidios, ethical storytelling would have also included information about victims' lives, about state structures that sanction such violence, and about anti-violence activism (such as the Ni Una Más movement) that has resulted in legal, political, and radical change. Thus, storytelling is the canvas where critical health communication praxis can occur.

This work is crucial because, as Finnegan (2018) argues, scholars, activists, legislators, and authorities have an ethical obligation to continue to demand justice for victims of feminicide. Such calls are becoming more popular alongside parallel coverage of women's rights and anti-feminicidal activism. Holling's (2014) research illustrates how feminicidio testimonios denounce state violence and invite listeners to identify with the testimonio and thus position themselves against such violence. By transitioning individuals from listeners to witnesses, individuals are involved in a transformative process that functions "as both a 'response-ability'" (Oliver, 2015) to violence and as a means to construct witnesses" (Holling, 2014, p. 315). Feminicidio testimonios are relational in that they hold "open the possibility of connections based on shared commitments to social justice and resistance to gender violence in light of women's vulnerability" (Holling, 2014, p. 317). Holling's (2014) feminicidio testimonio and Tait's (2011) view of moral responsibility in journalistic contexts elicit calls for moral involvement on behalf of readers, listeners, and constructors of the stories alike.

Recommendations for Communication Researchers and Practitioners

Given the urgency of the problem, I conclude with recommendations for scholars, journalists, and public health practitioners. The actions of these groups in this arena are intertwined.

First, journalists could consider implementing more trauma-informed journalism practices in their news coverage, which highlights the role of witnessing, emotions, and memorialization. Research illustrates how journalists in Mexico, for example, are aware of the organizational and disciplinary structures that limit their coverage of feminicidios and are actively exploring strategies to subvert such coverage limitations (Hernández, 2023b).

Additionally, health communication research has established the importance of thematic framing to raising attention to the structural sources of illness, risk, and death (Bhalla et al., 2019; Gounder & Ameer, 2018; Vardeman-Winter, 2017; Zoller & Casteel, 2022). Journalists could utilize more thematic (versus episodic) frames in their coverage. Thematic frames are critical because they link the violence to larger social and structural contexts, raise awareness in viewers, and work to promote social response (Sela-Shayovitz, 2018). Similarly, journalists could use connection frames in their coverage, which link abstract concepts to concrete events, actions, or outcomes (Below et al., 2008; Bouzerdan & Whitten-Woodring, 2018). Doing so would more explicitly link feminicidal acts of violence against women to larger conversations about violations of human rights, violence as a global public health epidemic, and other important contexts.

Menon et al. (2020) also highlight the importance of coverage that focuses less on the brutal violence inflicted upon victims and more upon the services available for individuals who might currently be facing gender violence. They assert that victims' and survivors' safety, right to dignity, and confidentiality are values that should be prioritized and considered alongside other dominant news values.

Public health scholars and practitioners can also be mindful of how media coverage of feminicidios and violence against women shapes the creation, deployment, and implementation of public health programs. News framing of violence against women importantly impacts both public knowledge and attitudes about public health concerns, as well as policy understandings and reactions to such concerns (Owusu-Addo et al., 2018). Health communication scholarship can participate in larger journalism discourses about violence against women (McCartan et al., 2015). As Carlyle et al. (2014) note, "By better understanding the interplay of media, public, and policy agendas, perhaps violence prevention researchers can find a way to restructure the debate that moves forward the public health agenda of violence prevention across all relationships in productive ways" (p. 2412).

Ultimately, in the complex web of news values, violence, and news coverage of feminicidios, I argue that critical health communication researchers can play an important role in developing a higher moral standard that reconsiders dominant practices related to the role of objectivity in news coverage of violence, the inclusion of visual spectacle (particularly in images of extreme violence, brutality, and dismemberment), and memorialization of the victim past her last moments. Only then can we further interrogate the impacts and outcomes of discursive violence and re-envision the intertwined praxis of critical health communication and trauma-informed journalism as a route to better health interventions.

References

Agnew, H. R. (2015). Reframing 'Femicide': Making room for the balloon effect of drug war violence in studying female homicides in Mexico and Central America. *Territory, Politics, Governance, 3*(4), 428–445.

Andelsman, V., & Mitchelstein, E. (2019). If it bleeds it leads: Coverage of violence against women and sexual and reproductive health in Argentina from 1995 to 2015. *Journalism Practice*, 13(4), 458–475.

Below, A., & Whitten-Woodring, J. (2008). Global warming heats up: Climate change, connection frames and the US policy agenda. American Political Science Association Annual Meeting, *Boston*, August 2008.

Bhalla, N., O'Boyle, J., & Haun, D. (2019). Who is responsible for Delhi air pollution? Indian newspapers' framing of causes and solutions. *International Journal of Communication*, 12, 41–64.

Bouzerdan, C., & Whitten-Woodring, J. (2018). Killings in context: An analysis of the news framing of femicide. *Human Rights Review*, 19, 211–228.

Bovee, W. G. (1991). The end can justify the means--but rarely. *Journal of Mass Media Ethics*, 6(3), 135–145.

Brüggemann, M. (2014). Between frame setting and frame sending: How journalists contribute to news frames. *Communication Theory*, 24(1), 61–82.

Butler, J. (2004). *Precarious life: The powers of mourning and violence*. Verso.

Butler, J. (2016). *Frames of war: When is life grievable?* Verso.

Carlyle, K. E., Scarduzio, J. A., & Slater, M. D. (2014). Media portrayals of female perpetrators of intimate partner violence. *Journal of Interpersonal Violence*, 29(13), 2394–2417.

Corona, I. (2012). Over their dead bodies: Reading the newspapers on gender violence. In H. Dominguez-Ruvalcaba & I. Corona (Eds.), *Gender violence at the U.S.-Mexico border: Media representations and public response* (pp. 104–127). University of Arizona Press.

Correia, A., & Neves, S. (2024). Newspaper headlines and intimate partner femicide in Portugal. *Social Sciences*, 13(3), 1–16.

Croteau, D., & Hoynes, W. (1997). *Media/society: Industries, images, and audiences*. Pine Forge.

Dominguez-Ruvalcaba, H., & Corona, I. (2012). *Gender violence at the U.S.-Mexico border: Media representation and public response*. University of Arizona Press.

Entman, R. M. (1993). Framing: toward clarification of a fractured paradigm. *Journal of Communication*, 43, 51–58.

Finnegan, N. (2018). *Cultural representations of feminicidio at the US-Mexico border*. Routledge.

Fregoso, R., & Bejarano, C. (2010). Introduction: A cartography of feminicide in the Américas. In R. Fregoso & C. Bejarano (Eds.), *Terrorizing Women: Feminicide in the Américas* (pp. 1–42). Duke University Press.

Fregoso, R. L. (2000). Voices without echo: the global gendered apartheid. *Emergences: Journal for the Study of Media & Composite Cultures*, 10(1), 137–155.

Fregoso, R. L. (2023). *The force of witness: Contra feminicide*. Duke University Press.

García, E. T., & Villanueva, O. M. M. (2020). Víctimas y victimarios de feminicidio en el lenguaje de la prensa escrita mexicana. *Comunicar: Revista científica iberoamericana de comunicación y educación*, 63, 51–60.

Gillespie, L. K., Richards, T. N., Givens, E. M., & Smith, M. D. (2013). Framing deadly domestic violence: Why the media's spin matters in newspaper coverage of femicide. *Violence against Women*, 19(2), 222–245.

Godoy-Paiz, P. (2012). Not just "another woman": Femicide and representation in Guatemala. *The Journal of Latin American and Caribbean Anthropology*, *17*(1), 88–109.

Gounder, F., & Ameer, R. (2018). Defining diabetes and assigning responsibility: How print media frame diabetes in New Zealand. *Journal of Applied Communication Research*, *46*(1), 93–112.

Green, M. A. (2022, November 29). A woman is a victim of femicide in Latin America every two hours. *Wilson Center*. Retrieved from https://www.wilsoncenter.org/blog-post/woman-victim-femicide-latin-america-every-two-hours.

Hardin, M., & Whiteside, E. (2009). Framing through a feminist lens: A tool in support of an activist research agenda. In P. D'Angelo & J. A. Kuypers (Eds.), *Doing news framing analysis: Empirical and theoretical perspectives* (pp. 312–330). Routledge.

Hernández, L. H. (2023a). *Narcoviolence, necropolitics, and feminicidios: Intersectional Praxis & media ethics reflections*. Paper presented at the 2023 National Communication Association convention.

Hernández, L. H. (2023b). When objectivity isn't enough: A case study on Feminicidios, violence against women, and anti-violence activism. In H. Schmidt (Ed.), *Issues facing contemporary American journalism* (pp. 61–67). Routledge.

Hernández, L. H., & De Los Santos Upton, S. (2018a). *Challenging reproductive control and gendered violence in the Américas: Intersectionality, power, and struggles for rights*. Lexington Books.

Hernández, L. H., & De Los Santos Upton, S. (2018b). Intersections of gender, sexuality, culture, and blame: An analysis of Latin American news discourses about feminicidios. [Conference Paper Presentation.] NCA 2018 *Convention, SLC, UT, USA*.

Hernández, L. H., De Los Santos Upton, S., & Diaz, A. (2020). *Media ethics and news coverage of violence in Latin American contexts: A case study on feminicidios and violence against women*. Paper presented at the 2020 National Communication Association convention.

Hernández, M. (2023). Covering *Feminicidios*: How Mexican journalists fight to improve representation of violence against women. *Journalism Practice*, *19*(6), 1215–1238. https://doi.org/10.1080/17512786.2023.2251983

Herscovitz, H. (2023). The judge and the influencer: Race, gender, and class in Brazilian news coverage of violence against women. In A. J. Baker, C. González de Bustamante, & J. E. Relly (Eds.), *Violence against women in the global south: Reporting in the #MeToo era* (pp. 85–111). Palgrave.

Holling, M. A. (2014). "So my name is Alma, and I am the sister of...": A feminicidio testimonio of violence and violent identifications. *Women's Studies in Communication*, *37*(3), 313–338.

Iyengar, S. (1991). *Is anyone responsible? How television frames political issues*. University of Chicago Press.

Lagarde y de los Ríos, M. (2010). Preface: Feminist keys for understanding feminicide. In R. Fregoso & C. Bejarano (Eds.), *Terrorizing women: Feminicide in the Américas* (pp. xi–xxviii). Duke University Press.

Lozano, N. (2019). *Not one more! Feminicidio on the border*. The Ohio State University Press.

Macfarlan, T. (2018, April 10). Outbreak of 'womb raiders' in Mexico: A SECOND female killer is arrested for murdering a pregnant woman, cutting her baby out and claiming it as her own. *Daily Mail*. Retrieved from https://www.dailymail.co.uk/news/article-5598311/Outbreak-murders-pregnant-women-unborn-child-cut-womb-Mexico.html

McCartan, K. F., Kemshall, H., & Tabachnick, J. (2015). The construction of community understandings of sexual violence: rethinking public, practitioner and policy discourses. *Journal of Sexual Aggression, 21*(1), 100–116.

McCue, D. (2023). *Decolonizing journalism: A guide to reporting in Indigenous communities*. Oxford University Press.

Menon, V., Pattnaik, J. I., Ipsita, J., & Padhy, S. K. (2020). Role of media in preventing gender-based violence and crimes during the COVID-19 pandemic. *Asian Journal of Psychiatry, 54*, 1–2.

Meyers, M. (1994). News of battering. *Journal of Communications, 44*(2), 47–63.

Mindich, D. T. Z. (1998). *Just the facts: How "objectivity" came to define American journalism*. NYU Press.

Montiel Valle, D. A., & Martin, Z. C. (2023). Entangled with the necropolis: A decolonial feminist analysis of femicide news coverage in Latin America. *Feminist Media Studies, 23*(3), 1222–1237.

Morgan, J., & Simons, M. (2017). Changing media coverage of violence against women: The role of individual cases and individual journalists. *Journalism Practice, 12*(9), 1165–1182.

Oliver, K. (2015). Witnessing, Recognition, and Response Ethics. *Philosophy & Rhetoric, 48*(4), 473–493. https://doi.org/10.5325/philrhet.48.4.0473

Owusu-Addo, E., Owusu-Addo, S. B., Antoh, E. F., Sarpong, Y. A., Obeng-Okrah, K., & Annan, G. K. (2018). Ghanaian media coverage of violence against women and girls: Implications for health promotion. *BMC Women's Health, 18*, 1–11.

Palazzolo, K. E., & Roberto, A. J. (2011). Media representations of intimate partner violence and punishment preferences: Exploring the role of attributions and emotions. *Journal of Applied Communication Research, 39*(1), 1–18.

Peters, J. D. (2001). Witnessing. *Media, Culture & Society, 23*(6), 707–723.

Pröll, F., & Magin, M. (2022). Framing feminicides—A quantitative content analysis of news stories in four Colombian newspapers. *Journalism and Media, 3*(1), 117–133.

Radford, J., & Russell, D. E. (1992). *Femicide: The politics of woman killing*. Twayne Pub.

Richards, T. N., Kirkland Gillespie, L., & Dwayne Smith, M. (2011). Exploring news coverage of femicide: Does reporting the news add insult to injury? *Feminist Criminology, 6*(3), 178–202.

Rodriguez, C. (2015). Exploring journalism and justice. *Medium*. Retrieved from https://medium.com/@genjustice/exploring-journalism-904962562993.

Russell, D. E. H., & Harmes, R. H. (2001). *Femicide in global perspective*. Columbia University.

Savage, M. W., Scarduzio, J. A., Lockwood Harris, K., Carlyle, K. E., & Sheff, S. E. (2017). News stories of intimate partner violence: An experimental examination of participant sex, perpetrator sex, and violence severity on seriousness, sympathy, and punishment preferences. *Health Communication, 32*(6), 768–776.

Scheufele, D. A. (1999). Framing as a theory of media effects. *Journal of Communication, 49*, 103–122. https://doi.org/10.1093/joc/49.1.103

Sela-Shayovitz, R. (2018). 'She knew he would murder her': The role of the media in the reconstruction of intimate femicide. *Journal of Comparative Social Work, 13*(1), 11–34.

Simons, M., & Morgan, J. (2017). Changing media coverage of violence against women: Changing sourcing practices? *Journalism Studies, 19*(8), 1202–1217.

Statista. (2022). Femicide rate in selected countries in Latin America in 2022. Retrieved from https://www.statista.com/statistics/1102327/femicide-rate-latin-america-by-country/.

Statista. (2024). Femicide in Latin America – Statistics & facts. Retrieved from https://www.statista.com/topics/6437/femicide-in-latin-america/#topic Overview.

Stevenson, M. (2018, April 5). Mexico shaken by killings of 3 pregnant women. *AP.* Retrieved from https://apnews.com/general-news-b7742c7bd84f49049b6caa9a99e052bb.

Sutherland, G., McCormack, A., Easteal, P., Holland, K., & Pirkis, J. (2016). Media guidelines for the responsible reporting of violence against women: A review of evidence and issues. *Australian Journalism Review, 38*(1), 5–17.

Taccini, F., & Mannarini, S. (2024). News media representation of intimate partner violence: A systematic review. *Sexuality Research and Social Policy, 22,* 252–267. https://doi.org/10.1007/s13178-023-00922-z

Tait, S. (2011). Bearing witness, journalism and moral responsibility. *Media, Culture & Society, 33*(8), 1220–1235.

Taylor, R. (2009). Slain and slandered: A content analysis of the portrayal of femicide in the news. *Homicide Studies,* 13, 21–49.

Tuchman, G. (2000). The symbolic annihilation of women by the mass media. In L. Crothers and C. Lockhart (Eds.) *Culture and politics: A reader* (pp. 150–174). Palgrave Macmillan.

United Nations. (2021a, November 24). The pandemic in the shadows: Femicides or feminicides in 2020 in Latin America and the Caribbean. Retrieved from https://www.cepal.org/en/notes/pandemic-shadows-femicides-or-feminicides-2020-latin-america-and-caribbean.

United Nations. (2021b, November 24). ECLAC: At least 4,091 women were victims of femicide in 2020 in Latin America and the Caribbean, despite greater visibility and social condemnation. Retrieved from https://www.cepal.org/en/pressreleases/eclac-least-4091-women-were-victims-femicide-2020-latin-america-and-caribbean-despite.

Valkenburg, P. M., Semetko, H. A., & De Vreese, C. H. (1999). The effects of news frames on readers' thoughts and recall. *Communication Research,* 26(5), 550–569.

Vardeman-Winter, J. (2017). The framing of women and health disparities: A critical look at race, gender, and class from the perspectives of grassroots health communicators. *Health Communication, 32*(5), 629–638.

Wallace, L. R. (2023). *The view from somewhere: Undoing the myth of journalistic objectivity.* University of Chicago Press.

World Health Organization. (2024, March 25). Violence against women. Retrieved from https://www.who.int/news-room/fact-sheets/detail/violence-against-women#:~:text=Globally%20as%20many%20as%2038,sexual%20violence%20are%20more%20limited.

Wright. (2011). Necropolitics, narcopolitics, and femicide: Gendered violence on the Mexico- U.S. Border. *Signs: Journal of Women in Culture and Society, 36*(3), 707–731.

Zelizer, B. (1998). *Remembering to forget: Holocaust memory through the camera's eye*. University of Chicago Press.

Zoller, H. M., & Casteel, D. (2022). #March for our lives: Health activism, diagnostic framing, gun control, and the gun industry. *Health Communication, 37*(7), 813–823.

4

GOD, COUNTRY, AND FAMILY

A Risk Orders Theory Approach to Deconstructing Health Messages About Family Planning in the Latine Community

Kimberly Field-Springer and Julee Tate

Risk orders theory makes theoretical contributions to critical health communication by considering higher level, taken for granted risk constructions that implicate systems of power. Risk orders theory is a framework for revealing how patterns of communication form the byproducts of institutionalized risk discourses which create the "risk society," or macro-social processes manifested by neoliberalism, postmodernity, and reflexive modernity (Beck, 1992, 2008; Giddens, 1990). The disintegration of spatial and temporal dimensions of how we identify, define, and manage risks that we ourselves produce is examined in discourse. Fundamental to risk orders theory is how the patterns of consequences penetrate private and public spheres affecting all of us, and these byproducts create social stratifications influencing political reformations (Beck, 1992). Risk orders theory is both a theoretical framework and method for deconstructing language and talk about risk constructions, exposing how knowledge(s) implicate institutions and systems of power.

Risk orders theory is a three-tiered framework. First-order risks examine the negotiation, maintenance, and creation of risks understood from the exchange of meanings among *experts, media sources,* and *publics* (Berger & Luckmann, 1967). Risk decisions are born within social systems and are embedded with probabilistic and evaluative orientations we attach to our risk constructions (Babrow, 1992). Moral values influence and are influenced by risk discourse. In identifying a risk, we ask ourselves if the risk is likely to occur and if it is desirable—we orient toward meanings and decisions based upon what we are capable of reconciling when it comes to divergent truth claims about risks (Babrow, 1992). Scientists disagree over facts and these disagreements are political (Beck, 1992; Kuhn, 1962). We experienced this struggle in real-time during the pandemic as scientific and layperson communities considered which interventions to prioritize in the prevention and treatment of COVID-19 (Field-Springer et al., 2024). This situation led to what World Health Organization (WHO) (2022) referred to as the infodemic—the spreading of misinformation, disinformation, and conspiracy theories on social media sites. Discord grew among segments of the public who uncritically embraced misinformation over science in the face of increasing distrust of science, medical institutions, and health interventions. Antivaccination discourses were informed by distrust in the state guided by neoliberal values of freedom, autonomy, and choice. These publics refused a vaccination even when they witnessed a loved one suffer. Those who chose to get vaccinated often relied on science and medical innovations. For these publics, risks were weighed against the desire to lessen personal illness if diagnosed as well as communal and social responsibilities to protect those at-risk (Bates et al., 2023). We negotiate risks, selectively elevate some risks over others, and shape understandings of risk through the negotiation of shared meaning. Social constructionist perspectives attend to the relationships among individuals, their social groups, and risk perceptions, revealing values, morals, and ideologies embedded in risk constructions.

First-Order Risks. First-order risks highlight the negotiation of truth claims and power dynamics embedded within public health discourse about risks illustrating how power struggles over values and morals can undermine trust in public health information. First-order risks illustrate the complex negotiation of competing truth claims, including who has the power to construct and contest claims. A Foucauldian approach dissects risk constructions by considering how power is constituted through taken for granted assumptions that form "regimes of truth" (Foucault, 1973, 1980). Public health interventions introduce risk taxonomies where knowledge, experience, and training have become a specialized trade and imposed upon by the body politic (Foucault, 1973; Lupton, 1995). Postmodern perspectives hold that "power relations are always implicated with knowledge and that no knowledge, therefore, can be said to be neutral" (Lupton, 2013, p. 39). Power struggles over truth evolve and change. According to a study conducted by the Pew Research Center, public positive trust in science declined from 73% pre-COVID-19 to 57% post-pandemic (Tyson & Kennedy, 2023). The circulation of misinformation and disinformation during the COVID-19 pandemic contributed to diminished trust in public health. Furthermore, a risk orders theory analysis of antivaccination discourse exposed how inaccurate information triggered a surge of unsubstantiated practices such as Hydroxychloroquine and Ivermectin to treat COVID-19 infection (Field-Springer et al., 2024). Medical expertise became irrelevant for many people.

Striley and Field-Springer (2014) argued that "To say a risk is socially constructed is not to say it is imaginary" (p. 553). Together, we make sense, manage, and negotiate meanings to determine how to live with risks. Ultimately, talk about risk *does* something. At this level, morality, values, and beliefs are exposed from the disentanglement of discourse about risks used to tame anxiety, fear, threats, and uncertainties about how to live in a risk-averse world. How are risk knowledge(s) prioritized over alternative meanings, and in what ways is language used to support arguments? How are values, morality, rules, norms, and belief systems intertwined within these risk constructions? Who is permitted to define a risk and what implications does this have for delegitimizing alternative meanings of risk in relation to one's subjectivity, positionalities, and identity formations? First-order risks expose values, morals, and belief systems embedded within risk discourses. First-order risk constructions beget higher-order constructions of risks informed from an ontological level by how we decide to live with risks and create narratives originating from moral panic and anxieties (Sastry & Lovari, 2016; Striley & Field-Springer, 2014, 2016). As we discuss next, second-order risks reveal how *talk* about risks create ontological insecurities.

Second-Order Risks. Second-order risks examine the interpretive meanings associated with our cautionary practices of risk avoidance or enactment. Decisions to adopt or reject risk practices form "additional threats" that engender both psychological and social implications because we may internalize guilt, shame, and/or blame ourselves and/or feel ostracized, judged, and/or excluded by others. There are three types of second-order risks: moral, social, and identity risks.

Moral risks involve how values embedded within risk discourses are associated with societal norms that make us feel good or bad about our risk behaviors. For instance, morality is engrained within messages advanced by breastfeeding advocates who promote "breast is best," consequently if a mother chooses not to breastfeed, they may be considered morally *bad* (Striley & Field-Springer, 2014). During the pandemic, values embedded in moral risks adopted by those spreading antivaccination misinformation prioritized religion and neoliberal ideals over science (Field-Springer et al., 2024). Moral risks are intricately tied to personal and societal belief systems about how one values risk practices. Moral risks are threats to our sense of goodness (Striley et al., 2022; Striley & Field-Springer, 2014, 2016). Risk constructions are muddled by moral judgments. By identifying moral risk constructions, values attached to bias, judgment, and stigma implicit in risk discourse are exposed. Meanings of risk are informed by the self and reinforced from the surveillance of institutionally defined and bound behaviors affecting our systems of beliefs. These belief systems are also policed by others.

Social risks are dangers that others will act on negative judgments which become threats to our relationships (Striley & Field-Springer, 2014, 2016). Social risks are perceptions of acceptance or rejection from others based on risk practices. Social risks entail the policing of moral behaviors (Striley & Field-Springer, 2014). Mothers who chose formula over breastfeeding face consequences of social rejection from other mothers who champion "breast is best," including the policing of who is permitted to enter the realm of "motherhood" (Striley & Field-Springer, 2014). To combat vaccination hesitancy, risk messaging during the pandemic relied on social conformity appeals such as, "we are in this together," and "do it for your community." Social risks are threats to our sense of belonging due to some action or inaction in relation to first-order risk constructions.

Identity risks are the third type of risk associated with second-order risks. Identity risk is the threat that we might lose some aspect of our self (Striley & Field-Springer, 2016). Identity risks are tied to the roles and occupations we adopt in the world. We are obliged in some ways to act within the rules governed by duties and responsibilities defined by societal norms and maintained through institutional systems of power (e.g., family, friendships, intimate relationships, occupations). Identity risks are intricately tied to both hidden and concealed positionalities in the world (e.g., gender, age, race, and class) shaped by our risk practices and ideologies informed by politics, religion, education. For instance, those who valued conservative ideologies were more inclined to believe that COVID-19 was a conspiracy, more likely to circulate disinformation, and less likely to trust medical institutions and interventions, including getting vaccinated (Field-Springer et al., 2024). Identity risks are connected to how one's sense of self is either affirmed or disconfirmed in discourse.

Second-order risks are not mutually exclusive and may conflict with one another creating contradictions in how we reconcile risk practices. For moral risks, how do people prioritize what they value as a good or bad risk? How does fear or apathy in relation to first-order risks expose positive, negative, or neutral values attached to moral risk frameworks? In what ways do individuals internalize guilt, shame, and/or blame from moral risk frameworks and how does this inform practices of denial leading to inaction versus fear leading to action? How do social norms influence feelings of exclusion, rejection, and/or judgments when understanding social risks? Individuals may choose to enact risky behaviors to avoid ostracism in a community even if this contradicts the seemingly impenetrable values in their moral risk frameworks. Finally, what does it mean to embody a risk?

What are implications for the self, agency, and identity formations in how we engage in or avoid cautionary risk practices? First- and second-order risks disclose communicative constructions constituted in discourse. As we discuss next, third-order risks examine how these constructions create patterns of communication that produce and (re)produce consequences of social risk practices.

Third-Order Risks. Whereas first-order risks stem from the philosophical orientations of strong constructionist perspectives of risk, third-order risks examine how first- and second-order risks create patterns impervious to change once institutionalized. Third-order risks are conceptualized within a weak constructionist perspective of risk. Third-order risks introduce ontological insecurity whereby patterns of risk knowledge(s) and behavior(s) potentially constrain or enable agency. Third-order risks compel us to ask how individuals are affected by biases, groups by health disparities, and societies by social injustices. Third-order risks include double-bind risks, agent constraining or enabling risks, and agency constraining or enabling risks.

Irreconcilable contradictions constitute double-binding risks. These patterns evolve from intractable second-order risk conflicts, making the choice between social or moral deviance incommensurable in certain circumstances. An example of an intractable circumstance is a college student who hid their COVID-19 vaccination status from family members who were antivaccination advocates, pitting moral risks against social risks. Agent-constraining risks inhibit our ability to define ourselves out of patterned ontological failures to conform. Agent-enabling risks are alternative risk discourses resisting patterns and, in turn, freeing ourselves from symbolic annihilation. Agency-constraining risks inhibit our imagination to act; agency is suppressed and domesticated into dominant ideologies where we either acquiesce or succumb to tactics institutionalized by systems of power. Agency-enabling is an act of resistance that may promote freedom to act and to imagine alternative risk practices.

Third-order risks are associated with ideological patterns of risk discourse and their consequences. For example, attention to third-order risks highlights how misinformation and disinformation take form. COVID-19 disproportionally affected marginalized groups in society. Members of the Latine community were four times more likely than any other group to become infected and two times more likely to die from COVID-19-related ailments. Social health determinants such as housing, work-related risks, lack of health insurance, and immigration status contributed to these risks (Sanchez et al., 2022). Risk values are thus politicized. For instance, those who have access to financial, educational, and medical resources experience fewer risks in capitalist societies (Douglas & Wildavsky, 1982).

Countries that favored free market policies were more accepting of casualties during COVID-19. In many of these countries, the political right emphasized civil liberties, government control, surveillance (Lesschaeve et al., 2021), and bodily autonomy (Field-Springer et al., 2024) over risks of illness and death. Third-order risks interrogate cultural ideologies of risk limiting or reimagining our abilities to conceptualize alternative realities (Field-Springer et al., 2024; Richardson, 2022). In the next section, we discuss abortion (mis) and disinformation as well as the risks associated with the lack of access to abortion resources.

Abortion Misinformation, Disinformation, and Stigmatization in the Latine Community

Communicative tropes concerning the polarizing nature of abortion discourse have been studied and well-documented (Condit, 1990), yet much has changed in the landscape of abortion discourse, resources, and practices in the United States. Risk orders theory is a critical health framework that can offer insight into the evolving truth claims and power structures informing the polarizing nature of women's reproductive health risk discourse. First-order risks expose how language is prioritized, legitimized, and applied within a particular risk construction. In anti-choice abortion discourse, it is often difficult to discern between medical facts and moral viewpoints. Anti-choice discourse often invokes morality by arguing that "abortion-harms-women" in ways that disregard the physical risks of carrying and delivering a child (Foster, 2021). Schmid et al. (2022) found that anti-choice discourse in newspaper coverage circulating in Alabama, Louisiana, and Mississippi framed abortion procedures as a *public health risk*. Motivated by state bans against elective abortion procedures during the COVID-19 pandemic, anti-choice advocates used the argument of abortion as a public health risk to promote their cause (Schmid et al., 2022). On the contrary, Watson (2018) argued that abortion is an essential healthcare need, not an elective or therapeutic procedure. Furthermore, Furgerson (2023) elucidated how anti-choice advocates relied on inaccurate scientific and medical language to campaign for heartbeat bills at six-weeks' gestation period, despite the fact the four chambers of a fetal heartbeat cannot medically be detected until after the 17-weeks' gestation period. Anti-choice discourses framed within the context of "abortion-harms-women" shapes cultural values of morality, stigmatization, and the sanctioning of deviant health behaviors hidden under the guise of protecting women (Saurette & Gordon, 2013).

The narrative framework that "abortion is a health and safety risk" carried over from *Planned Parenthood v. Casey* (1992), which permitted states to implement abortion regulations including 24-hour waiting periods. The ruling in this case further emboldened anti-choice advocates to argue abortion as a risky procedure. Targeted regulations of abortion providers (TRAP) laws permitted states to restrict abortion access by requiring informed consent, 24-hour waiting periods, counseling, and ultrasounds. The Supreme Court's majority argued that these provisions did not obstruct the undue burden rule, meaning that these regulations would not create a substantial obstacle for a person seeking an abortion. However, a study that investigated women's experiences of access to versus denial of an abortion found that women who were denied an abortion experienced more mental, physical, and economic risk factors (Foster, 2021). The restrictions did cause women to "turn away" from accessing an abortion often due to their financial circumstances, including the out-of-pocket cost for an abortion, mandatory waiting periods, and lack of transportation to an abortion clinic. For those able to access an abortion, the "turnaway study" found better mental health outcomes even if women had an emotional regret because the decision to have an abortion outweighed potential moral, social, and identity risks. For instance, women who had an abortion due to issues with their current partner or because they needed to care for their current children felt it was morally right based upon their family circumstances (Foster, 2021).

According to Watson (2019), access to abortion should be framed as a "moral good." Anti-choice discourse adopting morality arguments consequently produces patterns of stigmatization engendering a third-order, double-bind risk for those who pit moral risks based upon religious belief systems against social risks based upon reproductive justice. Almost half of abortions in the United States are patients under the poverty line and 73% of patients' reasons for abortion is that they cannot afford another child (Watson, 2019). Watson (2019) further articulates,

> Women have long been subjected to legal and social discrimination on the basis of their biological capacity for pregnancy. Today, the relatively new medical technologies of safe, effective contraception and abortion allow women to escape pregnancy's physical and social impact, and to come close to men's degree of sexual and reproductive freedom. Women cannot have social, economic, and interpersonal power comparable to men unless they can control whether and when they have children.
> *(Watson, 2019, p. 1197)*

Policies that impede women's access to abortion not only generate more health risks for the individual but also widen health inequalities that disproportionately affect those below the poverty level (Foster, 2021; Watson,

2018). In recent years, the argument for abortion access as a right, which views restricting that right as gender violence, has been successful in Latin American feminists' movements in Uruguay, Argentina, and Columbia (Fixmer-Oraiz & Murillo, 2023). Referred to as the green wave, the movement reinscribes the lack of abortion care to gendered violence and justice when access to reproductive health is limited (Fixmer-Oraiz & Murillo, 2023). Nonetheless, NARAL (2022) observed the need to remain vigilant in exposing misinformation circulating from Spanish-language influencers on social media who use religious ideology to propagate stigmatization embedded within anti-choice arguments.

Despite these concerns, shortly following the U.S. Supreme Court's decision to overturn *Roe v. Wade* (1973), abortion (mis) and disinformation spread on social media causing confusion and fear within Latine communities (Godoy, 2022a). Misinformation, according to the U.S. Surgeon General (2021) is categorized as false, inaccurate, or misleading, whereas disinformation is intended to deceive either to gain political power, disseminate conspiracy theories, and/or promote propaganda (Ball & Maxmen, 2020). Disinformation is more nuanced, complex, and prevalent in cross-language online messaging platforms (Chu et al., 2021; NARAL, 2022). Studies consistently report that those who reside in countries where politics are polarized by populist ideology are more likely to burrow themselves within peer networks online, distrust media, succumb to, and recirculate misinformation (Boulianne et al., 2022; Cheng et al., 2022).

According to Godoy (2022a), medical misinformation targeted toward the Latine community in the United States included incorrect information about the safety and legality of abortion, including assertions that abortion causes depression, cervical cancer, and infertility. Crisis pregnancy centers in rural Latine communities were predacious in driving medical disinformation (Godoy, 2022b). Social media from Spanish-language platforms, mainly Facebook and TikTok, vilified abortion providers, propagated medical disinformation, and advocated the narrative that *fetal personhood* begins at conception (NARAL, 2022). Findings of the NARAL (2022) study reported Spanish-language sites on Facebook and TikTok propagated (mis) and disinformation concealed in religiously charged narratives and anti-feminist messages. Abortion misinformation begins with the false premise that abortions are uncommon and are only carried out by morally deviant people, which is not the case, as nearly 25% of women in the United States have terminated a pregnancy at least once in their lifetime (Watson, 2018). Even more problematic is how inaccurate scientific and medical terminology related to abortion and other common procedures in anti-choice discourse lacked clarity and context regarding health risks which potentially can contribute to an increase in policies that criminalize abortion in a post-Roe America. In the following section, we apply risk orders theory to analyze (mis), and disinformation circulated by a popular influencer in the Latine community.

Responding to Spanish-Language Coverage of Abortion

Applying the critical health framework of risk orders theory (Striley & Field-Springer, 2014, 2016), our study explores the risk discourses of anti-abortion advocate, Eduardo Verástegui. Verástegui is an actor-turned-politician campaigning for *Movimiento Viva Mexico*. The actor has over 1.9 million followers on Facebook. Verástegui appeared in telenovelas on Mexican television and the popular television series, *Charmed*, nominated for several Teen Choice awards in the U.S. NARAL (2022) named Verástegui as an anti-choice activist who opposed Mexico's Supreme Court decision to decriminalize abortion. Verástegui was featured in several of the Susan B. Anthony Foundation super PAC political campaigns in Spanish-language media outlets. Susan B. Anthony is a pro-life non-profit organization in the United States that culturally appropriates feminism into messages advocating against abortion. These campaigns led with pro-natalist, religious, homophobic, and transphobic undertones and included messages that Kamala Harris supports infanticide and the message that abortion care endangers women. Verástegui's campaign targeted the U.S. Senate run-off in the state of Georgia with ads claiming that Democrats use taxpayer money to fund abortions up to the moment of birth (NARAL, 2022). Using risk orders theory as a framework for analysis, we explore themes which offer insight into Verástegui's anti-choice narratives.

The second author, who is a professor of Spanish and Latin American Studies, collected posts about abortion on Verástegui's Facebook feed from January 2022 through February 2024. A total of 25 single-spaced pages were used for analysis. Anti-choice campaign messages, sheathed in between weekly rosary prayers, flood Verástegui's Facebook page. Anti-choice messages in the *Movimiento Viva Mexico* campaign analyzed in the current study start in March of 2022 and include political messages targeted in the countries of Mexico, Argentina, and Columbia, as well as the state of Sinaloa in Mexico. The *Movimiento Viva Mexico* campaign posts appear with a logo accompanied with the hashtag #MovimientoVivaMexico. Risk orders theory, as lens for both analysis and theory, examines how (mis) and disinformation from an anti-choice advocate shape and reproduce cultural, societal, and political risk values. The following themes emerged in the discourse of Verástegui's posts: (a) the dangers of a mother's womb, (b) the golden rule, (c) if you are not with us, you are against us, (d) erasure of motherless women, and (e) God, country, family.

First-Order Risks: The Dangers of a Mother's Womb

First-order risks explore how claims are prioritized, legitimized, and circulated in context. At this level of analysis, we investigate what knowledge claims are materializing in anti-choice discourse. Verástegui's anti-choice messages used emotionally charged, medically inaccurate terms, and controversial images to propagate the "abortion is murder" trope, depicting women as devoid of agency. The *mother's womb* as a risk is a phrase used frequently in Verástegui's anti-choice messages. The medically accurate term is not womb, but uterus. Womb is a nontechnical term intended to arouse emotion and fear in anti-abortion discourse (Furgerson, 2023). First-order risks explore how meanings are emptied, adorned, altered, or signified to support an author's argument.

In March of 2022, the message targeted toward the Mexican state of Sinaloa includes a picture of a newborn accompanied with #AbortoNo "*NoAbortion,*" #DiputadosEstoyVivo "*CongressmenI'mAlive,*" and #DespenalizarEsPromover "*ToDecriminalizeIsToPromote.*" The newborn is personified with the expression, *I am alive*, urging members of parliament to say no to abortion. The last hashtag is warning that *if you decriminalize abortion, you are promoting abortion*. In another campaign post, Verástegui is pictured sternly gazing at the viewer pleading with Sinaloa representatives to vote in favor of life. On March 7, 2022, Verástegui posted:

> The life of babies in their mother's womb is at serious risk in Sinaloa. This Tuesday, March 8, the Congress of the state of Sinaloa will vote on a bill to decriminalize abortion up to 13 weeks of gestation. In other words, endorse abortion. Decriminalization has the effect of endorsement and approval, plain and simple. Thousands of Sinaloan babies will die if they approve it.

Medically inaccurate images of a newborn accompanied by morally driven messages evoke emotion and are intentionally misleading in the post. According to The American College of Obstetricians and Gynecologists (ACOG) (2024), following fertilization, which is the joining together of the egg and sperm, an embryo forms made up of biological cells, not a fully developed baby. The embryo is the official term for the process of development up to 8-weeks' gestation. A fetus develops at 9-weeks' gestation and beyond. Assigning moral agency to embryos or fetuses over a rational, biologically independent woman is unacceptable, and equates to forcing a woman to bear a child (Watson, 2019). The symbolization of life at conception "in their mother's womb" is depicted as a risk for Sinaloans.

Verástegui depicts a woman as devoid of agency as the womb is depicted as an inanimate object removed from an embodied, breathing human being. First-order risk constructions in the message rely upon medically inaccurate information that propagates the "abortion is murder" trope (Condit, 1990). First-order risk messages are not only misleading but deceptive especially as Verástegui espouses that "decriminalization" of abortion is the "endorsement and approval" of death.

On March 27, 2022, Verástegui, in a monologue video, pleads for solidarity with the pro-life #MarchaPorLaVida movement in Argentina #ArgentinaDesdeLaConcepcion. He said:

> You are facing in Argentina an increasing advance on the limits of conscientious objection. Those on the side of death are inciting more fear, more pressure, and more attacks. As much as here, in my country, Mexico, we need to work profoundly on the viable tools of legal judicial strategy. We need more pro-lifers in the field of politics, where an abortionist progressivism is advancing with unjust perversion that, far from protecting the human right to be born, to live, to enjoy a life project, doesn't just permit legal and free abortion, but even imposes it. Let us never tire of defending life. Let's go with all family, together.

Verástegui is galvanizing anti-abortion activists to stigmatize abortion-rights' activists as "on the side of death." The language "conscientious objection" is a term used when a health care professional refuses abortion care for reasons of religion, ethics, or moral beliefs. The Inter-American Commission on Human Rights (IACHR), which represents several Latin American countries, stated that health care workers who refuse abortion care based on conscientious objection are required to refer the patient without burden to another facility. Moral agency is once again focused on the "life project" of the unborn over the life project of a woman who is symbolically annihilated and devoid of agency, bodily autonomy, and ontological freedom to decide whether or not to bear a child. According to data from the United States in 2020, maternal mortality was 62% higher in states with abortion restrictions compared to states with abortion access and care (Hoyert, 2022). Childbirth is risky. Verástegui's truth claims obscure the experience of childbearing including the process of conceiving, deciding whether to become a parent, the nourishment of a fetus during pregnancy, health risks of carrying a fetus to term, and risks involved during labor and delivery.

Verástegui's posts illustrate first-order risk constructions using medically inaccurate information to minimize pregnancy complications and vilify life-saving abortion procedures, while falsely portraying embryos/fetuses as rational beings, ignoring the benefits of abortion in reducing maternal mortality. In the accounts featured below, first-order health risks are depicted with medically inaccurate information where complications of pregnancy are discounted. Verástegui's posts continue to crusade for the imagined risk to a future life project rather than the life project of a woman. He categorizes the embryo/fetus as a rational, sentient being when this is medically inaccurate. Access to abortion decreases maternal mortality. The risks from complications of pregnancy due to fatal birth defects screened early in pregnancy allow for the woman to receive life-saving medical intervention, like that of a dilation and evacuation procedure, which Verástegui vilifies.

On March 25, an image with four frames is posted to his account. The top left frame reads, "Life is not debated, it is defended. Today life is at risk. The manipulation of Beatriz's case in the Inter-American Court of Human Rights could impose the false right to abortion in our countries." Beatriz's case is central to the Inter-American court of Human Right's challenge to El Salvador's total abortion ban that criminalizes women. Salvadoran women have been convicted of homicide with sentences up to 40 years in prison, even women who miscarried both at home and in hospitals (Human Rights Watch [HRW], 2023). A woman, sentenced up to 30 years in prison in 2015 after her baby died in the hospital due to health complications three days following birth, was just released this year in El Salvador (Rocha, 2024). Beatriz's case was a high-risk pregnancy because the fetus showed signs of anencephaly at 11-weeks' gestation, a birth defect where the brain and skull are missing (ACOG, 2024). Anencephaly is considered a high-risk pregnancy because the medical condition, without intervention, could cause septic shock leading to a woman's death. However, El Salvador refused to abort the fetus. This refusal prompted provisional measures by the commission for Beatriz to receive the medical treatment needed to reduce risks of obstetrical hemorrhaging. Beatriz carried a non-viable fetus until she received an emergency C-Section at 26-weeks' gestation leading to a decline in her health. Access to abortion reduces maternal mortality and health complications while also protecting the life, liberty, autonomy, and human rights of a pregnant woman (HRW, 2023). To claim, as Verástegui does, that Beatriz's case was a manipulation of information is to deny scientific progress and medical institutions' conclusions that safe and legal abortions are necessary to reducing maternal mortality rates. On the right upper frame, Verástegui's post reads,

> This day is celebrated to remember and reaffirm that every life is valuable and that every conceived human being has the right to be born. In 1998, Argentina made the date official with the decree signed by then President Carlos Menem.

In 2020, however, Argentina relaxed abortion laws and abortion is currently legal up to 14-weeks' gestation. The bottom two posts feature a woman embracing a newborn and reads, "Let's defend life as a fundamental human right necessary to respect from the moment of conception until natural death" and March 25 is the celebration of the "day of the unborn child."

In February 2022, Verástegui shared a misleading post that falsely portrays an abortion procedure to incite fear, even though most U.S. medical abortions are safely performed with FDA-approved drugs up to ten-weeks' gestation. The post is an animated video he narrates called "the procedure." The video was originally created by Choice42, an anti-choice activist organization whose messages intentionally mislead people about medical terminations of pregnancy. The video exhibits a dilation and evacuation procedure which is rare and often performed after 14-weeks of gestation accompanied with Verástegui's voiceover, "the unvarnished truth of what abortion is: the murder of innocent babies." Over half of medical abortions in the United States, up to the year 2020, were performed by using the FDA approved drugs, Mifepristone and Misoprostol up to ten weeks of gestation (Ranji et al., 2023). Dilation and evacuation are commonly used procedures for miscarriage, stillbirth, and even fertility treatments (Furgerson, 2023), cases in which women chose to bear children. These videos are circulated with the nefarious intent to incite shock, shame, guilt, and fear much like displaying a fetus in a jar and laws that require a woman to listen to a fetal heartbeat prior to an abortion.

Second-Order Moral Risks: The Golden Rule

Second-order moral risks explore how risk language is intertwined with threats to our sense of goodness. Verástegui embeds risk perceptions within his Catholic religious beliefs. For example, he connects the Golden Rule to his argument that abortion is murder and those who commit the crime should be criminalized. Rather than treat others how you would want to be treated, Verástegui uses a double negative and his words have a punitive undertone. In February 2024, Verástegui posted:

> At some point in their life, some will ask: how is it possible that the aberration of abortion has been allowed? Could we really answer that we did everything in our power to save children from the crime of abortion? Respect for life is sacred. And each of us is responsible for standing up for the innocent who can't speak for themselves. Let's put the golden rule into practice. 'Don't do to others what you wouldn't want them to do to you. Treat others as you would like for them to treat you.'

Moral risks for Verástegui are imposed upon anyone who aborts an embryo/fetus. They are guilty, evil, and morally bad for committing a crime. Despite evidence showing that women who are unable to access abortion care experience negative outcomes, including poorer physical and mental health and barriers to socioeconomic and educational advancements (Foster, 2021), women who choose abortion are stigmatized as less than a woman, selfish, immoral, and evil by religious, pronatalist communities. Abortion rights proponents tend to police the borders of motherhood and value the moral agency of an embryo over that of a woman.

On September 6, 2023, the Supreme Court of Mexico voted to decriminalize abortion. Early the next morning, Verástegui posted "a special rosary" in which he called the Supreme Court of Mexico the "Supreme Court of Injustice." He said "el crimen del aborto," abortion is a crime and that it is time to call it by its name, "un crimen," a crime. He wrote, "That is what it is, a crime, the murder of an innocent baby who cannot defend himself. Who doesn't have a voice."

#MovimientoVivaMexico is Verástegui's political movement, and his platform is making abortion a crime. Moral risks assigned to women who abort as corrupt and evil beget the punitive sanctions exposed in second-order social risks.

Second-Order Social Risks: If You Are Not with Us, You Are Against Us

Second-order moral risks explore judgments of good and bad in our risk constructions, while second-order social risks explore the language used to create social sanctions. Verástegui's posts display homophobic and transphobic rhetoric, promote an outdated view of family, and inaccurately use the term "pro-abortion" instead of "pro-choice" creating social factions in opposition to abortion-rights activists, policy, and lawmakers who advocate access to abortion care. In May of 2023, Verástegui posted a video with the hashtag #ElPanhamuerto which shows the viewer images of politicians in Mexico who support access to abortion care. Xóchitl Galvez, former senator of the Mexican Republic posted,

> Abortion is an individual decision of the woman. If you make this determination, you should be accompanied, not judged. No more women should go to jail for deciding what happens to her. Global Day of Action for legal and safe abortion.

Verástegui responded, "Do you support Xóchitl? Then, do you support abortion? No? Then, it's not there. Don't get it wrong." He urged his followers not to support Xóchitl Galvez because of her views on abortion politics. In January of 2024, he wrote, "Claudia y Xóchilt are pro-abortion and pro-gender ideology. I am the only candidate who is a proven fierce enemy of these two plagues that only have the purpose of making our families sick." Verástegui's rhetoric vis-à-vis the family scattered throughout his posts exhibit homophobic and transphobic rhetoric and promotes an anachronistic vision of the family unit. Moreover, the term pro-abortion is inaccurate and should be replaced with pro-choice (Watson, 2018), as the terms incite different connotations.

Verástegui's anti-choice campaign messages –suggesting that if you vote to decriminalize abortion then you endorse abortion—impose a social sanction advancing the idea that if you are not with us, you are against us. In response to his Sinaloa anti-choice post on March 7, a commenter shared, "In favor of Life! No to Abortion! We ask on behalf of mothers that are about to abort that our Lord will enlighten them in their decision. Don't commit such a big sin. God bless them!" Another posted, "Don't even tell me which satanic party 'governs' in Sinaloa." His followers employ moral risks creating social norms and borders between sinners, mothers who terminate their pregnancy and the innocent, those who have no voice. On December 16, 2023, Verástegui posted:

> I will defend the lives of all Mexicans with my own life. Mainly, the lives of those who cannot defend themselves, of those who have no voice, the unborn children. I will defend the most important of all rights, the right to life, because without life, you cannot enjoy any other right. There will be no peace in Mexico as long as there is abortion, which is a crime, and the doctors who practice it, who are actually hitmen, should go to jail, first of all.

Social risks extend to not only women who terminate their pregnancy but also to lawmakers, and medical professionals who perform abortion care. Following the reversal of Roe v Wade in the United States, violence in protective abortion states rose dramatically from 2021 to 2022, most notably stalking increased 229% (Connolly, 2023). Social risks expose the boundaries of inclusion and exclusion in language, but Verástegui's discourse went further by inciting hostility toward social groups he not only excludes but condemns.

Second-Order Identity Risks: Erasure of Motherless Women

Second-order identity risks examine how risk constructions are linked with the roles we occupy and social positionalities. Verástegui argues against abortion under any circumstances by emphasizing the sanctity of all life, portrays the womb as a dangerous place, and pressures women to conform to traditional motherhood roles. Motherless women are erased in his risk constructions. In Verástegui's rosary posted on September 7, he wrote,

> It is neither right nor humane to kill a human being, much less a human being who cannot defend himself, a human being who has no voice. If all mothers' wombs were made of crystal and they could see the miracle growing within them, none of them would ever abort.

He then wrote that all life is equally valuable no matter how it is conceived. He makes no exceptions for abortion, "whether on a honeymoon, an unexpected pregnancy, an infidelity, or rape. All of those lives should be welcomed." Verástegui circles back again to the mother's womb as a threat. He wrote, "The womb of Mexican mothers is going to be the most dangerous place in all of Mexico. There will be more deaths there than in any part of Mexico." Identity risks are attached to cultural conceptions of motherhood and women are domesticated into the assigned role as a mother in a traditional family unit.

Even as Verástegui celebrates International Women's Day, he makes clear that, in his view, the identity of a woman is only made real through her ability to "mother." In his previous post as well as below, autonomy, self-resilience, agency, and empowerment are only realized in a woman's ability to procreate. He posted:

> Today is International Women's Day. And what I am moved to more than anything is a huge THANK YOU! First, to the woman who gave me life; to my sisters, for their love and their constant work on behalf of those they love and their way of building a world where we are all more brothers and sisters. Thank you to the mother of all, to Mary, model of woman, complete, prayerful, faithful, intelligent, the one who protects and shelters all of her children every day.

The concept of second-order identity risk explores how perceptions of risk are intertwined with societal roles and identity formations. Verástegui vehemently opposes abortion in all circumstances, underscoring the sanctity of life while positioning the womb as a perilous space, thereby coercing women to adhere to traditional motherhood ideals. Verástegui is a pronatalist whose identity of a woman is placed upon her ability to bear children. A woman's identity is fundamentally linked to her ability to procreate, celebrating motherhood as the essence of female identity, which marginalizes those who do not conform to these expectations, such as motherless women.

Third-Order Risks: God, Country, Family

Verástegui's use of rhetorical choices in his risk discourse creates the overarching ideological narrative: God, country, and family. His vision of government is clearly a theocracy, with Catholicism at the center of his religious and political ideals. The evils of abortion are situated in his constructions of moral, social, and identity risks and expose the ontological insecurities that lead to constraining third-order risk patterns. For example, first-order risk constructions form the scaffolding of medically inaccurate information which helps to support moral risks based upon religious tropes that assign personhood to an embryo. Forcing childbirth is immoral (Watson, 2019). First-order risk constructions in debating laws for abortion access and care are medically inaccurate, misleading, and deceiving. First-order risks unmask medically misleading language which gives rise to ontological insecurities revealed in second-order risk constructions. Second-order risk constructions lead to culturally constraining communicative patterns materialized in third-order risks discourse. Verástegui calls upon Mexico as a symbolic representation of motherhood and country enforced through both identity and social risk constructions. His oft repeated motto of the Conservative Political Action Convention (CPAC) is "God, Country, Family", which he repeats in Spanish in a video post: "Dios, Patria y Familia." In several politically driven posts, Verástegui's messages are situated within the rhetoric of tradition, family, and religion. On March 6, his post read:

> Nothing better than sharing projects and fighting spirit with good friends, who are also great leaders…And it is always a great moment to be able to talk and exchange ideas with The Kari Lake, Marjorie Taylor Greene, Eduardo Bolsonaro, Jair Messias Bolsonaro. The Latin American unity of those of us who defend and work for freedom and democracy in our people is key to stopping the systematic advance of left-wing progressivism. I have faith that, together, we can end socialism, a true cancer that destroys everything it touches, promotes abortion, the woke agenda and cultural Marxism.

Verástegui is pictured with Jair Bolsonaro, the equivalent of the Brazilian Donald Trump, and his son at CPAC in Washington D.C. Following this, on March 9, Verástegui posted a message for Mexico to do what Trump did in the United States, that is, elect "pro-life ministers to the Supreme Court of medical justice." Verástegui praises Trump's part in appointing anti-abortion advocates to the U.S. Supreme Court who voted to overturn Roe v. Wade. Verástegui pleads with Mexico to appoint Supreme Court judges to criminalize abortion.

Risk Orders Theory as a Critical Method to Examine Gender Reproductive Health Violence in the Circulation of (Mis) and Disinformation

Risk orders theory is a framework in response to the dominant techno-scientific and cognitive approaches that aim to measure and control risks, often assigning blame to individuals who deviate from societal health norms. Risk knowledge(s) is/are reduced to dangers by those with the power to identify, name, categorize, and prioritize risks. Realist perspectives take for granted power in defining the relationship between risk perceptions and risks constructions and are overly deterministic (Lupton, 2013). Conversely, risk orders theory combines a social constructionist and critical structuralist framework that guides one to interrogate knowledge(s) of risks including patterns of surveillance, conflict, and contradiction. Thus, risk orders theory is not apolitical, in that discourse is critically examined in relation to social actors' localized positions and capacity for agency to construct risks and act in a world that is continuously inducing moral panic and judgments. Risks are not discovered; they are produced and reproduced from our communicative interactions with each other.

By applying risk orders theory to analyze Verástegui's discourse, a popular anti-choice advocate in the Latine community, we identify medical messages that are inaccurate, confusing, and misleading circulating on social media. Risk orders theory exposes the political constructions concealed within Verástegui's motto, "God, country, and family." Verástegui's perspectives advance conservative political ideologies at the expense of a woman's ontological freedom. Silence on the topic of abortion is exercising a privilege and ignoring the "needs of women is not apolitical, it is abandonment" (Watson, 2018, p. 215). We urge the public to combat disinformation with medically accurate evidence demonstrating that access to abortion care reduces health risks for a woman and to contest ideological risk constructions that constrain a woman's bodily autonomy and sovereignty. Medical inaccuracies met without resistance harm pregnant people's healthcare agency and these knowledge(s) of risks become weaponized delimiting possibilities for alternate realities. Risk discourse has hidden implications for reproductive justice and, if left uncontested, can lead to the creation of cultural patterns that inscribe inequitable and unsafe health practices. Applying risk orders theory to public interpretations of risks highlights the importance of combating medically inaccurate misinformation and ensuring that health policies are based on accurate, evidence-based information. This approach emphasizes the need to protect women's health by challenging political ideologies that promote unsafe and inequitable health practices.

References

Babrow, A. S. (1992). Communication and problematic integration: Understanding diverging probability and value, ambiguity, ambivalence, and impossibility. *Communication Theory, 2*(2), 95–130. https://doi.org/10.1111/j.1468-2885.1992.tb00031.x

Ball, P., & Maxmen, A. (2020). The epic battle against coronavirus misinformation and conspiracy theories. *Nature, 581*, 371–375. https://doi.org/10.1038/d41586-020-01452-z

Bates, B. R., Finkelshteyn, S., & Odunsi, I. A. (2024). 'We were having a rather long conversation about the uproar': Memorable messages about COVID-19 vaccinations in a mostly young, white sample. *Journal of Communication in Healthcare, 17*(2), 143–153. https://doi.org/10.1080/17538068.2023.2223437

Beck, U. (1992). *Risk society: Towards a new modernity* (M. Ritter, Trans.). Sage. (original work published 1986).

Beck, U. (2008). *World at risk*. Polity Press.

Berger, P. L., & Luckmann, T. (1967). *The social construction of reality: A treatise in the sociology of knowledge*. Anchor Books.

Boulianne, S., Tenove, C., & Buffie, J. (2022). Complicating the resilience model: A four-country study about misinformation. *Media and Communication, 10*(3), 169–182. https://doi.org/10.17645/mac.v10i3.5346

Cheng, Z., Zhang, B., & Gil de Zúñiga, H. (2022). Antecedents of political consumerism: Modeling online, social media and WhatsApp news use effects through political expression and political discussion. *The International Journal of Press/Politics, 28*(4), 995–1016. https://doi.org/10.1177/19401612221075936

Chu, S. K. W., Xie, R., & Wang, Y. (2021). Cross-language fake news detection. *Data and Information Management, 5*(1), 100–109. https://doi.org/10.2478/dim-2020-0025

Condit, C. (1990). *Decoding abortion rhetoric: Communicating social change*. University of Illinois Press.

Connolly, C. (2023, May 11). Violence against abortion providers continue to rise following Roe reversal, new report finds. Retrieved from https://prochoice.org/violence-against-abortion-providers-continues-to-rise-following-roe-reversal-new-report-finds/.

Douglas, M., & Wildavsky, A. (1982). *Risk and culture: An essay on the selection of technological and environmental dangers*. University of California Press.

Field-Springer, K., Striley, K., Byerly, J., Simmons, N., Ferrell, T., & Quigley, S. (2024). 'Are you vaccinated? Yeah, I'm immunized': a risk orders theory analysis of celebrity COVID-19 misinformation. *Journal of Communication in Healthcare, 17*(4), 317–327. https://doi.org/10.1080/17538068.2024.2320984

Fixmer-Oraiz, N., & Murillo, L.M. (2023). "The term 'Life' should return to us": Learning from Latin America's green wave. *Women & Language, 46*, 275–283.

Foster, D. G. (2021). *The turnaway study: Ten years, a thousand women, and the consequences of having—or being denied—an abortion*. Simon and Schuster.

Foucault, M. (1973). *The birth of the clinic: An archaeology of medical perception* (A. Sheridan, Trans.). Vintage Books.

Foucault, M. (1980). *Power/knowledge: Selected interviews and other writings 1972–1977*. Vintage Books.

Furgerson, J. (2023). A working glossary of key terms in the abortion discourse. *Women & Language, 46*, 259–265.

Giddens, A. (1990). *The consequences of modernity*. Stanford University Press.

Godoy, M. (2022a, August 13). The Latino community is facing issues with misinformation on abortions. Retrieved from https://www.npr.org/2022/08/13/1117347604/the-latino-community-is-facing-issues-with-misinformation-on-abortions

Godoy, M. (2022b, November 3). Doctors and advocates tackle a spike of abortion misinformation– in Spanish. Retrieved from https://www.npr.org/sections/health-shots/2022/11/03/1133743997/doctors-and-advocates-tackle-a-spike-of-abortion-misinformation-in-spanish

Hoyert, D. L. (2022). Maternal mortality rates in the United States, 2020. *NCHS Health E-Stats*. https://doi.org/10.15620/cdc:113967

Human Rights Watch. (2023, March 23). El Salvador: Court hears case on total abortion ban. https://www.hrw.org/news/2023/03/23/el-salvador-court-hears-case-total-abortion-ban.

Kuhn, T. S. (1962). *The structure of scientific revolutions* (3rd ed.). University of Chicago Press.

Lesschaeve, C., Glaurdić, J., & Mochtak, M. (2021). Health versus wealth during the covid-19 pandemic: Saving lives or saving the economy? *Public Opinion Quarterly, 85*(3), 808–835. https://doi.org/10.1093/poq/nfab036

Lupton, D. (1995). The imperative of health: Public health and the regulated body. Sage.

Lupton, D. (2013). *Risk* (2nd ed.). Routledge.

NARAL (2022). *Translating abortion disinformation: The Spanish-language anti-choice landscape*. United States. Retrieved from https://www.prochoiceamerica.org/wp-content/uploads/2022/05/Translating-Abortion-Disinformation-The-Spanish-Language-Anti-Choice-Landscape.pdf

Planned Parenthood of Southeastern Pennsylvania v. Casey is 505 U.S. 833 (1992). https://supreme.justia.com/cases/federal/us/505/833/

Ranji, U., Diep, K., & Salganicoff, A. (2023, November 21). *Key facts on abortion in the United States*. Kaiser Family Foundation. Retrieved from https://www.kff.org/womens-health-policy/issue-brief/key-facts-on-abortion-in-the-united-states/

Richardson, E. (2022). Postscript: COVID-19 and the path forward. In G. L. Wright & L. Hubbard (Eds.), *The pandemic divide: How COVID increased inequality in America* (pp. 295–300). Duke University Press.

Rocha, L. (2024, January 17). El Savador woman freed after abortion conviction. *BBC*. Retrieved from https://www.bbc.com/news/world-latin-america-68014699.

Roe v. Wade, 410 U.S. 113 (1973). https://supreme.justia.com/cases/federal/us/410/113/

Sanchez, M., Dipietro, M., Babiinski, l L., Amendum, S. & Knnotek, S. (2022). Latine immigrant parents and their children in times of COVID-19: Facing inequities together in the "Mexican Room" of the New Latino South. In G. L. Wright & L. Hubbard (Eds.), *The pandemic divide: How COVID increased inequality in America* (pp. 231–255). Duke University Press.

Saurette, P., & Gordon, K. (2013). Arguing abortion: The new anti-abortion discourse in Canada. *Canadian Journal of Political Science/Revue canadienne de science politique, 46*(1), 157–185. https://doi.org/10.1017/S0008423913000176

Sastry, S., & Lovari, A. (2016). Communicating the ontological narrative of Ebola: An emerging disease in the time of "Epidemic 2.0." *Health Communication, 32*, 329–338. https://doi.org/10.1080/10410236.2016.1138380

Schmid, A. T., Veldhouse, A., & Payam, S. (2022). A press(ing) issue: analysing local news coverage of abortion in the US South during the COVID-19 pandemic. *Culture, Health & Sexuality, 25*, 1–15. https://doi.org/10.1080/13691058.2022.2164064

Striley, K., & Field-Springer, K. (2014). The bad mother police: theorizing risk orders in the discourses of infant feeding practices. *Health Communication, 29*, 552–562. https://doi.org/10.1080/10410236.2013.782225

Striley, K., & Field-Springer, K. (2016). When it's good to be a bad nurse: Expanding risk orders theory to explore nurses' experiences of moral, social and identity risks in obstetrics units. *Health, Risk & Society, 18*, 77–96. https://doi.org/10.1080/13698575.2016.1169254

Striley, K., Tenzek, K. E., & Field-Springer, K. (2022). Difficult dialogues about death: Applying risk orders theory to analyse chaplains' provision of end-of-life care. *Health, Risk & Society, 24*(3–4), 167–185. https://doi.org/10.1080/13698575.2022.2056582

The American College of Obstetricians and Gynecologists. (2024). *Dictionary*. https://www.acog.org/womens-health/dictionary

Tyson, A., & Kennedy, B. (2023, November). *Americans trust in scientists, positive views of science continue to decline*. Pew Research Center. Retrieved from https://www.pewresearch.org/wp-content/uploads/sites/20/2023/11/PS_2023.11.14_trust-in-scientists_REPORT.pdf.

U.S. Surgeon General. (2021). *A community toolkit for addressing health misinformation*. Retrieved from https://www.hhs.gov/sites/default/files/health-misinformation-toolkit-english.pdf.

Watson, K. (2018). *Scarlet A: The ethics, law, and politics of ordinary abortion*. Oxford University Press.

Watson, K. (2019). Abortion as a moral good. *The Lancet, 393*(10177), 1196–1197.

World Health Organization. (2022). *Infodemic*. Retrieved from https://www.who.int/health-topics/infodemic#tab=tab_1.

5
COMMUNICATING STRUCTURAL VIOLENCE

A Case Study of Entertainment Establishment Women Workers in Kathmandu, Nepal

Iccha Basnyat

> Sometimes, my mind does not work, and I become restless. I felt lonely and bad. I felt that it would be better to die than to live sometimes. Again, I thought to myself that dying does not do any good; it is a life of two days; there are some friends and enemies. If something happens to me, then society will look down on me and will spit on my body. They would think I did something wrong, so I attempted such a bad thing. And my family would also be more miserable. I thought that so many people were suffering more than I did. I feel like that and comfort myself, 'I have hands and legs to work, and then I have the world.' And I comfort and convince my friends who have low self-esteem and attempt such things [suicide].

This excerpt reflects deep emotional distress and a struggle with suicidal thoughts born out of working in an entertainment establishment. She is one of the many participants who shared their feelings of loneliness and despair leading to increased psychological distress. In this excerpt, she also shared about talking herself out of self-harm because of the societal stigma and the impact it may have on her family. Despite experiencing such intense distress, she focuses on her self-worth as a form of resilience to survive working as an entertainment establishment worker. Stigmatization, increased mental health struggles, and deteriorating physical health are experienced by women working in entertainment establishments. In Asia, entertainment establishments comprise guest houses, hotels, massage parlors, spas, exotic dance bars, singing-dancing performance bars, and small eateries where services range from companionship and entertainment

DOI: 10.4324/9781003426530-6
This chapter has been made available under a CC BY-NC-ND license.

to sex work (Ghimire et al., 2020; Lim et al., 2019). In Nepal, "Adult Entertainment Sector" (AES) is an umbrella term used by policymakers, researchers, donors, and practitioners to refer to these entertainment establishments (Oosterhoff et al., 2022).

Entertainment establishments are clandestine nighttime industries with questionable labor practices and unequal power relations between the owners/managers and customers, primarily men, which creates vulnerabilities for the women working within them (Basnyat, 2020; Basnyat & Pal, 2025). In Asia, the influx of women into these establishments has been driven by migration patterns looking for employment, income disparities, and increasing sexual demand from heterosexual men (Lim et al., 2019). For example, in China (Kelvin et al., 2013), Laos (Phrasisombath et al., 2012), and Singapore (Wong et al., 2012), a substantial number of female migrants are employed in entertainment establishments. Women employed in entertainment establishments frequently encounter professional exploitation, sexual harassment, verbal abuse, objectification, and commodification of their bodies, mainly from heterosexual men, including both employers and customers (Basnyat, 2020; Majic, 2014; Mavin & Grandy, 2013). Furthermore, women working in these establishments also encounter gender-based discrimination and harassment, which can be exacerbated by societal norms that stigmatize their work. Women workers are often labeled as immoral and face heightened risks of abuse without adequate protection (Basnyat, 2020). This includes increased vulnerability to STIs/HIV, stigma, sexual assault, marginalization, ostracism, exploitation, and harassment, coupled with psychological and emotional strain and limited access to preventive measures (Choudhury et al., 2015; Kelvin et al., 2013; Maticka-Tyndale et al., 2002; Nemoto et al., 2008; Seib et al., 2009; Wong et al., 2012). These negative impacts underscore the adverse impacts on entertainment establishment women worker's health and well-being.

Entertainment establishments are important sites for examining the everyday operation of structural violence. In this setting, structural violence is communicated through discriminatory language, threat of job loss, exploitation of labor, stereotyping, shaming, and labeling (Basnyat, 2017; Basnyat & Pal, 2025). Thus, structural violence is deeply embedded in the experiences of women working in entertainment establishments, shaping their health and well-being through systemic inequalities and communicative practices that perpetuate harm. In this chapter, I use the concept of *structural violence* to emphasize a need for health communication to move beyond individual-level theorization and consider health and communication as embedded within a system. This chapter begins by discussing the concept of structural violence. Then, the chapter transitions to a discussion lived experiences of women workers in entertainment establishments to understand how structural violence is normalized. Through a critical health communication perspective, this chapter illustrates the everyday communicative acts such as verbal threats and demeaning women that perpetuate structural violence. This chapter also highlights women's voices to emphasize the importance of critical health communication perspectives emerging from the Global South.

Structural Violence

Structural violence is a term coined by Galtung (1969). Structural violence refers to practices that violate human rights but do so as an invisible, indirect, and insidious process that is embedded within structures (Hamed et al., 2020). Structural violence is built into social configurations—economic, political, legal, religious, and cultural—that stop individuals, groups, and societies from reaching their full potential due to unequal power and, consequently, unequal life chances (Galtung, 1969). For Galtung, structural violence equates to social injustices that create unnecessary and avoidable suffering (De Maio & Ansell, 2018). As opposed to personal and physical violence, structural violence is indirect and hidden because it is built into systems of unequal power and, consequently, unequal life chances (De Maio & Ansell, 2018; Galtung, 1969). For example, #MeToo and Black Lives Matter movements are responses to violence embedded into our social systems that has and continues to cause harm to specific groups of people (Basnyat & Zhao, 2023). Although Galtung's work focused on peace and conflict research, the concept of structural violence has been broadened to include fields like anthropology and sociology. Paul Farmer (1996), a medical anthropologist and physician, expanded the concept of structural violence into healthcare, arguing that diseases and health are not solely biological but also shaped by social structures. For example, structural violence frequently manifests as barriers to healthcare, adverse treatment by healthcare workers, and heightened stigma and discrimination (Basnyat, 2017; Basnyat & Zhao, 2023).

Farmer (1996) describes structural violence as a socially structured pattern of collective social actions against human dignity, such as poverty, gender and social inequalities, racism, and human rights abuse. Specifically, Farmer et al. (2006) argue that structural violence constitutes social arrangements that put individuals and populations in harm's way, i.e., *structural* because social arrangements are embedded in our social world's political and economic organization and *violent* because social arrangements cause injury to people. For example, lack of access to resources, stable jobs, poor health care access, and discrimination create unequal life chances and increase harm to individuals and communities while normalizing this suffering (Basnyat, 2017). Furthermore, Farmer (2004) argues that structural violence inevitably means poorer health and a shorter life. For example, if someone dies from preventable diseases such as tuberculosis or autoimmune deficiency syndrome (AIDS) when advanced medications are available, that is a form of structural violence in healthcare (Ho, 2007). Farmer (2003) argues that structural violence is embedded in societal institutions, including healthcare, leading to widespread and often invisible forms of suffering. Thus, structural violence involves everyday forces that indirectly shape individuals' experiences, adversely impacting their health and well-being (Nandagiri et al., 2020).

Structural violence provides a much-needed nuanced way to explore health inequalities built into unequal social systems (Basnyat, 2017). Critical health communication, primarily from the Global South, has engaged in some exploration of structural violence. For example, Zhao and Basnyat (2021) examined the relationship between structural violence and agency in the context of Chinese reproductive health discourse. Dutta (2020) examined the interplays between structural violence and communicative inequality amidst the COVID-19 outbreak in migrant worker dormitories in Singapore. Both studies evaluated the role of communication in constituting and reinforcing systems of trauma, poverty, marginalization, and inequality that negatively impact health. Both studies also demonstrate the need for more research examining structural violence through the lens of critical health communication. This lens helps health communication move beyond individual responsibility to examine the broader systems that create and sustain suffering (Basnyat & Pal, 2025). By integrating critical health communication with structural violence, we can uncover how structures contribute to the health disparities of entertainment establishment workers.

Lived Experiences, Structural Violence, and Health Communication

Critical health communication provides a lens for understanding how entertainment establishments are structures that create harm to the women workers, reinforced through discourses that devalue their dignity. Structural violence manifests in the persistent marginalization of these workers, making them vulnerable to mental and physical health struggles while denying them the necessary support and protection. Drawing on the lived experiences of women workers in entertainment establishments, this analysis illustrates how structural violence is communicatively normalized, leading to increased mental stress and poor health outcomes for women working in these spaces. First, I briefly explain my research methods before sharing insights from the workers.

I conducted thirty-five semi-structured in-depth interviews after obtaining the Institutional Review Board approval from the Nepal Health Research Council (NHRC), a government body in Nepal, and the University's IRB. I collaborated with Kumudini, a local non-governmental organization (NGO) in Kathmandu that focuses on rescuing, rehabilitating, and reintegrating women and children who have been exploited, abused, or trafficked. Kumudini and I collaborated to develop an interview guide. We pilot-tested this guide with women working in entertainment establishments. Further, under Kumudini's advisement to ensure participant safety and avoid drawing unwanted attention, interviews were conducted by two women from partner NGOs who had prior relationships with the establishments' owners through providing counseling and skills training to women workers and could, therefore, enter the workspace discreetly. Interviews were scheduled at times and locations convenient for the participants to maintain privacy and encourage open sharing of their experiences. Participants were informed that they could withdraw from the interview at any time without losing their compensation. All participants completed the interviews, which lasted one-and-a-half to two hours each. The interviews were conducted in Nepali and later translated into English.

I determined that data saturation had been achieved at thirty-five interviews after the initial analysis did not reveal new categories or dimensions beyond those already identified (Choudhury et al., 2015). The participants ranged in age from 18 to 34 ($M = 24.77$, $SD = 4.36$) and came from 22 of Nepal's 75 districts, representing various ethnicities and castes. Their educational attainment varied from no formal education to completion of 10th grade; approximately one-third were uneducated, one-third had completed 5th grade, and one-third had education up to 10th grade. Monthly income varied from 3,000 rupees (~30 USD) without tips to between 10,000 rupees (~97 USD) and 25,000 rupees (~240 USD) with tips. The participants' official jobs were waitressing or singing or dancing (non-exotic), though the majority of the participants were waitresses.

I used thematic analysis to identify, scrutinize, and report patterns without trying to fit the data into a pre-existing coding frame. First, I reviewed the transcripts line-by-line during open coding, breaking down the data into smaller parts for comparison and further analysis (Corbin & Straus, 2015). This resulted in 100 pages of phrases, words, and sentences. Next, I conducted axial coding (Corbin & Strauss, 2015) by grouping the open codes into five broad categories. Finally, I performed selective coding to refine the categories further and better understand structural violence. During this stage, I refined categories and selected illustrative quotes (Corbin & Strauss, 2015). I also engaged in discussions with my collaborators to ensure an accurate reflection of the data. Although I was not able to conduct formal "respondent validation" (Anderson, 2010) to let participants provide feedback, I constantly sought clarification during the data collection and reading of the transcripts to ensure that participants' opinions and experiences were accurately interpreted.

The findings reveal that structural violence in entertainment establishments operates through coercive communication, forcing women into risky behaviors like smoking and drinking to keep their jobs. Employers and customers use threats, financial incentives, and emotional coercion to normalize exploitation, worsening women's physical and mental health. Gendered power imbalances leave women vulnerable to harassment due to the need to work and stigma, further reinforcing their marginalization. Ultimately, these exploitative labor conditions highlight systemic inequalities that perpetuate harm under the guise of employment. From a critical communication perspective, this reveals how communicative practices normalize exploitation, making structural violence an everyday experience.

Coercive Communication as Structural Violence

Structural violence is embedded within entertainment establishments where managers and customers pressure women to conform to harmful practices. Communication practices that threaten job security have led women to engage in risky behavior such as heavy smoking and alcohol consumption. Mentions of drinking refer to alcohol. Rekha explained: "If we refrain from drinking, he [manager] tells us to leave the job as he can find some other to replace. Why should people like you work here, he will say." Thus, women workers unwillingly have to engage in risky behaviors to keep their jobs. For example, Seema picked up smoking on her job because her employer insisted she smoke with the clients: "Before smoking, I did not have chest pains, and I did not get cold and cough so often." Similarly, Rukmani shared:

> I never used to drink but I have to drink because of my work. Drink a little, they [the employer] urged, and I started to drink. They [the employer] say if you do not drink then there is no business and how can we pay you? I slowly started with one or two glasses but gradually it became a habit to drink.

Statements like "If you do not drink, then there is no business, and how can we pay you?" are coercive communication, with employers increasing profits by forcing women to engage in behavior that negatively impacts their health. Both Rekha and Rukmani's experiences about being forced to smoke and drink to keep their jobs reveal an exploitative structure within entertainment establishments. Similarly, Resha shared:

> Not all owners are good. Some tell you to drink so that business goes well. They insist that we drink [alcohol] as we work. So, we may have to drink even if we do not want to. If we do not, they do not give us our salary, but if we drink, we receive it on time.

These forms of structural violence are manifested through coercive communication, such as withholding salary or threats of being fired, in turn normalizing harmful health behaviors. Rupa explained:

> A: It is daily now. It is our work. It is needed to drink daily.
> Q: What do you mean by saying it is needed to drink?
> A: We get a separate commission from [selling] wine. If we drink wine, we get a commission of hundred fifty rupees. If a customer drinks one glass of wine, and when the customer pays seven or eight hundred rupees, we also get a commission of that glass of wine, one hundred and fifty rupees.

Women are incentivized to drink with the customer, causing harm to the women for profit gain. The denial of salary unless the women smoke and drink to increase sales exemplifies how structural violence operates through unequal power relations, where employers manipulate the women's financial needs to enforce exploitative practices. The inability to assert personal boundaries or preferences due to the fear of losing their job illustrates how structural violence operates within this space, such that the women feel compelled to comply. To earn an additional three hundred rupees by drinking and selling a glass of alcohol, the women must put their health at risk. The ability to coerce the women workers to partake in risky behavior to increase sales for the business is the fundamental violence built into the system. In addition to managers, customers also engaged in coercive language. Rima explained:

> They [customers] told me to have a drink. I do not drink and do not like it. They said, 'Everyone drinks, so why do you not drink, big person? You do not want to be friends with us; now you are superior to us.' All asked me to drink, and I did that behavior.

Exploitive and coercive communication from customers is an everyday experience for women. This unhealthy expectation is built into the social practices that marginalize those who work in entertainment establishments, reinforcing gender inequalities and normalizing the exploitation of women. For example, the use of coercive language such as "*Why do you not drink, big person?*" and "*Now you are superior to us*" pressures the women to conform by communicating hostility toward women who choose not to partake in drinking and smoking. Retna summarizes this:

> Sometimes, they [customers] force us by saying, 'Please sit and eat. Otherwise, I will not talk with you,' or 'It would not be fun if you do not drink. It will be good.' Sometimes, I get confused and do not know how to convince them that I do not feel it. Even if I do not feel like drinking or sitting with them, the boss asks us to.

Coercion language used by customers, such as employing emotional manipulation and guilt to engage in unhealthy behaviors, exemplifies structural violence. This dynamic reflects a broader system of gendered power imbalance in entertainment establishments, where women's autonomy is undermined in favor of male customers' desires. Furthermore, the employer reinforces this structural violence by compelling workers to comply, regardless of their personal comfort or well-being. "*Sometimes, I get confused and do not know how to convince them I do not feel it*" indicates the precious and vulnerable positions of the women workers. Ruma also shared:

> We have to give continuous singing and dancing performances and may not have permission to take a break. When you feel tired and try to sit, you may face verbal abuse, humiliation, and domination from the boss.

The continuous performance coupled with abuse exemplifies an exploitative work environment, where coercive communication such as "*verbal abuse, humiliation, and domination*" forces the women to work until physical and psychological exhaustion, putting their health and well-being at risk. Structural violence operates through everyday interactions, leading to psychological distress, diminished personal autonomy, and potential long-term health consequences.

In addition, the women's vulnerability to managers and customers leaves them open to sexual harassment. For example, Resha said: "They [customers] are usually drunk and behave and touch inappropriately. That makes me feel bad. Even if we do not want to [go with them], the owner tells us to go." Being exposed to humiliation and demeaning experiences in their workplace and tolerating such behavior is expected of the women to increase sales for the business. Coercive communication within entertainment establishments demonstrates the everyday manifestation of structural violence in labor practices and exacerbates gendered vulnerabilities. The power to dictate compliance with customer demands reflects the everyday experience of the structural violence of women working in entertainment establishments. Coercive communication that pressures women to comply with practices that damage their physical and mental health due to fear of loss of a job, loss of income, differential treatments, and social pressure are all embedded in violence within this structure, i.e., entertainment establishment.

Deteriorating Physical Health as Structural Violence

Structural violence is reflected in the deteriorating health of the women in entertainment industries as a result of these practices. Seema, for example, said: "I have headaches and cannot get up in the morning. I go for morning walks; otherwise, my hands and feet swell, and I do not have money for treatment." Furthermore, she also highlighted this: "I have seen these things develop into bad habits and friends fall under the addiction of tobacco and alcohol." Seema is dealing with health issues as a consequence of engaging in heavy drinking and smoking in her job, and she also notes that such behavior is widespread among women working in the entertainment establishment. Surya also echoed this:

> It has impacted me because before smoking, I did not have chest pain and did not have colds or coughs so often. When I started smoking, for the first year, I did not have any complaints. Nowadays, I smoke a lot, and with my son growing up, tension is increasing.

Structural violence is evident in the direct link between the pressure in the workplace and the uptake of risky behavior, leading to adverse health outcomes.

Other job demands also led to health problems. For example, Sneha shared:

> When I started to work in this sector, due to lack of sleep and no proper timing for food, I got many health problems like stomach pain. Mostly uterus related. To be healthy means, it is necessary to eat on time and sleep on time to have enough sleep.

Sneha links her stomach pain and uterus-related issues to a poor working environment that puts demands on the women, compromising their health without ensuring support and protection for them. This is reflective of the everyday existence of structural violence within the work environment that harms women. Similarly, Snow said:

> For me, when I started to work in this sector, due to lack of sleep and no proper timing for food, it led to many health problems. I smoke a lot, and I have bad chest pain. Now, I am feeling constant pain, and if I do not smoke at night, I feel less pain.

Physical alignments attributed to increased smoking and drinking due to demands made of the women and increased mental stress such as depression, isolation, and anxiety due to working in entertainment establishments are harmful practices that are undermining the health and well-being of the women. Such practices are embedded and normalized within the structure, where the violence that is causing harm to the women remains invisible.

In addition to the impact on physical health, Surya and Shilpa note how health concerns are exacerbated by worry about family responsibilities. Shilpa said: "If I get ill, who will look after me? If anything happens to me, then who will look after my child? I get stressed because of it." Supriya also shared that poor health can lead to a decreased ability to care for their children properly and described how that pressure led to mental health challenges:

> When I am in tension, I lose my appetite, do not talk with others, and like to stay alone. I feel relaxed after crying. I used to do that. I have seen my friends using rough [vulgar] words, and they shout when they are tense.

Supriya's response to coping with structural violence within her work has been withdrawal, changes in her eating habits, and living with psychological stress. Negative health outcomes due to experiences of everyday structural violence in entertainment establishments underscore the embedded unequal power dynamics and inequalities impacting women. Structural violence operating through entertainment establishments has created a burden on women without adequate social, physical, or mental health support.

Gendered Labor as Structural Violence

Structural violence operates within a patriarchal society by limiting women's access to resources and assistance, making them more vulnerable to economic exploitation. A lack of support exacerbates the mental stress and anxiety of working in a nighttime industry. Parvathi, for example, stated: "I do not get help from anyone, and there is no place to get help, either. Because of that, I get stressed and am already stressed now thinking about it." Parvathi is referring to a lack of support in her life that necessitates doing this type of work, and she is also noting that due to this type of work, she also cannot get any support. The absence of support systems further entrenches their marginalization, reinforcing their dependence on precarious employment. The isolation felt by women working in the entertainment establishment is further exacerbated by the fear of revealing to others where they work. Priya explained:

> I have a daughter and need to educate her. Later, she may come to know about my work, as I have to work until late at night, which is not nice. She will come to know even if I try to hide. I thus wish that she did not know about it.

Priya is concerned about her daughter finding out where she works due to the stigma associated with entertainment establishments. Priya notes that she cannot talk freely about the challenges of their hard work due to this stigma: "We have worked hard for our livelihood, and it does not make any difference to be frank with anyone." Shanti shared more about how stigma silences the women:

> We could not show our work in front of society, and I felt bad about that. I joined this work when I had a hard time and problems. I had not studied enough for other job [types]. I had enough food and clothes when I reached this place [job], so I was happy about that. The only thing was that we could not show our work openly.

Shanti's statement highlights structural violence by pointing to how unequal access to education perpetuates socioeconomic disparities, preventing her from accessing stable and respected employment. Further, the gendered moral judgments placed upon the work that they can access exacerbate their social exclusion, making it harder for them to seek support or alternative employment opportunities. This can lead to psychological harm, as Pari shared:

> This sorrow is a test taken by god. We should not commit suicide. I try to convince them [other workers], telling them that the sorrows we face now are because of our previous deeds [referring to karma]. I have learned this from priests to whom I go sometimes.

"This sorrow" refers to Pari's mental anguish, which she reframes as a *"test taken by God"* highlights the toll of structural violence. Karma is a

cultural and religious concept that connects one's current life experience with deeds from the previous life, which provides a way to cope with the psychological impact of structural violence experienced by women working in entertainment establishments. Instead of addressing systemic inequalities, gendered stigma often left women to internalize their struggles as personal shortcomings. This approach further obstructs structural change. Further, sexual harassment and objectification faced by women reflect violence embedded into the system that puts women in harm's way due to the power imbalance and gender inequalities. Pema shared:

> Sometimes, someone comes, and they start touching as soon as they arrive. They ask straight away if you will spend the whole night and how much it is. That affects me negatively and intensely; my mind becomes tense, and I feel very bad. I think how awful it is to be born a girl child in this world.

The feeling that it is *"awful to be born a girl child"* underscores the existence of gender inequality exploited within entertainment establishments. This also reveals the deep-seated despair caused by systemic gender discrimination. Similarly, Puma said:

> The waitress confronts more problems than the stage performer. The customer approaches near and tries to touch, literally touching. But we need to tolerate it, which is our obligation. I felt so bad and uneasiness. I regret working in such a place.

The "need to tolerate" and "our obligation" highlight the unequal power and normalization of inappropriate behavior, leading Puma to feel *"bad and uneasiness"* and *"regret"* her work. This illustrates how structural violence is entrenched in systemic gender oppression. Lack of boundaries and expectation of tolerance are examples of structural violence that the women are enduring. Structural violence is revealed through the support of behaviors and environments that subject women to unwanted advances and coercion to comply with unwanted behaviors such as excessive drinking and smoking. Feeling *tense* and *bad*, as well as experiencing harassment, reflects how structural violence can create psychological harm to women working in entertainment establishments.

Conclusion

This chapter discusses structural violence within entertainment establishments from a critical health communication lens. By focusing on the intersection of structural violence and communicative practices, this chapter contributes to a more nuanced understanding of health disparities and advocates for addressing the root causes of inequality. Women's lived experiences highlight the role of communication in reinforcing structural violence, adversely impacting their health and well-being. Lived experiences of the women highlight that structural violence not only inflicts harm but also creates environments where unequal power and exploitative practices become normalized. Women's lived experiences reveal the intricate ways in which structural violence intersects with their daily lives and health outcomes. Communication in the form of social pressure, coercion, and coercive language sustains and reinforces structural violence. Communication practices contribute to normalizing structural violence, which in turn negatively impacts the health and safety of workers. These communicative practices are an everyday experience of violence for these women. *Coercive communication* demonstrates how structural violence is embedded within entertainment establishments, demanding that women comply with practices that increase physical and psychological health risks to them. Communication strategies that coerce women to engage in unhealthy behavior in order to keep their jobs reinforce inequalities and normalize harmful practices. Coercive communication operates as structural violence that created a false dichotomous choice between their health and their livelihood by pressuring the women to adopt unhealthy behavior in order to keep their jobs and earn money. When unhealthy behaviors are normalized and expected performance within the job, it is difficult for women to resist; this exploitative practice is an everyday aspect of structural violence.

Coercive communication has led to chronic health problems for women, underscoring the manifestation of structural violence within entertainment establishments. Deteriorating *physical health* and increased experience of *psychological harm* result from systemic inequalities that leave women working within entertainment establishments without support. Structural violence results from the normalization of working conditions that have negatively impacted the mental, emotional, and physical health of the women. Entertainment establishments systemically neglect the health of the women and prioritize profits. Further, the entertainment establishments systemically reinforce social and economic inequalities that disadvantage marginalized individuals and communities by offering low pay and jeopardizing opportunities for economic advancement.

Gendered labor reveals how women in entertainment establishments are subjected to objectification and harassment as a normalized part of their work. In this sense, structural violence is embedded in the norms and practices that undervalue the dignity and rights of the women generally, and particularly those working in these establishments. Structural violence thus perpetuates gendered vulnerabilities and psychological distress. Women's economic precarity undermines resistance to exploitative working conditions. The women sustain physical and psychological harm within a system that continuously marginalizes and devalues their labor. Thus, structural violence manifests through discourses that create and reinforce gender and economic inequality, inadequate social support systems, and poor working conditions for women.

This chapter continues the shift in health communication research and practice, moving from individual-level approaches to those considering the broader structural context. Traditional health communication research often focuses on individual behavior change, neglecting the systemic factors contributing to health disparities. By incorporating critical perspectives such as structural violence, researchers can better understand how systemic inequalities and communicative practices contribute to health inequities. For example, expectations of excessive drinking and smoking while facing verbal abuse highlight how structural violence is deeply embedded into systems where communication perpetuates harm and inequality. This shift is essential for developing more effective policies and interventions addressing health inequalities' root causes. Furthermore, research from the Global South provides valuable insights for health communication. Specifically, critical health communication perspectives must be incorporated into the analysis of structural violence. By focusing on everyday communicative practices that perpetuate structural violence, this chapter calls for policies, research, and interventions to develop more comprehensive strategies to combat health inequities and promote social justice.

References

Anderson C. (2010). Presenting and evaluating qualitative research. *American Journal of Pharmaceutical Education*, 74(8), 141. https://doi.org/10.5688/aj7408141

Basnyat, I. (2017). Structural violence in healthcare: Lived experience of street-based female commercial sex workers in Kathmandu. *Qualitative Health Research*, 27, 191–203. https://doi.org/10.1177/1049732315601665.

Basnyat, I. (2020). Exploring interlinkages of gender, power & health in the entertainment establishment based bars and restaurant settings in Kathmandu Nepal. *Qualitative Health Research*, 30, 1409–1418. https://doi.org/10.1177/1049732320913854.

Basnyat, I., & Pal, M. (2025). "Oh! She works in such a place": Intersections of dirty work & stigma in Dohori entertainment establishments in Kathmandu, Nepal. *Communication Monographs*. https://doi.org/10.1080/03637751.2025.2461155

Basnyat, I., & Zhao, X. (2023). Structural violence. In Ho, E., Bylund, C., van Weert, J., Basnyat, I., Bol, N., & Dean M. (Eds.), *The international encyclopedia of health communication*. Wiley Publishing. https://doi.org/10.1002/9781119678816.iehc0978

Choudhury, S. M., Erausquin, J. T., Park, K., & Anglade, D. (2015). Social support and sexual risk among establishment-based female sex workers in Tijuana. *Qualitative Health Research*, 25(8), 1056–1068. https://doi.org/10.1177/1049732315587282

Corbin, J., & Strauss, A. (2015). *Basics of qualitative research*. Sage Publications.

De Maio, F., & Ansell, D. (2018). "As natural as the air around us": On the origin and development of the concept of structural violence in health research. *International Journal of Health Services*, 48(4), 749–759. https://doi.org/10.1177/0020731418792825

Dutta, M. J. (2020). COVID-19, authoritarian neoliberalism, and precarious migrant work in Singapore: Structural violence and communicative inequality. *Frontiers in Communication*, 5, 58. https://doi.org/10.3389/fcomm.2020.00058

Farmer, P. (1996). On suffering and structural violence: A view from below. *Daedalus*, 125(1), 261–283.

Farmer, P. (2003). *Pathologies of power: Health, human rights, and the new war on the poor*. University of California Press.

Farmer, P. (2004). An anthropology of structural violence. *Current Anthropology*, 45(3), 305–325.

Farmer, P. E., Nizeye, B., Stulac, S., & Keshavjee, S. (2006). Structural violence and clinical medicine. *PLoS Medicine*, 3(10), e449. DOI: 10.1371/journal.pmed.0030449

Galtung, J. (1969). Violence, peace and peace research. *Journal of Peace Research*, 6, 167–191.

Ghimire, A., Samuels, F., & Bhujel, S. (2020). *The gendered experiences of adolescent girls working in the adult entertainment sector in Nepal*. Report. London: Gender and Adolescence: Global Evidence. https://gage.odi.org/wp-content/uploads/2020/11/The-gendered-experiences-of-adolescents-girls-working-in-the-adult-entertainment-sector-in-Nepal_final.pdf

Hamed, S., Thapar-Björkert, S., Bradby, H., & Ahlberg, B. M. (2020). Racism in European health care: structural violence and beyond. *Qualitative Health Research*, 30(11), 1662–1673. https://doi.org/10.1177/10.1177/1049732320931430

Ho, K. (2007). *Structural violence as a human rights violation*. University of Essex Press.

Kelvin, E. A., Sun, X., Mantell, J. E., Zhou, J., Mao, J., & Peng, Y. (2013). Vulnerability to sexual violence and participation in sex work among high-end entertainment centre workers in Hunan Province, China. *Sexual Health*, 10(5), 391–399. https://doi.org/10.1071/SH13044

Lim, R. B. T., Tham, D. K. T., Cheung, O. N., Adaikan, P. G., & Wong, M. L. (2019). A public health communication intervention using edutainment and communication technology to promote safer sex among heterosexual men patronizing entertainment establishments. *Journal of Health Communication*, 24(1), 47–64. https://doi.org/10.1080/10810730.2019.1572839

Majic, S. (2014). Beyond "victim-criminals" sex workers, nonprofit organizations, and gender ideologies. *Gender & Society*, 28(3), 463–485. https://doi.org/10.1177/0891243214524623

Maticka-Tyndale, E., Lewis, J., Clark, J. P., Zubick, J., & Young, S. (2000). Exotic dancing and health. *Women & Health*, *31*(1), 87–108. https://doi.org/10.1300/J013v31n01_06

Mavin, S., & Grandy, G. (2013). Doing gender well and differently in dirty work: The case of exotic dancing. *Gender, Work & Organization*, *20*(3), 232–251. https://doi.org/10.1111/j.1468-0432.2011.00567.x

Nandagiri, R., Coast, E., & Strong, J. (2020). COVID-19 and abortion: Making structural violence visible. *International Perspectives on Sexual and Reproductive Health*, *46*(Supplement 1), 83–89. https://doi.org/10.1363/46e1320

Nemoto, T., Iwamoto, M., Colby, D., Witt, S., Pishori, A., Le, M. N.,... & Giang, L. T. (2008). HIV-related risk behaviors among female sex workers in Ho Chi Minh City, Vietnam. *AIDS Education and Prevention*, *20*(5), 435–453. https://doi.org/10.1521/aeap.2008.20.5.435

Oosterhoff, P., Snyder, K., & Sharma, N. (2022) Getting work: The role of labour intermediaries for workers in Nepal and the international 'Adult Entertainment Sector,' IDS Working Paper 580, *Brighton: Institute of Development Studies*. https://doi.org/10.19088/IDS.2022.075

Phrasisombath, K., Thomsen, S., Sychareun, V., & Faxelid, E. (2012). Care seeking behaviour and barriers to accessing services for sexually transmitted infections among female sex workers in Laos: a cross-sectional study. *BMC Health Services Research*, *12*(1), 1–9. https://doi.org/10.1186/1472-6963-12-37

Seib, C., Fischer, J., & Najman, J. M. (2009). The health of female sex workers from three industry sectors in Queensland, Australia. *Social Science & Medicine*, *68*(3), 473–478. https://doi.org/10.1016/j.socscimed.2008.10.024

Wong, M. L., Chan, R., Tan, H. H., Yong, E., Lee, L., Cutter, J.,... & Koh, D. (2012). Sex work and risky sexual behaviors among foreign entertainment workers in urban Singapore: findings from Mystery Client Survey. *Journal of Urban Health*, *89*(6), 1031–1044. https://doi.org/10.1007/s11524-012-9723-5

Zhao, X., & Basnyat, I. (2021). Lived experiences of unwed single mothers: exploring the relationship between structural violence and agency in the context of Chinese reproductive health discourse. *Health Communication*, *36*(3), 293–302. https://doi.org/10.1080/10410236.2019.1683953

Advocacy, Activism, and Social Change

6

CRITICAL PRAGMATISM AND THE POLITICS OF THE POSSIBLE

Communicating for Critically Holistic Health in the Workplace and Beyond

Heather M. Zoller

Critical health communication draws attention to the political negotiation of meaning related to health and illness at personal, cultural, and policy levels (Khan, 2014; Lupton, 1994; Zoller & Dutta, 2008; Zoller & Kline, 2008). Contrasting with post-positivist and normative research, critical perspectives elucidate relationships among communication and both overt and hidden social conflicts marking the status quo, with a goal of achieving participatory and democratic social change (Sastry et al., 2021; Waitzkin, 1983).

I investigate power and resistance through critical and poststructural lenses. These traditions elucidate how communication ideologically naturalizes and reifies sectional interests as universal (Fraser, 1990/91; Giddens, 1979; Said, 1978). Gramsci's (1971) theorizing of hegemony explicates how dominant groups promote consent to inequitable relationships by leading subordinate groups to adopt taken-for-granted "common sense" meaning systems that support dominant interests. These relationships of dominance and subordination are linked to intersecting constructions of difference including gender, class, race/ethnicity, sexuality, ability status, and country of origin (Basnyat, 2017; Dillon & Basu, 2013; Pal et al., 2023). Critical poststructural perspectives (e.g., Bakhtin, 1981; Foucault, 1980) view power and knowledge as mutually constitutive. Feminist and decolonial research, for example, recovers epistemological erasures wrought by patriarchal and colonial logics and techniques (Hernández & De Los Santos Upton, 2019; Pal et al., 2023).

These critical communication perspectives tie cultural and ideological domination to material and embodied practices. For example, Foucauldian biopower highlights the role of discourse in embodied governance strategies aimed at managing population health (Dempsey & Gibson, 2017; Zoller, 2003a). In addition to consent processes, ideological domination is intertwined with coercive power (Dempsey et al., 2022; Zoller & Ban, 2024). For example, recent theorizing of necropolitics and necrocapitalism highlights the institutional calculus of life and death in carceral, military, and corporate apparatus that render certain bodies as outside the protection of the state and therefore killable (de Souza, 2022; Dempsey et al., 2022; Ganesh, 2018; Mbembe, 2019).

Linking Counter-Hegemony and Social Change to Critical Pragmatism

Operating through seduction or coercion, hegemony draws our attention to the ways that dominant interests structure the status quo so that subordinated groups' everyday assumptions, goals, and activities support elite interests (Hardy & Phillips, 2004). Yet Gramsci's theorizing dialectically highlights the role of communication in resisting and transforming relationships of consent. As an active negotiation between dominant and marginalized groups, resistance entails struggles over the shape and limits of power, potentially contributing to transforming power inequities through counterhegemony (Gramsci, 1971; Lupton, 1995; Parker, 2003).

Despite detractors who equate critical theorizing with problem-focused and problem-focus (Bisel et al., 2020), critical scholars seek to not only *identify* power inequities but also to *change* them. Disrupting hegemonic discourses creates opportunities to communicatively challenge and reformulate the relations of power that undermine health. Given that power operates in part by colonizing meaning systems and identities, promoting emancipatory social change through open communication entails not only facilitating expression of voice but also reclaiming hidden conflict by considering whose interests are expressed in discourse (Conrad, 2011; de Souza, 2019; Deetz, 1992). This dialogic process facilitates the construction of more inclusive systems of meaning that can forge new social orders. Moreover, achieving counterhegemony requires a multifrontal approach that brings together disparate groups into unifying, solidarity frames (Anderson, 2023; Gramsci, 1971).

Drawing from Gramsci, I focus on health activism and community organizing as routes to counter-hegemony. Additionally, my approach to activism is influenced by *critical pragmatism*. Jettisoning pragmatism's association with expediency (Leonhirth, 2001), this perspective promotes solidarity building as a route to undermine hegemony (Rorty, 1989). In particular, critical pragmatism prioritizes contextualized and experimental forms of social change that widen the scope of democratic participation

(Ray, 2004; Reed et al., 2022; Shuler & Tate, 2001). Dewey theorized these improvisational efforts as social intelligence; the search to "... find new imaginative ways to challenge and dismantle existing power structures" (Kadlec, 2008, p. 55).

Focusing on embodied experimentation challenges critical researchers who embrace *orthodoxies* privileging certain social arrangements (e.g., socialism, welfare capitalism, anarchy). Critical pragmatism's social constructionist and contingent worldview highlights the emancipatory potential in rejecting dogma (and realist ontologies more generally): "Agency presupposes a world that is always evolving. No guarantees. No fixed truths. Just the fragile attempts of finite creations to flourish in an environment that impinges upon them daily" (Glaude, 2007, p. 25). In the face of flux and precarity, organizing resistance is thus a continual process of improvisational action, assessment, and adjustment, consonant with Weick's sensemaking theory (Glaude, 2007).

Critical pragmatism balances a hermeneutic of suspicion regarding power relations with a more affirmative stance toward social change. Reflecting on pragmatism's spirit of realistic hope, Eddie Glaude Jr. (2007) connected John Dewey's theorizing with James Baldwin's efforts to reconstitute the promise of democracy while continually confronting "evils" such as sexism, racism, and slavery's legacies.

I believe my approach to critical theorizing makes at least three key contributions to health communication. First, Gramscian ideological critique deconstructs reified assumptions undergirding the status quo, opening discursive closures for dialogue and change. Second, poststructural and dialectical theorizing highlights the communicative constitution of agency and resistance in limiting the inequitable exercise of power. Third, critical pragmatism promotes embodied, experimental forms of praxis as routes to social change. In the next section, I demonstrate how the communicative constitution of health and illness ideologically enables and constrains new and emancipatory forms of health organizing.

Dominant Ideologies in Defining Health and Attributing Illness

Health communication scholars need to consider how dominant interests shape and are shaped by our definitions of health and illness attributions. Health discourses are constitutive of organizing, and recursively, organizing shapes the biological, material, and symbolic conditions for health. Illness attributions are a key mechanism in this mutual process. Discourses diagnosing the causes of illness are ideologically linked with dominant beliefs about the "proper organization of society" (Tesh, 1994, p. 8) including social hierarchies and economic relationships (see also Rosner & Markowitz, 2024; Zoller & Sastry, 2016). Although attributions are based in part on evolving scientific understanding, "diagnostic frames" involve selections and deflections of reality that organize certain responses and suppress others (Kirkwood & Brown, 1995). This is the case because (a) multiple factors (agents, environments, hosts) interrelate to produce health and disease, and (b) symbolic systems translate certain dis-ease states into recognized "illnesses" to be addressed.

Western discourses tend to emphasize individualistic causes of illness and organize biomedical interventions aimed at the individual body. For example, U.S. health systems have privileged technocratic versus political interventions, spurred by germ and genetic theories of illness (Tesh, 1994). The biomedical focus, while important, overlooks the need to prevent illness by addressing more fundamental sociopolitical causes of illness (McKnight, 1988; Obinna, 2021).

Western public health efforts, despite focusing on population-level illness prevention, also tend to reinforce individualistic diagnostics (Knight et al., 2016). Many nineteenth century health reformers adopted personal behavior attributions that reinforced dominant class ideologies, blaming high illness rates among working class and low-income (often immigrant and minoritized) people on the choices and moral failings of those groups (Waitzkin, 1983). These theories were self-justifying as they affirmed the moral superiority of white, usually Protestant, upper-class groups (Tesh, 1994). Contemporary lifestyle attributions similarly reinforce the status quo by drawing attention away from the political/structural factors that most strongly predict health status and life expectancy, including income, social status, and access to resources (Phelan et al., 2010).

Although lifestyle attributions are appealing in part because they seem to be "objective" and apolitical, critical health communication research has shown in practice how lifestyle discourses politically undercut structural and cultural interventions. For example, I described how workplace health promotion (WHP) and occupational safety and health (OSH) initiatives reinforce health risks by diagnosing the worker rather than work as the problem and locus of intervention (Zoller, 2003a). Programs encourage workers to change their "lifestyles" and/or safety behaviors rather than alter workplace sources of illness. Polluters and their supporters use lifestyle theories to deflect action on environmental toxin exposures, which are born disproportionately by low-income and minoritized groups (Zoller, 2012). Campaigns persuading people to avoid soda and fast food (Ahn, 2015) reify industry profits (Ban, 2016; Crawford, 1977; Freudenberg, 2014). Critical researchers also elucidate how governmental, philanthropic, and business initiatives impose Western lifestyle attributions on the global south, justifying neoliberal social and economic interventions that cut health-protective social programs and regulations (de Souza et al., 2008; Olufowote et al., 2017; Sastry & Dutta, 2013; Zoller, 2008).

Challenging Diagnostic Reductionism

Dialectically, movements have organized to resist and rearticulate these dominant diagnostic discourses. As a graduate student, I examined how the World Health Organization's (WHO) "Healthy Cities/Healthy Communities" initiative challenged medical and lifestyle reductionism. Drawing from the burgeoning bio-psycho-social model, advocates situated health as a positive state of physical, mental, and social well-being and not just the absence of disease. Drawing insights from the social ecological model of health, Healthy Cities materials depicted a "mandala" that nests health within community, cultural, economic, political, and environmental influences. The initiative promoted intersectoral organizing to address these interrelated factors (Hancock, 1993). The "social determinants" movement represented another holistic approach that focused on non-medical health influences (McKnight, 1988; Niederdeppe et al., 2008). Advocates also broadened wellness and holistic health to include spiritual along with mental, biological, and social well-being (Geist-Martin & Scarduzio, 2011; Zook, 1994).

Despite the challenge to medical reductionism, unfortunately, the critical potential of these models was blunted. Wellness promotion is usually targeted at upper-middle class and wealthy audiences with access to resources, making already healthy people better off (Fujishiro et al., 2022). "Social determinants" often translate into a multicausal web of unprioritized illness factors, allowing scholars, practitioners, and politicians to choose seemingly "apolitical" and less expensive interventions (Tesh, 1994; Zoller, 2005b). It seems easier and less controversial to create a behavior change campaign than to change social conditions that produce inequalities (Lupton, 1995).

By contrast, "fundamental cause" theories attribute preventive illness to political structures including access to resource access (income/wealth, education, communication infrastructure) and social status (including ethnicity, nationality, sexuality, and other differences). These factors are the primary predictors of health status and longevity (Kennedy et al., 1998; Marmot & Bell, 2012; Pickett & Wilkinson, 2015). Our income and social status influence whether we have the resources to protect our health and avoid risk (e.g., working conditions and environmental exposures). In addition to resource access, social marginalization creates physical and mental health stressors (Obinna, 2021). More broadly, having control over our lives predicts our physical and mental health status (Marmot & Theorell, 1991, Kennedy et al., 1998). Therefore, relations of power ultimately underlie the matrix of factors that produce illness (i.e., genetics, lifestyles, environment, germs, and micro-organisms).

Diagnostic Discourses and Health Disparities

Increasing attention to social causes has spurred more research into health disparities. Yet here too health communication needs to consider how we attribute the causes of those disparities. When scholars acknowledge differential rates of morbidity and mortality among social groups, I see at least four different causal attributions that organize different responses (see Table 5.1).

One approach, *Ignoring Sociopolitical Contexts*, acknowledges disparities in disease rates among social groups, but attributes those differences to biological, behavioral, or cultural characteristics of members of those groups (Lupton, 1995). As a result, solutions largely ignore underlying political factors, such as lifestyle campaigns persuading people to eat better without reference to barriers groups face in doing so (Heuman et al., 2013; Snyder, 2007). This approach stigmatizes by "blaming the victims" for higher illness rates (see for discussion Davis & Quinlan, 2017; Gerbensky-Kerber, 2011; Vardeman-Winter, 2017; Zoller, 2003b). These attributions overlook the fact that people who have higher incomes and higher social status (e.g., majority ethnicity, non-immigrants, cisgender people) have better health outcomes and longer life expectancy than people with lower incomes and lower social status, *even when engaging in the same health behaviors* (e.g., smoking, sedentary habits) (Benach et al., 2013; Sabanayagam & Shankar, 2012).

TABLE 6.1 Diagnosing and Addressing Disparities

	Acknowledges Disparities	*Change Locus*	*Intervention Orientation to Sociopolitical Contexts*
Disregarding Disparities	No	None	None
Ignoring Sociopolitical Context	Yes	Individual	Ignores
Individually Adapting to Sociopolitical Contexts	Yes	Individual	Adaptation
Collectively Reforming Sociopolitical Contexts	Yes	Collective	Reform
Collectively Transforming Sociopolitical Contexts	Yes	Collective	Transformation

A second approach, *Individually Adapting to Sociopolitical Contexts*, acknowledges structural factors that produce disparities and promotes individual-level accommodations to those structures. For example, health educators might provide information to low-income groups about purchasing more nutritious food at a low cost (e.g., eating frozen vegetables) (see Gillies et al., 2021). These efforts help people manage their health within structures of inequality in the short-term, but place the onus for change on individuals and leave overarching social systems in place. Moreover, these discourses may still attribute the causes of disparities to group characteristics such as lack of knowledge/health literacy (see for example Nutbeam, 2000).

A third approach, *Collectively Reforming Sociopolitical Contexts*, diagnoses structural and political causes of disparities and prioritizes collective changes within existing systems (e.g., economic systems, policy frameworks, and corporate power). Reform is associated with incremental change. For example, food pantries and governmental food benefits make food available in the short-term but leave larger food system inequities in place (de Souza, 2019; Ivancic, 2017; Okamoto, 2017). Similarly, attributing health disparities to lack of health insurance and promoting increased access (du Pre & Overton, 2022) focuses on treatment versus prevention and stops short of transforming medical care systems (Kennedy et al., 1998).

A fourth approach, *Collectively Transforming Sociopolitical Contexts*, attributes disparities to access to power and resources and prioritizes collective efforts to transform those sociopolitical conditions (e.g., Fundamental Causes) (Phelan et al., 2010). While there is no definitive distinction between reformative and transformative change, the latter seeks to more fundamentally alter existing conditions and the power relations undergirding them (Zoller, 2005a). For example, food system transformations include promoting a right to food, local ownership, and environmental sustainability (see Dempsey, 2024; LeGreco & Douglas, 2021). Transforming political contexts entails altering structural barriers such as poverty and racism.

A few points about these four orientations are in order. The first is that the link between diagnostic discourses and corresponding solutions often hinges on how researchers and practitioners define "modifiable" risk factors. Many scholars acknowledge structural and social causes of disparities but equate "modifiable" factors with individual choices (see for example Bezzina et al., 2024; Liang & Beydoun, 2019; Mundra et al., 2023). This discourse ideologically reifies existing social conditions (e.g., economic arrangements and environmental exposures) as unchangeable.

The adaptive and transformative perspectives push health advocates to consider a broader range of factors as communicatively modifiable.

Secondly though, we need to further investigate relationships among individual and collective efforts as well as adaptative, reformative, and transformative approaches to change. As I alluded to above, critical scholars are concerned that adaptive reforms undermine the potential for transforming social structures (e.g., a food pantry alleviates immediate hunger, thereby leaving in place gendered and racialized neoliberal government and corporate policies that leave minoritized groups without adequate income or access to affordable food). Indeed, I consistently advocate for transforming the root causes of health disparities including corporate/"commerciogenic" sources of illness (Freudenberg, 2014; Zoller, 2016). However, building a multifrontal resistance movement with and for marginalized groups involves balancing short-term needs with longer-term change (see, for example researchers drawing from the culture-centered approach [CCA] such as Dillon & Basu, 2013; Dutta & Kaur-Gill, 2018). We need to more thoroughly assess when reformist advocacy *contributes to* larger social changes and when it *impedes* them. As a critical pragmatist, I view these not as philosophical questions but empirical questions to investigate in practice.

A Critically Holistic Health Framework: Redefining the Possible Through Activism

To do so, I investigate two innovative, experimental activist initiatives that change the workplace as a path to worker and community well-being, one emphasizing Collective Reform and the other Collective Transformation. Although neither explicitly frames their efforts as health activism, they holistically address structural factors that influence health, redefining what counts as modifiable in more collective terms. I first describe how the reform-oriented multistakeholder agricultural initiative Equitable Food Initiative (EFI) inspired the Critically Holistic framework for health. I then describe how the 1worker1vote union cooperative movement reflects and extends the Critically Holistic framework in seeking to fundamentally transform economic systems.

The Critically Holistic Model of Workplace Health Promotion: EFI

EFI is a multistakeholder initiative aimed at improving working conditions for agricultural workers in Mexico, Canada, Peru, and the United States (Zoller et al., 2023). Oxfam organized the initiative with human rights, labor, and environmental advocates such as the Farm Labor Organizing

Committee, Farmworker Justice, and the Pesticide Action Network, as well as agricultural operations and retailers including Costco and Whole Foods. Voluntary standards address worker health and safety, the social environment (e.g., discrimination, harassment), as well as remuneration, time off, and other benefits. Workers are trained in occupational and food safety practices. Certified farms sell produce with the EFI label. EFI's primary innovation is to place workers on teams with management to elicit employee concerns and address standards on an everyday basis. This differs from third-party certification efforts relying on periodic inspection (Brown & Getz, 2008). While not designed as a public health intervention, the initiative promotes healthy work, with implications for organizing public health more broadly.

My co-authors and I theorized the *Critically Holistic and Worker-Centered Framework* of health based on EFI's standards and practices of the certified farms we evaluated (Zoller et al., 2023). Critical Holism conceptualizes the physical, mental, and social/spiritual aspects of health but differs from other holistic work-health models such as Working Well (Geist-Martin & Scarduzio, 2011) and the U.S. Centers for Disease Control (CDC)'s Total Worker Health initiative (Schill & Chosewood, 2013) in several ways. First, the framework expands "holistic" health to prioritize economic issues (including pay and benefits) as well as environmental health risks (including worker, consumer, and public toxin exposures). Second, Critical Holism prioritizes structural interventions that promote safe, equitable, and healthy working conditions (particularly outside of white-collar settings) rather than worker behaviors and choices (see also Harrison & Stephens, 2019). This focus on working conditions integrates occupational health and safety and WHP along with organizational policies and cultural practices (e.g., hiring decisions, time off, racial and sexual harassment). Third, the model promotes worker voice as a direct component of good health and structural mechanisms promoting attention to worker's needs.

Critical Holism was inspired by EFI's standards protecting workers' physical health (e.g., ensuring access to water, safety equipment) as well as mental and social health (e.g., addressing racial and sexual harassment, conflict management, and team communication). Certified farms also addressed workers' economic standing by improving pay and income stability through training and job enrichment. One farm integrated economics into WHP programming by highlighting government housing supports and other economic assistance in addition to lifestyle information. EFI also inspired the Critically Holistic model by promoting the safe use of agricultural chemicals to reduce environmental illness sources for workers, fenceline neighbors, and consumers. The initiative further protects consumer health by training and empowering workers to improve food safety and reduce food-borne illness.

EFI inspired the model's focus on substantive employee voice as key to worker well-being. Unlike third-party verification efforts with limited and often announced external inspections, EFI places workers on teams with management to promote continual standards compliance as well as elicit and respond to employee concerns. When paired with external certification, the teams promote long-term attention to worker voice. Without that structural mechanism, employee participation can be harnessed to serve managerial goals (Stohl & Cheney, 2001). Participation should be central to any model of health given that control over our lives is a key contributor to the health-wealth gradient (Fujishiro & Heaney, 2009; Marmot & Bell, 2012).

Discussion

The Critically Holistic model challenges existing WHP and wellness promotion efforts that focus on white collar work and target workers rather than working conditions. The model reconfigures lifestyle-focused initiatives by articulating the responsibility of employers to provide safe and equitable (physical, mental, social, economic, and environmental) working conditions. The model conceptualizes holism to encompass external health effects including fenceline communities and consumers. Furthermore, by addressing working conditions among precarious, contingent and im/migrant workforces, the model locates the causes of health disparities within work processes and not social groups (Fujishiro et al., 2022).

This approach points to the critical role of work in influencing health and health disparities (Ahonen et al., 2018; Basnyat, 2017; Basu & Dutta, 2008; Cao & Wang, 2021; Dutta & Kaur-Gill, 2018). The framework also has broader implications. EFI's growth and impact (https://equitablefood.org/our-impact/) demonstrates the feasibility of modifying the structural causes of illness and promoting substantive participation around decisions that influence health.

At the same time, the initiative is limited. EFI can be considered "Collective Reform" because it ultimately leaves managerial power in place (Brown & Getz, 2008; van den Akker et al., 2024). The model is not designed to directly challenge the extractive nature of the corporate food system, neoliberal privatization, or the concentration of profits within monopoly agriculture. Taking a critical pragmatic orientation, my colleagues and I recognized those limitations (as a more immediate response to current constraints) while also considering how this experimentation *could inspire larger changes* (Zoller et al., 2023). We discussed how the leadership team model has been re-applied by activist labor movements including the Immokalee Workers' Fair Food Fight and observed that holistic improvements in work hours, income, and physical health facilitate larger political participation and advocacy by workers (see, for example, Khan in this volume).

This critical pragmatist viewpoint embraces innovation as a source of hope and a catalyst for change. However, critical pragmatism is not about accepting inadequate compromises; thus, a part of my research goal was to compare EFI's approach with more transformative organizing.

Collective Transformation Through the Union Cooperative Movement

The second project exemplifies how a Critically Holistic framework translates to broader scale changes supporting health. The 1worker1vote union cooperative movement, like EFI, is not explicitly designed around public health goals. The union cooperative movement reconfigures work as a part of larger economic transformations. The movement's vision is to create democratic worker ownership among those previously marginalized from the economy while meeting social and environmental needs. Yet, their efforts drive changes that can reduce health disparities, prevent illness, and promote well-being for cooperative workers and the larger community.

First, the movement reflects the Critically Holistic framework by promoting workers' physical, mental, and social health. As I indicated earlier, a critical approach acknowledges that economic well-being is foundational to holistic health. Worker-owned cooperatives support economic health by sharing profits among workers as dividends (Battilani & Schröter, 2012; Cheney et al., 2014). Furthermore, 1worker1vote can reduce health disparities because it seeks to create wealth for the structurally marginalized, including women, immigrants, racial minorities, low-income, and LGBTQ groups.

Second, the movement exemplifies Critical Holism by promoting democratic governance, which has numerous implications for holistic health. Cooperative collective decision-making builds meaningful relationships among workers, thereby strengthening social capital with positive effects on physical, social, and mental health (Majee & Hoyt, 2010; Morris et al., 2013). To aid this process, Co-op Cincy, a founding cooperative incubator in the 1worker1vote network, promotes cultural cohesion through conflict management and team-building skills. The movement further organizes a mutually supportive local and national network to enhance worker solidarity building and share resources for sustainable cooperative development.

In addition to promoting social ties, democratic decision-making facilitates control over work. Democratic voice gives workers greater control over physical, mental, and social working conditions (although the pressures of business can be a limiting factor). For example, Co-op Dayton, a part of 1worker1vote, is investigating how to promote wellness and stress reduction among worker-owners. Participants are discussing how to go beyond coping to re-organize workplace stressors. Their newsletter (9/16/24) encouraged workers to "Set boundaries that honor your needs and promote self-care" as well as "Choose yourself and prioritize your well-being and happiness" along with "Challeng[ing] yourself to embrace growth and step outside your comfort zone."

The movement takes a structural approach to power and voice that goes beyond EFI's leadership teams. In addition to giving workers a vote on major organizational decisions, the movement addresses managerial power by affiliating workers with labor unions that bargain for their interests. Unionization prevents management from eroding worker voice and interests through cooperative degeneration.

This approach reflects a third way that movement extends the Critically Holistic health framework, which is by seeking to transform not just the workplace but larger economic, political, and social equities that impinge on health. The network organizes around Mondragon cooperative values, which prioritize social transformation and solidarity building (Zoller, 2024). Worker ownership is conceived as an alternative to capitalist extraction and income inequality. Moreover, reinvigorating the labor movement is a key way to raised standards for all working people (Witherell, 2013). Although advocates acknowledge when unions have failed women and minoritized groups, they highlight historical solidarities among civil rights, union, and cooperative movements in promoting social and economic equity. For example, their Worker Owner Workbook links the movement to the socialist cooperative activism of W.E. DuBois, the Brotherhood of Sleeping Car Porters (BSCP), and the Montgomery Bus Boycott.

The movement's vision of economic and social transformation holistically enhances the health and well-being of the community. The dual mission of cooperatives (creating successful businesses and quality, democratic jobs) increasingly extends to serving community social justice goals (e.g., food and health care access) and replacing extractive practices with environmental sustainability (Cheney et al., 2014). For example, Co-op Cincy's farm and food hub, Our Harvest, partners with government and community programs (including Supplemental Nutrition Access Program) to offer affordable food for low-income residents (Zoller, 2023). Our Harvest's August 2024 newsletter described efforts "establishing Mini farmers' markets" in retirement facilities and food-insecure neighborhoods ... additionally, we'll be enrolling customers in Produce Perks, a program that provides free produce dollars to stretch their food budgets further." The newsletter observed that, "every decision is made with integrity and care for both our workers and the environment." The network's advocacy resists thus reconnects commerce with community and environmental health.

Discussion

The critical pragmatic lens highlights how the union cooperative movement's experimentation resists hegemonic, extractive capitalism and demonstrates the "practicality" of Collective Transformation. Although 1worker1vote would not typically be construed as a health social movement, the movement advocates for holistic changes in the sociopolitical roots of preventable illness and health disparities for workers and society more broadly.

In a keynote address to the Associação Brasileira de Pesquisadores de Comunicação Organizacional de Relações Públicas (ABRAPCORP), I argued that 1worker1vote's efforts are critical to preventing the next pandemic. Increasing income and reducing social inequality reduces stress and improves physical health in ways that reduce vulnerability to infectious illness (Stillwaggon, 2006). In addition, income inequality is associated with increases in political partisanship and extremism, which in turn fuels the spread of disinformation and conspiracy theories that reduce support for government and public health interventions (Gollust et al., 2017; Hopp et al., 2020; Osmundsen et al., 2021; Winkler, 2019). Responses to the Covid pandemic crystalized the need to address and prevent "infodemics." Furthermore, disinformation and conspiracy theorizing drives hate and divisions across gender, sexuality, race, and nationality differences (van Prooijen & Douglas, 2018) in ways that undermine collective commitments to public health. Efforts like the union cooperative movement to increase people's sense of economic security and social connectedness are thus critical to pandemic prevention. Furthermore, environmentally sustainable businesses can reduce our exposure to novel illnesses, resulting from our incursions into wild spaces. This movement can by no means solve all these problems, but it demonstrates significant pathways toward addressing them.

Conclusion: Promoting Critically Holistic Health Through Transformative Change

One important goal of this volume is to demonstrate the centrality of critical perspectives to the health communication discipline. The ideological analysis of diagnostic health discourses showed that all health communication efforts are political. Therefore, scholars drawing from multiple perspectives and methodologies need to interrogate the relations of power embedded in taken-for-granted assumptions the role of communication in reducing preventable illness and health disparities. All prevention-oriented scholars, and not just critical ones, must account for how our attributions of causality drive interventions that reinforce or resist social and political inequities.

My approach to critical and pragmatist theorizing highlighted the mutual communicative constitution of health and organizing, demonstrating that changing our conceptualization of health can transform health communication theorizing and practice. The Critically Holistic framework recognizes and prioritizes *changing* the fundamental sociopolitical conditions that underlie health risks. What if health communication re-centered its efforts from individual behavior change to creating safe work in supportive communities and sustainable and equitable economies? Changing the focus of our health education, campaigns, community organizing, and policy advocacy would be not just ethical but more effective in reducing preventable illness.

It is not tenable for scholars to acknowledge sociopolitical barriers to good health but *Ignore* them in designing solutions. In addressing health disparities, the field can begin to grapple more explicitly with how to link *Individual Adaptation* and *Collective Reform* to *Collective Transformation*. The two cases described here pragmatically demonstrate that collective change is practical and not just an abstract ideal.

Whereas the breadth of many holistic/wellness orientations (multicausal webs) can lead to privileging individualistic interventions appropriate to more powerful groups, the Critically Holistic framework connects physical, social, and mental health to relations of power. The model encourages us to pay more attention to the role of communication in promoting "control of life" related to work, income, and environmental decision-making. Focusing on work and related sociopolitical conditions as a major driver of health disparities reduces the stigmatizing victim-blaming inherent to individual and group-based explanations.

Moreover, while it might be daunting, the framework's breadth is crucial as we find ourselves promoting health in the face of global, intertwined crises (e.g., misinformation and disinformation prospering in new digital environments, the growth of hate discourse, anti-government extremism and partisanship along with economic disparities, climate change, and environmental degradation). Using transmission models of communication to encourage individualistic changes is not adequate for this task. In the face of these critical issues, yet more research on whether gain or loss frames encourage 10% more U.S. citizens to eat vegetables is not an effective use of our time. If the discipline is to play a meaningful role in protecting public health, we need more communicative insights into advocacy for democratic, equitable, and sustainable social change.

Thus, I hope that this chapter spurs greater theoretical and practical debates about approaches to communication and social change. Reflecting the critical pragmatist lens, in place of abstract theorizing, I grounded the discussion in the experimental organizing of EFI and the union cooperative movement. Moreover, rather than treat different approaches in competitive, zero-sum terms, the critical pragmatist lens encourages us to consider how different efforts can build toward transformation. For example, we can explore how critical, dialogic education (Asante, in press; Freire, 1973; Papa et al., 2006), advocacy by health professionals and "grasstops" NGOs (see Carter, this volume), as well as grassroots/subaltern activism and alternative organizing (Basu & Dutta, 2008; González-Agüero et al., 2020; LeGreco & Douglas, 2021) can work together to achieve change.

For critical scholars in particular, the pragmatic orientation can prevent us from spiraling into arguments based in orthodoxies about the best way to achieve change (e.g., only socialism, government intervention, or cultural change). By embracing more-than and both-and logics over binaries, we investigate how a multitude of experimental efforts (e.g., private, governmental, union, grassroots, corporate) can synergize to promote emancipatory changes. I find that it is sometimes easier for critical scholars to agree on problems with the status quo than to formulate alternatives. It can also be easy to fall into cynicism, continually focusing on seemingly promising efforts actually reproduce neoliberal capitalist relationships. Although it is crucial to consider hegemonic influences on resistance efforts, promoting counterhegemonic praxis requires building realistic hope for transformational change (Zoller, 2024). Critical pragmatism can help us sidestep a communicative trap in which embodied, existing alternatives for change are continually named as inadequate or compromised, leaving ambitious visions to be viewed as impractical, impossible, or always on the horizon.

In closing, I would note that health communication scholars of all theoretical and methodological traditions can make significant contributions to advocacy for policies and practices that promote healthy and equitable economies in sustainable environments. The invisibility of public health successes creates a paradox in which reducing illness and death actually leads to reduced investments and actions because the risks (e.g., measles) are no longer viewed as problems. At a time when the very notion of government and public commitments are called into question in many places, we need to be proactive in demonstrating the power of democratic collective changes, both small and large, to promote well-being and improve the lives of the public.

References

Ahn, S. J. (2015). Incorporating immersive virtual environments in health promotion campaigns: A construal level theory approach. *Health Communication*, *30*(6), 545–556. https://doi.org/10.1080/10410236.2013.869650

Ahonen, E. Q., Fujishiro, K., Cunningham, T., & Flynn, M. (2018). Work as an inclusive part of population health inequities research and prevention. *American Journal of Public Health*, *108*(3), 306–311. https://doi.org/10.2105/ajph.2017.304214

Anderson, B. (2023). The role of public relations in a counterhegemony: A case study of the 1968 poor people's campaign. *Public Relations Review*, *49*(4), 102363. https://doi.org/10.1016/j.pubrev.2023.102363

Asante, G. (2025). Rethinking (LGBT) empowerment: Exploring the potential of community-based participatory research project among human rights NGOs in Ghana. *Journal of Applied Communication Research*, *53*(2), 91–112. https://doi.org/10.1080/00909882.2025.2470232.

Bakhtin, M. M. (1981). *The dialogic imagination*. The University of Texas Press.

Ban, Z. (2016). Delineating responsibility, decisions and compromises: a frame analysis of the fast food industry's online CSR communication. *Journal of Applied Communication Research*, *44*(3), 296–315. https://doi.org/10.1080/00909882.2016.1192290

Basnyat, I. (2017). Theorizing the relationship between gender and health through a case study of nepalese street-based female sex workers. *Communication Theory*, *27*(4), 388–406. https://doi.org/10.1111/comt.12114

Basu, A., & Dutta, M. J. (2008). Participatory change in a campaign led by sex workers: Connecting resistance to action-oriented agency. *Qualitative Health Research*, *18*(1), 106–119. https://doi.org/10.1177/1049732307309373

Battilani, P., & Schröter, H. G. (2012). *The cooperative business movement, 1950 to the present*. Cambridge University Press.

Benach, J., Malmusi, D., Yasui, Y., & Martínez, J. M. (2013). A new typology of policies to tackle health inequalities and scenarios of impact based on Rose's population approach. *Journal of Epidemiology and Community Health*, *67*(3), 286–291. https://doi.org/10.1136/jech-2011-200363

Bezzina, A., Clarke, E. D., Ashton, L., Watson, T., & James, C. L. (2024). Workplace health promotion programs targeting smoking, nutrition, physical activity, and obesity in men: A systematic review and meta-analysis of randomized controlled trials. *Health Education & Behavior*, *51*(1), 113–127. https://doi.org/10.1177/10901981231208396

Bisel, R. S., Kavya, P., & Tracy, S. J. (2020). Positive deviance case selection as a method for organizational communication: A rationale, how-to, and illustration. *Management Communication Quarterly*, *34*(2), 279–296. https://doi.org/10.1177/0893318919897060

Brown, S., & Getz, C. (2008). Privatizing farm worker justice: Regulating labor through voluntary certification and labeling. *Geoforum*, *39*(3), 1184–1196. https://dx.doi.org/10.1016/j.geoforum.2007.01.002

Cao, A., & Wang, M. (2021). Exploring the health narratives of chinese female migrant workers through culture-centered and gender perspectives. *Health Communication*, *36*(2), 158–167. https://doi.org/10.1080/10410236.2019.1669269

Cheney, G., Santa Cruz, I., Peredo, A. M., & Nazareno, E. (2014). Worker cooperatives as an organizational alternative: Challenges, achievements and promise in business governance and ownership. *Organization, 21*(5), 591–603. https://doi.org/10.1177/1350508414539784

Conrad, C. (2011). *Organizational rhetoric: Strategies of resistance and domination*. Polity.

Crawford, R. (1977). You are dangerous to your health: The ideology and politics of victim blaming. *International Journal of Health Services, 7*(4), 663–680. https://doi.org/10.2190/YU77-T7B1-EN9X-G0PN

Davis, C. S., & Quinlan, M. M. (2017). Communicating stigma and acceptance. In J. Yamasaki, P. Geist Martin, & B. Sharf (Eds.), *Storied health and illness* (pp. 191–220). Waveland Press.

Deetz, S. (1992). *Democracy in an age of corporate colonization: Developments in communication and the politics of everyday life*. State University of New York Press.

Dempsey, S. (Ed.). (2024). *Organizing eating: Communicating for equity across U.S. food systems*. Routledge.

Dempsey, S., & Gibson, K. E. (2017). Food, biopower, and the child's body as a scale of intervention. In P. Marcell & F. Bosco (Eds.), *Food and place: A critical introduction* (pp. 253–269). Rowman & Littlefield.

Dempsey, S. E., Zoller, H. M., & Hunt, K. P. (2022). The meatpacking industry's corporate exceptionalism: Racialized logics of food chain worker disposability during the COVID-19 crisis. *Food, Culture & Society, 26*(3), 571–590. https://doi.org/10.1080/15528014.2021.2022916

de Souza, R. (2019). *Feeding the other: Whiteness, privilege, and neoliberal stigma in food pantries*. MIT Press.

de Souza, R. (2022). Communication, carcerality, and neoliberal stigma: The case of hunger and food assistance in the United States. *Journal of Applied Communication Research, 51*(3), 1–18. https://doi.org/10.1080/00909882.2022.2079954

de Souza, R., Basu, A., Kim, I., Basnyat, I., & Dutta, M. J. (2008). The paradox of "fair trade:" The influence of neoliberal trade agreements on food security and health. In H. M. Zoller & M. J. Dutta (Eds.), *Emerging perspectives in health communication* (pp. 411–430). Routledge.

Dillon, P., & Basu, A. (2013). Preventing HIV/AIDS through a culture-centered health campaign: The Sonagachi HIV/AIDS Intervention Program. In M. J. Dutta & G. Kreps (Eds.), *Reducing health disparities: Communication interventions* (pp. 113–132). Peter Lang.

du Pre, A., & Overton, B. C. (2022). *Communicating about health* (6th ed.). Oxford Press.

Dutta, M., & Kaur-Gill, S. (2018). Precarities of migrant work in Singapore: Migration, (im)mobility, and neoliberal governmentality. *International Journal of Communication, 12*, 4066–4084.

Foucault, M. (1980). *The history of sexuality: An introduction* (R. Hurley, Trans.; Vol. 1). Vintage.

Fraser, N. (1990/91). Rethinking the public sphere: A contribution to the critique of actually existing democracy. *Social Texts, 25/26*, 56–80.

Freire, P. (1973). *Education for critical consciousness*. Seabury Press.
Freudenberg, N. (2014). *Lethal but legal: Corporations, consumption and protecting public health*. Oxford University Press.
Fujishiro, K., Ahonen, E. Q., & Winkler, M. (2022). Investigating employment quality for population health and health equity: A perspective of power. *International Journal of Environmental Research and Public Health*, *19*(16), 9991. https://www.mdpi.com/1660-4601/19/16/9991
Fujishiro, K., & Heaney, C. A. (2009). Justice at work, job stress, and employee health. *Health Education & Behavior*, *36*(3), 487–504. https://doi.org/10.1177/1090198107306435
Ganesh, S. (2018). Logics of mobility: Social movements and their networked Other. *International Journal of Communication*, *12*(14). https://ijoc.org/index.php/ijoc/article/view/9660
Geist-Martin, P., & Scarduzio, J. (2011). Working well: Reconsidering health communication at work. In T. L. Thompson, R. Parrott, & J. F. Nussbaum (Eds.), *Handbook of health communication*, 2nd edition (pp. 117–131). Lawrence Erlbaum.
Gerbensky-Kerber, A. (2011). Grading the "good" body: A poststructural feminist analysis of body mass index initiatives. *Health Communication*, *26*(4), 354–365. https://doi.org/10.1080/10410236.2010.551581
Giddens, A. (1979). *Central problems in social theory: Action, structure and contradiction in social analysis*. University of California Press.
Gillies, C., Super, S., Te Molder, H., de Graaf, K., & Wagemakers, A. (2021). Healthy eating strategies for socioeconomically disadvantaged populations: A meta-ethnography. *International Journal of Qualitative Studies on Health and Well-being*, *16*(1), 1942416. https://doi.org/10.1080/17482631.2021.1942416
Glaude, E. S. (2007). *In a shade of blue: Pragmatism and the politics of Black America*. University of Chicago Press. https://www.press.uchicago.edu/Misc/Chicago/298248.html
Gollust, S. E., Barry, C. L., & Niederdeppe, J. (2017). Partisan responses to public health messages: Motivated reasoning and soda taxes. *Journal of Health Politics, Policy, & Law*, *42*(6), 1005–1037.
González-Agüero, M., Vargas, I., Campos, S., Farías Cancino, A., Quezada Quezada, C., & Urrutia Egaña, M. (2020). What makes a health movement successful? Health inequalities and the insulin pump in Chile. *Critical Public Health*, *32*(2), 1–12. https://doi.org/10.1080/09581596.2020.1808190
Gramsci, A. (1971). *Selections from the prison notebooks* (Q. Hoare & G. N. Smith, Trans.). International Publishers.
Hancock, T. (1993). The evolution, impact and significance of the healthy cities/Healthy communities movement. *Journal of Public Health Policy*, *14*(1), 5–17. https://doi.org/10.2307/3342823
Hardy, C., & Phillips, N. (2004). Discourse and power. In D. Grant, C. Hardy, C. Oswick, & L. L. Putnam (Eds.), *The Sage handbook of organizational discourse* (pp. 299–316). Sage.
Harrison, M. A., & Stephens, K. K. (2019). Shifting from wellness at work to wellness in work: Interrogating the link between stress and organization while theorizing a move toward wellness-in-practice. *Management Communication Quarterly*, *33*(4), 616–649. https://doi.org/10.1177/0893318919862490

Hernández, L. H., & De Los Santos Upton, S. (2019). Critical health communication methods at the U.S.-Mexico border: Violence against migrant women and the role of health activism [conceptual analysis]. *Frontiers in Communication, 4.* https://doi.org/10.3389/fcomm.2019.00034

Heuman, A. N., Scholl, J. C., & Wilkinson, K. (2013). Rural hispanic populations at risk in developing diabetes: Sociocultural and familial challenges in promoting a healthy diet [article]. *Health Communication, 28*(3), 260–274. https://doi.org/10.1080/10410236.2012.680947

Hopp, T., Ferrucci, P., & Vargo, C. J. (2020). Why do people share ideologically extreme, false, and misleading content on social media? A self-report and trace data–based analysis of countermedia content dissemination on Facebook and Twitter. *Human Communication Research, 46*(4), 357–384. https://doi.org/10.1093/hcr/hqz022

Ivancic, S. R. (2017). Gluttony for a cause or feeding the food insecure? Contradictions in combating food insecurity through private philanthropy. *Health Communication, 32*(11), 1441–1444. https://doi.org/10.1080/10410236.2016.1222562

Kadlec, A. (2008). Critical pragmatism and deliberative democracy. *Theoria, 117,* 54–80. https://doi.org/10.3167/th.2008.5511704

Kennedy, B., Kawachi, I., & Prothrow-Stith, D. (1998). Income distribution, socioeconomic status, and self rated health in the United States: Multilevel analysis. *British Medical Journal, 317*(7163), 917–921. https://doi.org/10.1136/bmj.317.7163.917

Khan, S. (2014). Manufacturing consent?: Media messages in the mobilization against HIV/AIDS in India and lessons for health communication. *Health Communication, 29*(3), 288–298. https://doi.org/10.1080/10410236.2012.753139

Kirkwood, W. G., & Brown, D. (1995). Public communication about the causes of disease: The rhetoric of responsibility. *Journal of Communication, 45*(1), 55–76. https://doi.org/10.1111/j.1460-2466.1995.tb00714.x

Knight, E. K., Benjamin, G. D., & Yanich, D. (2016). Framing social determinants of health within the professional public health community: Research translation and implications for policy change. *Journal of Applied Communication Research, 44*(3), 256–274. https://doi.org/10.1080/00909882.2016.1192291

LeGreco, M., & Douglas, N. (2021). *Everybody eats: Communication and the paths to food justice.* UC Press.

Leonhirth, W. (2001). William James and the uncertain universe. In D. K. Perry (Ed.), *American pragmatism and communication research* (pp. 89-). Laurence Earlbaum.

Liang, H., & Beydoun, M. A. (2019). Modifiable health risk factors, related counselling, and treatment among patients in health centres. *Health & Social Care in the Community, 27*(3), 693–705. https://doi.org/10.1111/hsc.12686

Lupton, D. (1994). Toward the development of critical health communication praxis. *Health Communication, 6*(1), 55–67. https://doi.org/10.1207/s15327027hc0601_4

Lupton, D. (1995). *The imperative of health: Public health and the regulated body.* Sage Publications.

Majee, W., & Hoyt, A. (2010). Are worker-owned cooperatives the brewing pots for social capital? *Community Development, 41*(4), 417–430. https://doi.org/10.1080/15575330.2010.488741

Marmot, M., & Bell, R. J. P. h. (2012). Fair society, healthy lives. *Public Health*, *126*, S4–S10.

Marmot, M., & Theorell, T. (1991). Social class and cardiovascular disease: The contribution of work. In J. J. T & G. Johansson (Eds.), *The psychosocial work environment: Work organization, democratization and health* (pp. 21–48). Baywood.

Mbembe, A. (2019). *Necropolitics*. Duke University Press. https://doi.org/10.1215/08992363-15-1-11

McKnight, J. (1988). Where can health communication be found? *Journal of Applied Communication Research*, *16*(1), 39–43.

Morris, J. C., Gibson, W. A., Leavitt, W. M., & Jones, S. C. (2013). *The case for grassroots collaboration: Social capital and ecosystem restoration at the local level*. Lexington Books.

Mundra, A., Kalantri, A., Jakasania, A., Sathe, H., Raut, A., Maliye, C., Bahulekar, P., Dawale, A., Paradkar, R. J., Siriah, S., Kumar, S., Gupta, S. S., & Garg, B. (2023). Vitalizing community for health promotion against modifiable risk factors of noncommunicable diseases (V-CaN) in Rural Central India: Protocol for a hybrid type II implementation effectiveness trial. *JMIR Research Protocols*, *12*, e42450. https://doi.org/10.2196/42450

Niederdeppe, J., Bu, Q. L., Borah, P., Kindig, D. A., & Robert, S. A. (2008). Message design strategies to raise public awareness of social determinants of health and population health disparities. *Milbank Quarterly*, *86*(3), 481–513. https://doi.org/10.1111/j.1468-0009.2008.00530.x

Nutbeam, D. (2000). Health literacy as a public health goal: A challenge for contemporary health education and communication strategies into the 21st century. *Health Promotion International*, *15*(3), 259–267. https://doi.org/10.1093/heapro/15.3.259

Obinna, D. N. (2021). Confronting disparities: Race, ethnicity, and immigrant status as intersectional determinants in the COVID-19 era. *Health Education & Behavior*, *48*(4), 397–403. https://doi.org/10.1177/10901981211011581

Okamoto, K. E. (2017). "It's Like Moving the Titanic:" Community organizing to address food (in)security. *Health Communication*, *32*(8), 1047–1050. https://doi.org/10.1080/10410236.2016.1196517

Olufowote, J. O., Aranda, J., Wang, G. E., & Liao, D. (2017). Advancing the new communications framework for HIV/AIDS: The communicative constitution of HIV/AIDS networks in Tanzania's HIV/AIDS NGO sector. *Studies in Media and Communication*, *5*, 79–92. https://doi.org/https://doi.org/10.11114/smc.v5i1.2390

Osmundsen, M., Bor, A., Vahlstrup, P., Bechmann, A., & Petersen, M. (2021). Partisan polarization is the primary psychological motivation behind politcal fake news sharing on Twitter. *American Political Science Review*, *115*(3), 999–1015. https://doi.org/10.1017/S0003055421000290

Pal, M., Cruz, J. l., & Munshi, D. (2023). Decolonizing knowledge: Cultural aspirations, political self-determination and social rights in knowledge making. In L. Tuhiwai Smith & D. Munshi (Eds.), *Organizing at the margins: Theorizing organizations of struggle in the global south* (1 ed., pp. 15–33). Palgrave Macmillan. https://doi.org/10.1007/978-3-031-22993-0

Papa, M., Singhal, A., & Papa, W. (2006). *Organizing for social change: A dialectic journey of theory and praxis*. Sage.
Parker, P. S. (2003). Control, power, and resistance within raced, gendered, and classed work contexts: The case of African American women. *Communication Yearbook, 27*, 257–291.
Phelan, J. C., Link, B. G., & Tehranifar, P. (2010). Social conditions as fundamental causes of health inequalities: Theory, evidence, and policy implications. *Journal of Health and Social Behavior, 51 Suppl*, S28–S40. https://doi.org/10.1177/0022146510383498
Pickett, K., & Wilkinson, R. (2015). Income inequality and health: A causal review. *Social Science & Medicine, 128*, 316–326. https://doi.org/10.1016/j.socscimed.2014.12.031
Ray, L. (2004). Pragmatism and critical theory. *European Journal of Social Theory, 7*(3), 307–321. https://doi.org/10.1177/1368431004044195
Reed, I. A., Gross, N., & Winship, C. (2022). Pragmatist sociology: Histories and possibilities. In N. Gross, I. A. Reed, & C. Winship (Eds.), *The new pragmatist sociology* (pp. 3–30). Columbia University Press.
Rorty, R. (1989). *Contingency, irony, and solidarity*. Cambridge University Press.
Rosner, D., & Markowitz, G. (2024). *Building the worlds that kill us: Disease, death, and inequality in American history*. Columbia University Press.
Sabanayagam, C., & Shankar, A. (2012). Income is a stronger predictor of mortality than education in a national sample of US adults. *Journal of Health, Population and Nutrition, 30*(1), 82–86. https://doi.org/10.3329/jhpn.v30i1.11280
Said, E. (1978). *Orientalism*. Pantheon.
Sastry, S., & Dutta, M. J. (2013). Global Health Interventions and the "Common Sense" of Neoliberalism: A Dialectical Analysis of PEPFAR. *Journal of International and Intercultural Communication, 6*(1), 21–39. https://doi.org/10.1080/17513057.2012.740682
Sastry, S., Zoller, H. M., & Basu, A. (2021). Editorial: Doing critical health communication: A forum on methods [editorial]. *Frontiers in Health Communication, 5*(144). https://doi.org/10.3389/fcomm.2020.637579
Schill, A. L., & Chosewood, L. C. (2013). The NIOSH Total Worker Health™ Program: An Overview. *Journal of Occupational and Environmental Medicine, 55*, S8–S11. https://doi.org/10.1097/jom.0000000000000037
Shuler, S., & Tate, M. (2001). Intersections of feminism and pragmatism: Possibilities for communication theory and research. In D. K. Perry (Ed.), *American pragmatism and communication research* (pp. 209–224). Lawrence Earlbaum Associates.
Snyder, L. B. (2007). Health communication campaigns and their impact on behavior. *Journal of Nutrition Education and Behavior, 39*(2, Supplement), S32–S40. https://doi.org/https://doi.org/10.1016/j.jneb.2006.09.004
Stillwaggon, E. (2006). *AIDS and the ecology of poverty*. Oxford University Press.
Stohl, C., & Cheney, G. (2001). Participatory processes/paradoxical practices. *Management Communication Quarterly, 14*(3), 349–407. https://doi.org/10.1177/0893318901143001
Tesh, S. N. (1994). *Hidden arguments: Politics, ideology and disease prevention policy*. Rutgers University Press.

van den Akker, A., Gilmore, A. B., Fabbri, A., Knai, C., & Rutter, H. (2024). Aligning rhetoric with reality: a qualitative analysis of multistakeholder initiatives in the global food system. *Health Promotion International*, *39*(6), daae165. https://doi.org/10.1093/heapro/daae165

van Prooijen, J. W., & Douglas, K. M. (2018). Belief in conspiracy theories: Basic principles of an emerging research domain. *European Journal of Social Psychology*, *48*(7), 897–908. https://doi.org/10.1002/ejsp.2530

Vardeman-Winter, J. (2017). The framing of women and health disparities: A critical look at race, gender, and class from the perspectives of grassroots health communicators. *Health Communication*, *32*(5), 629–638. https://doi.org/10.1080/10410236.2016.1160318

Waitzkin, H. (1983). *The second sickness*. The Free Press.

Winkler, H. (2019). The effect of income inequality on political polarization: Evidence from European regions, 2002–2014. *Economics & Politics*, *31*(2), 137–162. https://doi.org/https://doi.org/10.1111/ecpo.12129

Witherell, R. (2013). An emerging solidarity: Worker cooperatives, unions, and the new union cooperative model in the United States. *International Journal of Labour Research*, *5*(2), 251–268.

Zoller, H. M. (2003a). Health on the line: Identity and disciplinary control in employee occupational health and safety discourse. *Journal of Applied Communication Research*, *31*(2), 118–139. https://doi.org/10.1080/0090988032000064588

Zoller, H. M. (2003b). Working out: Managerialism in workplace health promotion. *Management Communication Quarterly*, *17*(2), 171–205. https://doi.org/10.1177/0893318903253003

Zoller, H. M. (2005a). Health activism: Communication theory and action for social change. *Communication Theory*, *15*(4), 341–364. https://doi.org/10.1111/j.1468-2885.2005.tb00339.x

Zoller, H. M. (2005b). Women caught in the multicausal web: A gendered analysis of Healthy People 2010. *Communication Studies*, *56*(2), 175–192. https://doi.org/10.1080/00089570500078809

Zoller, H. M. (2008). Technologies of neoliberal governmentality: The discursive influence of global economic policies on health promotion. In H. M. Zoller & M. Dutta (Eds.), *Emerging perspectives in health communication: Meaning, culture, and power* (pp. 390–410). Routledge.

Zoller, H. M. (2012). Communicating health: Political risk narratives in an environmental health campaign. *Journal of Applied Communication Research*, *40*(1), 20–43. https://doi.org/10.1080/00909882.2011.634816

Zoller, H. M. (2016). Health activism targeting corporations: A critical health communication perspective. *Health Communication*, *32*(2), 219–229. https://doi.org/10.1080/10410236.2015.1118735

Zoller, H. M. (2023). Addressing health inequalities through worker and consumer cooperatives: Co-op Cincy's organizing for food justice. In S. Dempsey (Ed.), *Organizing eating: Communicating for equity across U.S. food systems* (pp. 139–165). Routledge.

Zoller, H. M. (2024). Pragmatic utopianism in the union cooperative movement: (Dis)Organizing transformative social change. *Communication Monographs*, *92*(2), 1–29. https://doi.org/10.1080/03637751.2024.2399137

Zoller, H. M., & Ban, Z. (2024). Communication, power, and organizational politics. In D. M. Vernon & P. Marshall Scott (Eds.), *Organizational communication theory and research* (pp. 277–294). De Gruyter Mouton. https://doi.org/doi:10.1515/9783110718508

Zoller, H. M., & Dutta, M. J. (Eds.). (2008). *Emerging perspectives in health communication: Meaning, culture, and power*. Routledge.

Zoller, H. M., & Kline, K. N. (2008). Theoretical contributions of interpretive and critical research in health communication. In C. Beck (Ed.), *Communication yearbook* (Vol. 32, pp. 89–136). Routledge.

Zoller, H. M., & Sastry, S. (2016). Communicating the politics of healthcare systems. In J. Yamasaki, P. Geist-Martin, & B. F. Sharf (Eds.), *Storied health and illness: Communicating personal, cultural, and political complexities* (pp. 306–332). Waveland Press.

Zoller, H. M., Strochlic, R., & Getz, C. (2023). An employee-centered framework for healthy workplaces: Implementing a critically holistic, participative, and structural model through the Equitable Food Initiative. *Journal of Applied Communication Research*, *51*(2), 164–184. https://doi.org/10.1080/00909882.2022.2106579

Zook, E. G. (1994). Embodied health and constitutive communication: Toward an authentic conceptualization of health communication. In S. A. Deetz (Ed.), *Communication yearbook* (Vol. 17, pp. 378–387). Sage.

7
HIV INTERVENTIONS, COLLECTIVIZATION EFFORTS, AND CITIZENSHIP ON THE MARGINS OF THE STATE IN INDIA

Shamshad Khan

Substantial progress has been made over the past few decades in the global fight against HIV/AIDS. The most marked progress can be seen in the 51% drop in AIDS-related deaths since 2010, following a 69% decline since 2004 (UNAIDS, 2023). Yet there continues to be a lag in reduction of new HIV infections, with only 38% decline globally and even a much slower decline in Asia and the Pacific (only 14%) (UNAIDS, 2023). In India, the rate of decline has almost plateaued since 2015–2016 (National AIDS Control Organisation, 2023). Additionally, Eastern Europe and Central Asia have witnessed an increase of 49% in new HIV infections since 2010; and a similar increase in AIDS-related deaths has also been registered (UNAIDS, 2023). Thus, while noting the successes to date, The Joint United Nations Programme on HIV/AIDS (UNAIDS) has cautioned us against losing the gained momentum, particularly in the context of the recent decline in global funding for HIV/AIDS and the lack of political leadership that is desperately needed if we want to be on track to end HIV/AIDS as a major public health challenge by 2030 (UNAIDS, 2019).

With key marginalized populations (including female sex workers [FSWs], men who have sex with men, transgender people and those who inject drugs) bearing a disproportionate burden of the disease globally, the HIV epidemic particularly exposes fault lines in society including social and health inequities, marginalization, poverty, stigma, and discrimination (UNAIDS, 2023). For instance, India's HIV epidemic, the second largest in the world (after South Africa), remains highly concentrated in key affected populations (National AIDS Control Organisation, 2023). However, while such pockets of disease concentration make mitigation challenging, they

DOI: 10.4324/9781003426530-9
This chapter has been made available under a CC BY-NC-ND license.

also show us that the path to ending this epidemic lies in the collective power of people. Such change is only possible through community empowerment and mobilization that goes beyond neoliberal organizing to enable community members to deliberate, negotiate, resist, and confront power structures, along with well-supported public policies and political commitment (Basu, 2010; Basu & Dutta, 2007; Khan et al., 2019; Zoller, 2005).

In this chapter, I share findings from an ethnographic research study focused on understanding the impact of a community-led structural intervention (CLSI) program among the female, male, and transgender sex workers in the Mysore and Mandya districts of South India. Led by *Ashodaya Samithi* (a sex-worker collective), the CLSI project engaged in community-driven outreach and mobilization that aimed to reduce the risk of HIV and STI infections by addressing the social and structural contexts of their lives (including stigma, discrimination, and violence) and by creating an enabling environment and communicative networks and spaces that promoted access to and utilization of services. The CLSI project also engaged in community capacity building in CLSI programming and management through curriculum-based demonstrative learning that soon emerged as *Ashodaya* Academy—the first UNAIDS-recognized regional learning site on HIV in the Asia-Pacific region run entirely by sex workers (UNAIDS, 2009).

Drawing on detailed narrative accounts from the field, this chapter demonstrates that CLSI's collectivization created complex socialities and conditions of possibility for emergent forms of citizenship that were deeply empowering. More specifically, I argue that through their everyday communication, deliberation, resistance, and alliance building, the members of the *Ashodaya Samithi* began to see commonalities in their living and working conditions (as sex workers), which further united them to navigate risks, demand services, and expand their rights and freedoms while they promoted enhanced visibility, audibility, and recognition as citizens at local and global levels (Khan et al., 2019; Lorway & Khan, 2014).

Citizenship studies have challenged traditional notions of citizenship tied to the nation-state (Alexander, 1994; Isin & Turner, 2002). Critical scholars have argued that previous notions of citizenship (as legal rights and status emanating from the nation-state) assume 'universalism' and 'inclusion' while overlooking the systemic processes of exclusion and discrimination that render some groups as undeserving of social and political recognitions and thereby deem them as 'outsiders' (Isin & Turner, 2002: p. 6). A persistent focus in critical citizenship studies has been to make visible and address the injustices and inequities that happen in democratic states through processes of marginalization (Nordberg, 2006; Stavinoha, 2019). Alternative theorizing about citizenship calls for a critical examination of the social injustices and inequities arising from treating citizenship as an exclusionary category as well as efforts to redress these issues (Alexander, 1994; Atluri, 2012; Isin, 2012; Sabsay, 2012). Scholars have further argued that such endeavors require people's active participation in all matters that affect their everyday lives as well as grassroots activism, rather than just being 'dutiful' citizens (Kligler-Vilenchik, 2017).

Citizenship studies seek to understand the potential of communicative practices among marginalized people who struggle to be in the role of citizens through solidarity, empowerment, and community mobilization (Paz, 2019; Stavinoha, 2019). In the context of sex work and HIV/AIDS, for example, scholars have shown how organically formed community-led organizations presented "autonomous" rationality "parallel to and in spite of the mainstream discourse" (Basu, 2011, p. 392) as well as challenged unequal relations of power and control within the sex industry (Basu & Dutta, 2007, 2008). Such studies have approached community from a constitutive perspective, exploring how communication practices create interpretive communities and how participatory methodologies help unravel the processes and strategies employed by community members to co-create effective responses to health challenges (Basu, 2017; Underwood & Frey, 2007).

Several studies have examined the trajectory of fights for citizenship rights by marginalized communities, such as the "gender-variant communities," in post-colonial context in India (Dutta, 2012; Ghosh, 2022). They have argued that despite constitutional rights and the recent passing of Transgender Persons (Protection of Rights) Bill in 2019, the citizenship status of such groups has merely shifted from being 'illegal' to constrained or 'captive' (by dominant liberal notions of citizenship) to 'stranded' citizens. The advent of AIDS disease spurred demands for citizenship rights for these sexually dissident communities, but with limited success (Ghosh, 2022). Others have observed that attempts to legitimize and gain social inclusivity for sexual minorities in post-colonial India must transcend Eurocentric discourses of citizenship to speak to the intersections of local contexts of class/ caste and gender marginality (Dutta, 2012). Such studies have demonstrated the "messy entanglement of putatively universalizable and abstract norms and ideals of modern citizenship with particular histories and locations" (Dutta, 2012. p.141).

While these citizenship studies are valuable for their emphasis on local contexts, apart from Basu and Dutta (2007, 2008), their focus has not been on the communicative acts and agencies of these groups, nor have they foregrounded how these communities understand and view their own marginality and citizenship. Indeed, much scholarly work on citizenship is focused on extensive theorizing, while empirical and ethnographic studies in post-colonial contexts remain limited. There is thus a lack of understanding about the range of citizenship issues confronted by these communities, particularly when citizenship is promoted in reference to frameworks of heteronormativity and heteromasculinity (Alexander, 1994; Atluri, 2012). There is a need in critical health communication literature to examine the areas where political arenas of citizenship and sexuality overlap with post-coloniality.

In this context, it is important to ask: how do multiple forms of power and domination play out in the everyday lives of people who have experienced high levels of stigma and discrimination, and how do these groups, despite their marginalized status, understand and challenge these systemic oppressions (Basu, 2011, 2017; Basu & Dutta, 2011; Dutta & Basu, 2011; Dutta-Bergman, 2004; Zoller, 2005)? In other words, how are everyday communication practices of these sexually dissident communities implicated in the continual recreation of such political fields of domination and dissent? To this end, the current ethnographic study was designed to understand: (a) the conditions under which a highly participative sex-worker collective—*Ashodaya Samithi*—was formed in the state of Karnataka (India), (b) the experiences of its members as it related to forming the collective, and (c) how, collectively, they encountered and challenged relations of power and control while navigating health risks and asserting their rights and identities.

I begin by describing the study's research methodology. Drawing on the larger study, I describe how members of this collective encountered stigma, discrimination, and violence as they navigated risks and managed health and social issues. I also describe how members engaged individual and collective forms of resistance and alliance building to gain empowerment and work toward greater visibility and recognition of their rights and freedom. I conclude the chapter by discussing what I think communities are telling us about how to make HIV and other health interventions a success and the ways in which mutual recognition as citizens is meaningful to them in this process.

Methodology

Study Site: The Formation of the Ashodaya Samithi

In 2004, under the auspices of *Avahan* (a Bill & Melinda Gates Foundation HIV/AIDS initiative in India), a team of researchers from the university of Manitoba (Canada) and the staff of a local non-governmental organization (Karnataka Health Promotion Trust, KHPT) collaboratively launched a health intervention to address HIV and STI among the sex workers of

Mysore and Mandya districts of Karnataka (Reza-Paul et al., 2012). Using a peer outreach and participatory mapping approach, the intervention aimed to promote community capacity building to reduce HIV vulnerability in sex-worker population in a region where the rates were considerably high (Beattie et al., 2010; Beksinska et al., 2018). The intervention acted as a catalyst for the sex workers, spread across the two districts, to generate a feeling of community around common issues and shared experiences that went beyond healthcare and HIV, including violence, social stigma, housing needs, among others. Coming together to jointly address issues faced by them led to the formation of the *Ashodaya Samithi* in 2005, a sex worker-run community-based organization (CBO). From the start, *Ashodaya Samithi* recorded success both in terms of community engagement as well as in reducing the risk of HIV/STI infections. With increase in membership and participation, the collective grew, refining and building on its goals and priorities as deemed appropriate and relevant by the sex worker community (Navarrete Gil et al., 2021).

Critical Ethnography

As noted earlier, the goal of the current study was to document the formation and growth of *Ashodaya Samithi* to understand how sex workers, who were previously dispersed and unknown to each other, rallied around a set of common issues and actively participated to build a shared vision and a path of action for themselves. To foreground the experiences of the community in building a sex-worker collective from the ground up, we employed a critical ethnographic approach in our study. The foundational premise of this methodological approach includes reflective thinking, empirical inquiry, and iterative data collection that aims for transformative action. What makes critical ethnography distinct from conventional ethnography is that it strives to challenge the status quo and reveal underlying domain of assumptions and power relations—more than outlining the cultural context (of research) that often implies affirmation of prevailing sets of meanings (Thomas, 2003). Critical ethnography thus aims for a political purpose in that it "strives to unmask hegemony and address oppressive forces" (Crotty, 1998, p. 12). In this approach, researchers explore the local meanings within the larger context of structural inequities and power imbalances with the aim to reveal both the prevailing unjust status quo as well as the resistance (Crotty, 1998; Thomas, 2003). To do this, critical ethnography draws on participatory methodologies to foreground local narratives that reveal the lived experiences of people who are subjected to systemic inequities but are also the potential agents of social change.

Data Collection and Analysis

Ethnographic data collection involved a variety of sources that included (a) four months of observations at multiple intervention sites in the districts of Mysore and Mandya (e.g., solicitation sites, learning centers, drop-in centers, clinics, organizational meetings, and group activities of the *Ashodaya Samithi*); (b) semi-structured interviews ($n = 50$) with scholars and professionals who initiated the project, members of the targeted communities, service providers (e.g., counselors, managers, outreach workers), and members of *Ashodaya Samithi*; and (c) a document analysis of project proposals, progress reports, HIV/STI and behavioral surveillance data, learning and counseling materials, news reports, etc.

An ongoing collaboration with KHPT, a well-established health nonprofit organization working in the area for more than ten years, eased the way for the author to introduce the study to *Ashodaya* members. Drawing on participatory methodologies, the author attended a series of meetings with *Ashodaya* members to share details about the study and to seek their input in shaping the study. With initial feedback, an interview guide was prepared, which was further refined to include topic areas most relevant to their needs and experiences. Further, a few members, who were keen to learn about research, were trained by the author in the conduct of qualitative interviews. Together with trained community researchers, the author conducted a total of 40 interviews with *Ashodaya* members that included 23 interviews with FSWs, 11 with male sex workers (MSWs), and 6 with transgender sex workers. All participants, before consenting to the interview, were made aware about the voluntary nature of the participation and that a decision not to participate will not hinder any services they receive at the *Ashodaya*. The interviews were conducted in the local language (Kannada) either with help of a translator when the author conducted the interview or directly by a trained community member, with a choice provided to the interviewees. All interviews were audio-taped, with consent, and either transcribed or translated and transcribed in English.

The transcribed interviews were subjected to an inductive critical thematic analysis. Thematic analysis is "a method for systematically identifying, organizing, and offering insight into patterns of meaning (themes) across a data set" and is a flexible method that allows for research study goals to be explored in depth (Braun & Clarke, 2012, p. 57). A critical thematic analysis takes this approach a step further and allows researchers to identify the intersecting macro-forces that facilitate and constrain the everyday lives of the study participants. In this study, using an inductive thematic analysis approach, the interview transcripts were iteratively read and re-read to generate a set of initial codes that adequately reflected the emerging themes in the dataset. These codes were then reworked and refined to understand the recurring themes that also represented the broader social forces and the influence of dominant discourses on the narratives shared by the participants. The emerging refined set of codes was then inputted, and interview data was coded with the aid of NVivo 11 software.

The complete study dataset included site observational fieldnotes, interviews with key players associated with *Avahan* initiative and *Ashodaya Samithi*, interviews with service providers, as well as sex worker members of Ashodaya. While insights from the broader study dataset informs the analysis, this chapter draws primarily on interview data with FSWs, MSWs, and transgender members of *Ashodaya Samithi* (N=40). The study received ethics approval from the Simon Fraser University Research Ethics Board and from the local institutions.

Ashodaya *Member Participant Profile*

The average age of participants was 33 years, ranging from 21 to 46 years, with 16 participants having completed primary or secondary schooling, and two with a higher degree. In terms of marital status, most (87%) FSWs were married with children but few in the case of MSWs or the transgender participants.

Findings

Most interviewees conveyed genuine interest, enthusiasm, and passion for *Ashodaya Samithi* and a vision for the future as a sex worker's collective. In their narratives, participants make visible their lived experiences of marginalization, their efforts toward collective capacity building, and their everyday acts of communication through which they attempt to claim citizenship status in a way that is meaningful to them.

Transformation Within: Identity Consciousness

In talking about the formation of *Ashodaya Samithi*, several participants shared how it nurtured in them the desire to thrive and succeed that went beyond survival. Having led a life full of challenges due to systemic discrimination, these participants were struggling to survive and the founding of the *Ashodaya Samithi* provided them with much needed hope and energy.

> My life has seen many changes [since Ashodaya]. Before coming to Ashodaya...I did not have confidence that I will survive. Since I was a

sex worker, I had an assumption that sex worker has no value in society, nobody respects, and I was very tired with life and was not interested to live... Ashodaya helped me in getting back to my children ...in identifying myself as a sex worker. ...When I had lost hope of achieving anything in life, Ashodaya gave me a job and helped me in taking care of my children and helped me in identifying myself.

(FSW ID # 3)

We might be HIV positive any day, [but] we should have the confidence to survive...this confidence to live is given to us by Ashodaya.... Also taught us how to prevent HIV, by taking safety measures....

(Female sex worker ID # 5)

Low self-esteem and self-worth are associated with poor health outcomes among sex workers in a highly stigmatized profession with its everyday risks of violence (Beattie et al., 2010; Ekstrand et al., 2018). Particularly, MSWs and transgender sex workers struggled to come out in the open in a society governed by strict traditional gender norms that often led them to break away from their families (Bhutada et al., 2023; Huynh et al., 2018; Khan, 2020), with many sharing stories like, "my brother would hit me with a cricket bat...ask me to wear shirt-pant and not behave like a hijra... I ran away from home....slept in a railway station....people attacked me... it's been like that since then." For many, social ostracization had become part of their life and that is what they had come to expect. After coming together as a collective, many felt they had a chance to get back into society, which breathed new hope in their lives. For instance, the FSW quoted above managed to secure a job with connections made through *Ashodaya Samithi*. The position enabled her to resume the role of a "mother"—the duties of which are a significant marker of female citizenship, especially in a place like India that has historically defined womanhood and citizenship in traditional patriarchal/hierarchal ways (Khan et al., 2018). For most participants, sex work remained their primary occupation. Through *Ashodaya,* however, they were able to improve their 'workplace' environment and the prospects of earning more at their jobs. This aspect added significantly to their quality of life, as can be discerned from the following narrative:

Earlier, we did not have discipline when we went to a client. Now after coming here [Ashodaya]... [we learnt] how to go[behave], how to use the condoms and all the other things... [earlier] the girls [FSWs] would sleep on footpaths[sidewalk]... nor were they clean. Now that soap and shampoo is given here, they have a bath and rest. ... Before no one [client] would call us for even Rupees (Rs.)10. Now... they call us for... Rs.100, even for Rs.200. A lot of changes have taken place... [we learnt] we need to create a clean environment in the place we work.

(Female sex worker ID # 23)

If we use condoms and keep ourselves healthy, we can have sex in life [continue this profession] for 20 years instead of 10 years. We can also earn for 20 years and see some money[enjoy] in life and dress up like other people in society.

(Male sex worker ID # 5)

Living in poverty and financial crisis with no family support primarily drove most women and men to enter this profession; so, finding a way to enhance their earnings and making it more tolerable appealed to them. Further, with no education, financial or social security, including no permanent place to live, most participants were used to taking life a day at a time rather than to plan for the future. Through *Ashodaya* they learnt about options to bring stability and professionalism in their lives within broader societal frameworks.

We have a co-operative bank account [now]. Earlier we would spend our money by eating or drinking outside. If we had to open an account in the bank for ourselves, they would ask us for ID card, ration card and other documents. We were not able to open a bank account in our names as we live in rented [transitional] housing... Through *Ashodaya Samithi*, we opened a co-operative bank account...we got our PAN [identity]cards done, we are given applications for ration [food] card....

(Female sex worker ID # 3)

A recurring theme running across participants' narratives was the need to belong to society by other society members. This was a major undercurrent no matter what the focus of their story might be. They shared many instances of having faced myriad forms of stigma, discrimination, and violence in their lives from authority figures including police and health providers as well as through interactions with clients, brokers, romantic partners, family, and the broader community. Their primary reference to *Ashodaya Samithi,* thus, related to collectivized efforts toward empowerment and stigma mitigation to gain pride in their identity as a sex worker and the confidence to demand respect in the society.

Earlier we did not know anything about IPC 377A [gay criminalisation] ... we thought that the rights were only for the males and females...We now know about HIV and though we are transgender, we are also human beings, and we are part of the [society]…after forming the *Samiti*, our attitudes have changed…I know about my rights… I have also learnt about my property rights, and I have the courage to live happily and help others in the society…we are equal to others.

(Trans gender sex worker ID #1)

Despite the historical exclusions that sex workers (and particularly transgender communities) have faced within the government system and in the broader society, *Ashodaya*—as an organization that facilitates healthcare and well-being among its member sex workers—has in certain ways created a second chance for its members to belong and be part of the society, thereby opening up new life possibilities in the future, beyond despair and oppression. Further, becoming more literate in civil rights and entitlements transforms their willingness to accept their marginal positioning in the society. *Ashodaya* helped to cultivate this critical consciousness about their rights and their potential to transform their socio-economic destinies. Participating with the group helps build up their agency and stirs up the possibility of becoming full participating members of the society and rising out of the shadows of marginality.

Changes in Interactions with Police and Health Care System

The confidence instilled by *Ashodaya Samithi* spilled into their interactions with police and health care systems. Sex workers almost everywhere in the world are harassed by law enforcement agencies given their vulnerabilities, the stigma associated with the profession, and varying interpretations of their legal standing (Platt et al., 2018). But in Karnataka, the violence and harassment faced by sex workers is particularly well known (Bhattacharjee et al., 2016; Blanchard et al., 2018; Huynh et al., 2018). Fear of authorities, lack of family support, social stigma, and power imbalances have created age-old rifts in the relationships between sex workers and police. Yet these groups need the most protection given the dangers involved in sex trade. However, participants shared how over time, with knowledge and support from *Ashodaya,* they were able to bring a marked change in their relationship with police and in some cases even be able to ally with them.

> Earlier police would shout at us using dirty words, assault us, scold us by calling us *chakka*. [They would] ask us, "why do you behave like this? Why can't you be a man? Why are you doing this kind of job?" and we wouldn't know what to answer. We would take the beatings from them, and would take whatever they do…they would have free

sex, without using condoms...but after we formed an association, if the police arrest, we ask, "Why are you arresting us? Why are you doing this? What wrong did we do? ... Now we [even] sit with the same police and tell them about our HIV prevention program training, we tell the police about events happening at *Ashodaya*. What I feel is that our community members [sex workers] have also changed. We have also learnt to give respect to others in the society, to each other and then to ask for respect back....

(Male sex worker ID # 10)

Through empowerment, collectivization, and peer support, the sex workers attempted to overcome their fear of police harassment and even advance it to the level of having an open dialogue. Given an opportunity, they would try to share the initiatives (HIV and other social and financial schemes) undertaken by *Ashodaya* and to that extent attempt to make the police understand the social realities faced by the sex workers and the conditions associated with sex trade.

Their newly acquired confidence and pride in their identity also had an impact on encounters with the health care system, which like law enforcement agencies, they would avoid as much as possible.

We did not get treatment like this [clinic at *Ashodaya*] anywhere else. [Earlier] They [doctors in government hospitals] refused to even touch us.... A [HIV] positive patient is treated as an untouchable. Even the medicines were not given on a timely basis. But now, when a visiting card [reference from *Ashodaya*] is shown, we are getting a better treatment. We are having the confidence to go meet the doctor and share our problems.

(Female sex worker ID # 31)

Besides facilitating access to healthcare, *Ashodaya* provided participants with information to help reduce their risks to HIV. This information was perhaps available earlier but made more sense to them when delivered by a peer worker whom they trusted to know their day-to-day realities.

We cannot say that all of our community people are having safe sex, using condoms. If they get paid more, they will have sex without condoms and if others [health staff, media] advise them to use condoms, they will not listen. But, when I as a sex worker tell another sex worker [about condom use], she will think I am a sex worker and advising her, so she will listen to me. And I can explain with my example, about my past life and present status, then it will be easy for her to implement [use condoms] the same in her life.

(Male sex worker ID # 5)

Over the years, this area and the sex worker community have witnessed quite a few HIV prevention programs focused primarily on safe sex education and HIV treatment. But what stood out for the participants in case of *Ashodaya* was the comprehensive support received, addressing almost all challenges faced by them, even if directly not related to health or HIV.

Many *Samithi*'s [organizations] are working towards preventing HIV in Mysore, but... they[only] give condoms... in *Ashodaya* they conduct every program like HIV prevention, STI prevention, distribute condoms, referring from our [*Ashodaya*] clinic to other hospitals and also identify wherever there are other HIV patients and provide them with medicines... *Ashodaya Samithi* is also admitting our children in the hostel, and also once they identify girls below 18 years of age, they would not let them [do sex] work but send them home...so *Ashodaya Samithi* is doing all these kind of work, but other *Samithis* are not doing this.

(Female sex worker, ID # 13)

The ability and willingness of *Ashodaya* to address the diverse issues and challenges faced by the sex worker communities and to go beyond the narrow focus of HIV prevention was a driving force of the collective. This responsiveness resulted in not only growing membership but also active participation by the members.

A Step Beyond Citizenship and Toward Activism

The collective derived its strength not only from its comprehensive approach toward HIV prevention but also by bringing the different groups of sexual minorities together—be it FSW, MSW, or transgender sex workers—thereby providing them with a shared vision and a path to action. By providing a safe space, *Ashodaya*, performed a protective role for its members and fostered intimate solidarities. Members described a sense of recuperation from the loss of familial and community ties severed by stigmatization and ostracization. The organization both enhanced their recognition of the oppression they faced and offered some respite from discrimination and structural violence. The participants took pride in building collective consciousness, strength, and solidarities.

> We realized we cannot face them [society] all alone…[but] if we have a *Samithi* [collective] of our own, we can face anything. When thousands of us make a noise together our problems will be heard. Hence, we decided to form our own Samithi.
> *(Transgender sex worker ID#1)*

> We are 3000 sex workers in *Ashodaya* and this is our strength… And where we feel strong is the fact that our *Samithi* is working with all three categories like hijadas [transgender], men and women. This makes us feel very strong. There was nothing like this for the sex workers. Now, we have an opportunity to take leadership and ownership to work towards finding solutions to our problems. We have taken this as a challenge and moving ahead.
> *(Female sex worker ID # 2)*

An underlying sentiment running across most participants' narratives was the pride in forming and belonging to this collective. There was something about "becoming an *Ashodaya* sex worker" that raised the political consciousness and productivity of the group, especially in how it re-wrote the individual life experiences of its members as part of a larger forms of oppression facing the community. The members started relating to each other's experiences—feelings of oppression and the need for a respectful place in society—and the effect spiraled to go beyond local and even national boundaries.

> There were many *Samithis* which would come and go, but after formation of our *Samithi*, our community had a lot of empowerments. [Other] *Samithi* and NGOs… they will have targets to complete…they go after completing the work, but our *Ashodaya Samithi* is ongoing. The benefits and facilities should be provided to our community [sex workers], till their existence… our sex workers take initiative to provide information to another sex worker, to build up the capacity, community mobilization, all these programs are conducted differently. It is not only in Mysore [city], but in Rajasthan [a different Indian state] and at international levels…we are working everywhere…different countries have appreciated our *Ashodaya Samithi* 's work…have come identified our work. Also, people from here have gone there and worked, we joined with them.
> *(Male sex worker ID # 10)*

By pooling their experiences of discrimination, oppression, and stigmatization associated with their profession, the members were able to see the systemic inequities and structural violence in their lives—and developed feelings of empathy for all sex worker communities across provincial, national, and international boundaries. *Ashodaya,* by conducting programs that met the comprehensive needs of its members, raised forms of visibility and collective awareness that superseded the nation-state, and opened up new political terrain that allows people to feel affirmed that they have a political base or power to challenge and to assert their political legitimacy.

As noted earlier, contemporary and critical citizenship studies adopt a broader view of citizenship, going beyond the political and cultural authority of the nation-state, to recognize the political and social struggles of marginalized populations (Khan et al., 2019). *Ashodaya* members, after years of struggling alone as sex workers and with their marginalized sexual identities, started collectively demanding participation in social and cultural events that mattered hugely to them, particularly in the localized contexts.

> Earlier we would celebrate Republic Day [celebration of laying down of Indian constitution] in schools, but after coming to this sex work, we are not going anywhere [not able to attend celebrations], we have been cornered is what we would feel. But after forming our *Samithi*, we are conducting all programs happening in the society...we celebrate Independence Day, we celebrate festivals.
>
> *(Male sex worker ID # 10)*

> Nobody would keep a seat for us, nobody would call us saying come and sit down. Now there is Ashodaya, and Ashodaya invites us for everything, whether it is Chamundi pooja or Ganapathi festival [Hindu festivals] or going to any rally. Without any discrimination, all different sangha [associations], *Samithi*s join together and conduct programs and they invite us... to show that we are also human beings. They have showed us a good way in life.
>
> *(Female sex worker ID#9)*

In the context of India, religious and cultural festivals occupy an important part of people's lives and often it is in participation of these festivals that people gain or maintain their social legitimacy. These are the spaces and venues where forms of sociality and identities converge, and consciousness building is solidified—spaces that are often ignored in conventional understanding of citizenship. But taking the concept of citizenship beyond conventional understanding to incorporate struggles against systemic inequities clarifies how *Ashodaya* builds capacity and empowers its member to stand together in their fight for social justice, equity, and the ability to be a true citizen. In that sense, *Ashodaya* instilled seeds of activism in its members and pushed them to go beyond being 'dutiful' citizens and to demand their rightful place in society.

Discussion and Conclusion

Decades of the HIV/AIDS epidemic has shifted global responses, with a movement away from a biomedical and behavioral intervention approach aimed at individual level changes toward a more broad-based attempt at addressing the social drivers of the epidemic. Research has proven that those living on the margins of society, as a consequence of structural violence in their lives, are rendered most vulnerable to HIV. These social forces of inequity and marginalization need to be urgently addressed. As noted by UNAIDS (2019), "where there are inequalities, power imbalances, violence, marginalization, taboos, and stigma and discrimination, HIV takes hold" (p. 2) and any effort to end this epidemic has to keep the marginalized communities at the center as "politicians or public health officials… have little or no knowledge of the lives and experiences of the people they are charged to serve" (p. 14).

Sex worker communities have been targeted with top-down health campaigns of safe sex, condom use, and STI prevention with scant inclusion of their voices or attention to the contextual factors that shape their vulnerability to HIV. These campaigns have produced very limited success (Basu, 2010; Basu & Dutta, 2007; Khan, 2014, 2018; Khan et al., 2018). Although community capacity building and mobilization has become more central to HIV prevention programs, there remains a tendency toward narrow, top-down, targeted intervention even in a community-based approach to HIV. For example, George et al.'s (2015) study compared a CLSI among FSWs that acknowledged power inequality and structural discrimination as the underlying conditions of their HIV vulnerability and attempted to address them through peer worker support as opposed to another community-based intervention with a targeted approach where the goal was to increase the limited knowledge of FSWs and their access to healthcare through peer workers. The CLSI peer workers had a much broader mandate, going beyond providing condoms and health information to developing collective identity and capacity to deal with the challenges of their lives. In the TI approach, the peer workers (although from the community) had a narrow focus on promoting condom use and clinic access as well as recruiting members. This difference resulted in much lesser engagement by FSWs and less success (George et al., 2015). As noted by critical communication scholars, community engagement, mobilization, and change are more likely to result from participatory and organically-formed interventions (rather than top-down or targeted) that facilitate marginalized communities reflecting on their approach to health and the connections between structure and agency (Basu, 2010; Basu & Dutta, 2008; Dutta, 2007, 2010; Khan, 2014; Khan et al., 2019; Thaker et al., 2018).

Jana (2012) views community mobilization, particularly in marginalized sex worker communities, as largely a political and dynamic process which generates solidarity, collective bargaining power, and a demand for agency that extends much beyond health as "we cannot expect sex workers to mobilize around HIV concerns alone, as HIV tends to be rather low on their list of priorities" (p. 5). In my study, we found that for participants the unique aspect of *Ashodaya Samithi* was its umbrella feature, in that it addressed a variety of their needs and concerns ranging from their physical, financial, or emotional security to health care access. Moreover, the initiative promoted solidarity in working toward their political and social aspirations as full members of the society. And while at a cursory glance some of the narratives from the participants about *Ashodaya* may almost sound as testimonials for a program or agency, they depict the urgency felt in the sex worker community for an organization that reflects their needs and realities. *Ashodaya* seems to fulfill these needs greatly (even if not perfectly), and members do not want to risk losing this resource.

The participants showed an intense desire not only to gain better health but also to participate in society as respected members, feeling that through *Ashodaya Samithi* they had proven themselves to be responsible citizens and therefore earned social and political recognition. *Ashodaya*, thus, not only performed a protective role for its members but also as a collective, allowing the sex workers to be in a position to negotiate with local officials and entities (lodge owners, police officials, and to hospitals) to receive recognition as a legitimate group with responsibilities (i.e., health service delivery) conventionally under the jurisdiction of the state. Taking up responsibilities like the state (health, cooperative bank, education, etc.), was marginal work but quite central to the work of fighting the HIV epidemic.

Ashodaya, having organically grown within the community and based on local meanings and concerns, offered a comprehensive and meaningful response to HIV by addressing the varied social, economic, and political aspects of their vulnerability to HIV. It also enabled a deep sense of reflexivity among its members that made them think of sex work as a profession (as frequently noted by participants), taking a pride in their role and developing a sense of professionalism or almost an entrepreneurial approach to sex work and collectivization where they see themselves as responsible citizens (who assume responsibility for the health of themselves and others). By being a member of *Ashodaya Samithi,* they have come to realize more broadly the oppressive position in which they have been placed in society, and this realization and community solidarity, in time, turns them into a politically aware (for instance, showing solidarity with sex workers' plight beyond local boundaries) and "responsibilized" political force that is able to assert its own unified politics (as a definable social group with a unified identity) and legitimate social positioning. As some participants noted, just the mere mention of the name, *Ashodaya Samithi,* got police, health care officials, and nearby shop owners to take them respectfully as all of them were aware of *Ashodaya's* broader scope of work. So, while HIV prevention and increased health care access may have gotten the community together, the dynamic process of mobilization (growth in membership and engagement and broader mandate) led them to think of themselves as a politically and culturally viable entity that could challenge and change myriad forms of social oppression facing their disenfranchised group.

References

Alexander, M. J. (1994). Not just (any) body can be a citizen: The politics of law, sexuality and postcoloniality in Trinidad and Tobago and the Bahamas. *Feminist Review, 48,* 5–23. https://doi.org/10.2307/1395166

Atluri, T. (2012). The prerogative of the brave: Hijras and sexual citizenship after orientalism. *Citizenship Studies, 16*(5–6), 721–736. https://doi.org/10.1080/13621025.2012.698496

Basu, A. (2010). Communicating health as an impossibility: Sex work, HIV/AIDS, and the dance of hope and hopelessness. *Southern Communication Journal, 75*(4), 413–432. https://doi.org/10.1080/1041794x.2010.504452

Basu, A. (2011). HIV/AIDS and subaltern autonomous rationality: A call to recenter health communication in marginalized sex worker spaces. *Communication Monograph, 78,* 91–408. https://doi.org/10.1080/03637751.2011.589457

Basu, A. (2017). Reba and her insurgent prose: Sex work, HIV/AIDS, and subaltern narratives. *Qualitative Health Research, 27*(10), 1507–1517. https://doi.org/10.1177/1049732316675589

Basu, A., & Dutta, M. (2008). Participatory change in a campaign led by sex workers: Connecting resistance to action-oriented agency. *Qualitative Health Research, 18,* 106–119. https://doi.org/10.1177/1049732307309373

Basu, A., & Dutta, M. J. (2007). Centralizing context and culture in the co-construction of health: Localizing and vocalizing health meanings in rural India. *Health Communication, 21*(2), 187–196. https://doi.org/10.1080/10410230701305182

Basu, A., & Dutta, M. J. (2011). 'We are mothers first': Localocentric articulation of sex worker identity as a key in HIV/AIDS communication, *Women Health, 51,* 106–123. https://doi.org/10.1080/03630242.2010.550992

Beattie, T. S., Bhattacharjee, P., Ramesh, B. M., Gurnani, V., Anthony, J., Isac, S., Mohan, H. L., Ramakrishnan, A., Wheeler, T., Bradley, J., Blanchard, J. F., & Moses, S. (2010). Violence against female sex workers in

Karnataka state, south India: Impact on health, and reductions in violence following an intervention program. *BMC Public Health, 10*, 476. https://doi.org/10.1186/1471-2458-10-476

Beksinska, A., Prakash, R., Isac, S., Mohan, H. L., Platt, L., Blanchard, J., Moses, S., & Beattie, T. S. (2018). Violence experience by perpetrator and associations with HIV/STI risk and infection: a cross-sectional study among female sex workers in Karnataka, south India. *BMJ Open, 8*, e021389. https://doi.org/10.1136/bmjopen-2017-021389

Bhattacharjee, P., Isac, S., McClarty, L. M., Mohan, H. L., Maddur, S., Jagannath, S. B., Venkataramaiah, B., Moses, S., Blanchard, J., & Gurnani, V. (2016). Strategies for reducing police arrest in the context of an HIV prevention programme for female sex workers: evidence from structural interventions in Karnataka, South India. *Journal of the International AIDS Society, 19* (4 Suppl 3), 20856. https://doi.org/10.7448/IAS.19.4.20856

Bhutada, K., Chakrapani, V., Gulfam, F. R., Ross, J., Golub, S. A., Safren, S. A., Prasad, R., & Patel, V. V. (2023). Pathways between intersectional stigma and HIV Treatment engagement among men who have sex with men (MSM) in India. *Journal of the International Association of Providers of AIDS Care, 22*, 23259582231199398. https://doi.org/10.1177/23259582231199398

Blanchard, A., Nair, S. G., Bruce, S. G., Ramanaik, S., Thalinja, R., Murthy, S., Javalkar, P., Pillai, P., Collumbien, M., Heise, L., Isac, S., & Bhattacharjee, P. (2018). A community-based qualitative study on the experience and understandings of intimate partner violence and HIV vulnerability from the perspectives of female sex workers and male intimate partners in North Karnataka state, India. *BMC Women's Health, 18*(1), 66. https://doi.org/10.1186/s12905-018-0554-8

Braun, V., & Clarke, V. (2012). Thematic analysis. In H. Cooper, P. M. Camic, D. L. Long, A. T. Panter, D. Rindskopf, & K. J. Sher (Eds.), *APA handbook of research methods in psychology*, Vol. 2: *Research designs: quantitative, qualitative, neuropsychological, and biological* (pp. 57–71). American Psychological Association. https://doi.org/10.1037/13620-004

Crotty, M. (1998). *The foundations of social research: Meaning and perspective in the research process*. Sage Publications, Inc. https://doi.org/10.4324/9781003115700

Dutta, A. (2012). Claiming citizenship, contesting civility: The institutional LGBT movement and the regulation of gender/sexual dissidence in West Bengal, India. *Jindal Global Law Review, 4*(1), 110–141.

Dutta, M. J. (2007). Communicating about culture and health: Theorizing culture-centered and cultural sensitivity approaches. *Communication Theory, 17*(3), 304–328. https://doi.org/10.1111/j.1468-2885.2007.00297.x

Dutta, M. J. (2010). The critical cultural turn in health communication: Reflexivity, solidarity, and praxis. *Health Communication, 25*(6–7), 534–539. https://doi.org/10.1080/10410236.2010.497995

Dutta, M. J., & Basu, A. (2011). Culture, communication, and health: A guiding framework. In *The Routledge handbook of health communication* (pp. 346–360). Routledge.

Dutta-Bergman, M. J. (2004). An alternative approach to social capital: Exploring the linkage between health consciousness and community participation. *Health Communication, 16*, 393–409. https://doi.org/10.1207/s15327027hc1604_1

Ekstrand, M. L., Heylen, E., Mazur, A., Steward, W. T., Carpenter, C., Yadav, K., Sinha, S., & Nyamathi, A. (2018). The role of HIV stigma in ART adherence and quality of life among rural women living with HIV in India. *AIDS and Behavior, 22*(12), 3859–3868. https://doi.org/10.1007/s10461-018-2157-7

George, A., Blankenship, K. M., Biradavolu, M. R., Dhungana, N., & Tankasala, N. (2015). Sex workers in HIV prevention: From social change agents to peer educators. *Global Public Health, 10*(1), 28–40. https://doi.org/10.1080/17441692.2014.966251

Ghosh, B. (2022). State, citizenship and gender-variant communities in India, *Citizenship Studies, 26*(2), 127–145. https://doi.org/10.1080/13621025.2021.2024147

Huynh, A., Khan, S., Nair, S., Chevrier, C., Roger, K., Isac, S., Bhattacharjee, P., & Lorway, R. (2018). Intervening in masculinity: Work, relationships and violence among the intimate partners of female sex workers in South India. *Critical Public Health, 29*, 1–12. https://doi.org/10.1080/09581596.2018.1444266

Isin, E. F. (2012). Citizenship after orientalism: An unfinished project. *Citizenship Studies, 16*(5–6), 563–572. https://doi.org/10.1080/13621025.2012.698480

Isin, E. F., & Turner, B. S. (2002). *Handbook of citizenship studies*. SAGE Publications Ltd. https://doi.org/10.4135/9781848608276

Jana, S. (2012). Community mobilisation: myths and challenges. *Journal of Epidemiology and Community Health, 66*(Suppl 2), ii5. https://doi.org/10.1136/jech-2012-201573

Khan, S. (2014). Manufacturing consent?: Media messages in the mobilization against HIV/AIDS in India and lessons for health communication. *Health Communication, 29*(3), 288–298. https://doi.org/10.1080/10410236.2012.753139

Khan, S. (2020). Examining HIV/AIDS-related stigma at play: Power, structure, and implications for HIV interventions. *Health Communication, 35*(12), 1509–1519. https://doi.org/10.1080/10410236.2019.1652386

Khan, S., Lorway, R., Chevrier, C., Dutta, S., Ramanaik, S., Roy, A., Bhattacharjee, P., Misra, S., Moses, S., & Blanchard, J. (2018). Dutiful daughters: HIV/AIDS, moral pragmatics, female citizenship and structural violence among Devadasis in northern Karnataka, India. *Global Public Health, 13*(8), 1065–1080. https://doi.org/10.1080/17441692.2017.1280070

Khan, S., Lorway, R., O'Neil, J., Pasha, A., & Reza-Paul, S. (2019). Health communication and citizenship among sex workers in Mysore, India: Beyond "centers" and "margins". *Frontiers in Communication, 4*(62). https://doi.org/10.3389/FCOMM.2019.00062

Kligler-Vilenchik, N. (2017). Alternative citizenship models: Contextualizing new media and the new "good citizen". *New Media & Society, 19*(11), 1887–1903. https://doi.org/10.1177/1461444817713742

Lorway, R., & Khan, S. (2014). Reassembling epidemiology: Mapping, monitoring and making-up people in the context of HIV prevention in India. *Social Science & Medicine (1982), 112*, 51–62. https://doi.org/10.1016/j.socscimed.2014.04.034

National AIDS Control Organisation (2023). *Sankalak: Status of national AIDS & STD response* (5th ed.).

Navarrete Gil, C., Ramaiah, M., Mantsios, A., Barrington, C., & Kerrigan, D. (2021). Best practices and challenges to sex worker community empowerment and mobilisation strategies to promote health and human rights. In S. M.

Goldenberg et al. (Eds.), *Sex work, health, and human rights: Global inequities, challenges, and opportunities for action.* (pp. 189–206). Springer.

Nordberg, C. (2006). Claiming citizenship: Marginalised voices on identity and belonging. *Citizenship Studies, 10*(5), 523–539. https://doi.org/10.1080/13621020600954952

Paz, A. I. (2019). Communicating citizenship. *Annual Review of Anthropology, 48*(1), 77–93. https://doi.org/10.1146/annurev-anthro-102317-050031

Platt, L., Grenfell, P., Meiksin, R., Elmes, J., Sherman, S. G., Sanders, T., Mwangi, P., & Crago, A. L. (2018). Associations between sex work laws and sex workers' health: A systematic review and meta-analysis of quantitative and qualitative studies. *PLoS Med, 15*(12), e1002680. https://doi.org/10.1371/journal.pmed.1002680

Reza-Paul, S., Lorway, R., O'Brien, N., Lazarus, L., Jain, J., Bhagya, M., Fathima, M. P., Venukumar, K. T., Raviprakash, K. N., Baer, J., & Steen, R. (2012). Sex worker-led structural interventions in India: a case study on addressing violence in HIV prevention through the *Ashodaya Samithi* collective in Mysore. *Indian Journal of Medical Research, 135*, 98–106. https://doi.org/10.4103/0971-5916.93431

Sabsay, L. (2012). The emergence of the other sexual citizen: Orientalism and the modernisation of sexuality. *Citizenship Studies, 16*, 605–623. https://doi.org/10.1080/13621025.2012.698484

Stavinoha, L. (2019). Communicative acts of citizenship: Contesting Europe's border in and through the media. *International Journal of Communication, 13*, 1212–1230.

Thaker, J., Dutta, M., Nair, V., & Rao, V. P. (2018). The interplay between stigma, collective efficacy, and advocacy communication among men who have sex with men and transgender females. *Journal of Health Communication, 23*(7), 614–623. https://doi.org/10.1080/10810730.2018.1499833

Thomas, J. (2003). Musings on critical ethnography, meanings, and symbolic violence. In R. Clair (Ed.), *Expressions of ethnography: Novel approaches to qualitative methods* (pp. 45–54). State University of New York Press.

UNAIDS. (2009). UNAIDS Executive Director joins Chief Minister to launch Learning Site on HIV and sex work in Bangalore, India. October 12. Retrieved from: https://www.unaids.org/en/resources/presscentre/featurestories/2009/october/20091012bangalore

UNAIDS. (2019). *Communities at the centre: Defending rights, breaking barriers, reaching people with HIV services.* Retrieved from: https://www.unaids.org/en/resources/documents/2019/2019-global-AIDS-update

UNAIDS. (2023). *The path that ends AIDS: UNAIDS Global AIDS Update 2023.* Joint United Nations Programme on HIV/AIDS.

Underwood, E. D., & Frey, L. R. (2007). Communication and community: Clarifying the connection across the communication community. *Annals of the International Communication Association, 31*(1), 370–418. https://doi.org/10.1080/23808985.2007.11679071

Zoller, H. M. (2005). Health activism: Communication theory and action for social change. *Communication Theory, 15*(4), 341–364. https://doi.org/10.1111/j.1468-2885.2005.tb00339.x

8
NAVIGATING THE TERRAIN

Applying Critical Health Communication Methods to Participatory Action Praxis with Black Women Farmers

Andrew Carter

> *"Black women have solutions to poverty issues"*
> *"President Biden help us as we helped you"*
> *"America acts as if Black women don't exist"*
> *"Black children deserve sustainable life skill opportunities in agriculture"*
> *"No NWIAA, no Black farmers"*

These slogans were just a few of the several dozen signs that were printed and distributed to those in attendance on September 21, 2023 for the National Women in Agriculture Association's (NWIAA) "Equity and Inclusion" protest march in Washington, D.C. The marchers were flanked by a police escort and made stops for demonstrations at Capitol Hill, Department of Agriculture headquarters, and the White House. Participants represented leadership from the organization's 70+ national and international chapters in addition to various state policymakers and community activists. The primary goal of the "Equity and Inclusion" march was to generate public support for NWIAA's proposal to become a congressionally chartered organization and serve as a pilot program of 4-H (a U.S.-based network of organizations that develop citizenship, leadership, responsibility, and life skills of youth through experiential learning and a positive youth development approach) for Black youth in agriculture. In the organization's 15+ years of advocating for Black women farmers, this was the closest they had come to realizing their goal of securing sustainable government funding.

To date, NWIAA is one of the largest non-profits for Black women in agriculture nationally and incorporates a life-course perspective by

DOI: 10.4324/9781003426530-10
This chapter has been made available under a CC BY-NC-ND license.

connecting farming disparities to broader inequities in the food system. The organization is headquartered in Oklahoma City in the United States and comprises approximately 45,000 members across the United States, Caribbean, and Africa. I have collaborated with NWIAA since September 2021 as the academic partner in an academic-community partnership to highlight the lived experiences of its members and chapter leaders and serve as a political ally in its quest for policy change. This work aligns with my broader decade-long research agenda exploring how Black farmers challenge power inequities and structural barriers in agriculture occupations, in order to preserve their cultural legacies and address broader Black social and public health inequities. A throughline connecting this research is my use of critical methodologies and identity as a critical health communication (CHC) scholar-activist. In this chapter, I document my use of critical methods with NWIAA to center participant voices and interrogate power imbalances and political tensions when developing community solutions. I illuminate my findings through the lens of four conceptual anchors of the culture-centered approach (CCA) (i.e., participation, communication infrastructures, partnerships, and reflexivity; Dutta, 2018). This chapter contributes important insights and takeaways for practitioners seeking to develop and strengthen CHC partnerships and intervention models.

Context: Black Health and Farming Disparities

Black communities in the United States are disproportionately impacted by food system-generated health inequities (Odoms-Young & Bruce, 2018). In 2022, nearly 23% of Black individuals were considered food insecure. Black communities also experience food access disparities. According to the United States Department of Agriculture (USDA) Food Environment Atlas (2020), roughly one in five Black households resided in census tracts classified as food deserts. Diet-related chronic conditions, such as diabetes, hypertension, cardiovascular disease, certain cancers, all disproportionately impact Black individuals in comparison to their white counterparts (Abrahamowicz et al., 2023; Niakouei et al., 2020). While public health trends have shifted away from individual-level cause-and-effect rationale models to include social and structural determinants of health such as employment, housing, and built environment (Brown et al., 2019; Dankwa-Mullan et al., 2010), one potentially overlooked contributor to these inequities is the communicative erasure of the Black farming tradition and associated cultural foodways within mainstream discourses (Lunsford et al., 2021).

Black farming inequities in the U.S. trace back several decades (Hinson & Robinson, 2008). Since 1920, Black farmers have experienced significant land loss, with rates of nearly 50% every ten years, almost tripling the percentage of white farmers during the same period (Grant et al., 2012). Today, Black farmers account for less than 2% of the nation's farmers (48,697 producers) (USDA Natural Agricultural Statistics Service (NASS) 2017a). Black-operated farms represent just 0.5% of U.S. farmland (4.7 million acres), 0.4% of total agriculture sales ($1.4 billion), and are disproportionately small scale in comparison to white farms (USDA NASS, 2017a). Black farmers are particularly vulnerable to climate change impacts and have low political power to advocate for policies that support climate resilience (Akamani, 2021).

For Black women farmers, the current landscape is even bleaker. Despite record numbers of female farmers entering the agricultural industry over the past decade, most are white (95%; 1.1% Black, respectively; USDA NASS, 2017b) and non-operating landowners (513,000 white, 22,000 People-of-Color, respectively; Horst & Marion, 2019), reflecting marked disparities in access to inherited land and wealth and credit to purchase land. Several factors have contributed to this disparity, including prohibitive policy legislation (e.g., patriarchal and racist inheritance laws; Pilgeram et al., 2022), legacies of structural discrimination (e.g., 1999 Pigford v. Glickman USDA class action lawsuit settlement [Hinson & Robinson, 2008]), and combined racialized and gendered capitalism (e.g., land ownership disparities; Horst & Marion, 2019).

The eradication of Black women farmers represents more than a mere statistic or data footnote. These absences symbolize erasure of a rich cultural legacy responsible for upholding several Black sovereignty and community food security movements throughout history and linking together women's shared diasporic political legacies and agricultural contributions (Layman & Civita, 2022). The multigenerational advocacy efforts of NWIAA are situated within this context.

Why a Critical Communication Approach to Studying Food System-Generated Crises?

Against the backdrop of enduring social crises, including climate change, racial injustice, unfair labor practices, and pandemic outbreaks, among others, increased mainstream and scholarly attention has been given to how we collectively organize society and allocate resources (Alkon et al., 2020; Chancel, 2020). In the context of food systems, prevalent public health issues like food access and insecurity, increasing chronic disease rates, and environmental degradation are a result of structural injustices (e.g., food apartheid, cultural erasure of local food practices and meanings) that disproportionately impact communities of color and other marginalized groups (Gist-Mackey & Dougherty, 2023; Hunt, 2023). To meaningfully address these challenges requires innovative approaches that incorporate knowledge and theoretical models from non-dominant sectors and disciplines.

Until recently, communication research has not featured in these conversations, often being marginally positioned as a strategic tool of message dissemination by top-down knowledge brokers, such as the National Science Foundation, National Institutes of Health, and the Bill and Melinda Gates Foundation (Canfield, 2022). Consider Mohan Dutta's commentary in a 2020 research forum article in the *Journal of Applied Communication Research* on how scientists traditionally incorporate communication theory in development science and agriculture contexts.

> The development of the science of communication...has been centered on creating message dissemination frameworks that would diffuse the innovations/interventions created by scientists... In the context of food insecurity, it is the scientists that do the thinking and the communicators then come in to disseminate the accurate science to the audience based on the latest techniques/technologies of communication.
> *(Schraedley et al., 2020, p. 9)*

While this orientation persists in mainstream knowledge production enterprises, critical communication research increasingly views food systems not merely as platforms for message dissemination but as inherently communicative entities intertwined with political and power dynamics that "transect human and natural systems" and manifest "environments, social structures, and lived conditions, in fundamentally uneven ways" (Gordon et al., 2022, p. 2). Past studies in this domain have investigated the intersection of power, inequity, and communication across a variety of topics and contexts (see for example Clause, 2021; de Souza, 2019; Gordon et al., 2020; Zoller, 2024). These studies offer a critical foundation for exploring how food systems perpetuate structural communicative inequities that generate social, environmental, and public health risks. The methodological case study featured in this paper builds on this important critical work.

My Critical Orientation

I draw on varying critical lenses and methods as a primary compass for exploring issues of power and inequity in food systems across multiple ecological levels. For example, in my research exploring food access and alternative food networks in Memphis, Tennessee, I incorporated the theoretical and methodological underpinnings of nexus analysis (Scollon &

Scollon, 2007), a historical-ethnographic critical discourse analysis, to connect individual stories and everyday practices of patrons at two local farmers markets with distinct cultural histories to Memphis's racial history, food economy, and socio-spatial construction. At the level of food policy, Adele Hite and I employed rhetorical methods to adapt stasis theory to examine the embedded, ideological nature of scientific claims underpinning U.S. public health nutrition policy (see Hite & Carter, 2019). My research agenda has primarily centered on food production disparities and their impact on food access at the individual and community levels. Some of my research projects exploring African, Caribbean, and Black (ACB)[1] farming inequities in the United States (Carter & Alexander, 2020; Carter et al., 2024) and internationally (Carter, 2023) have incorporated various axioms of the CCA (Dutta, 2008).

The CCA is a useful lens for foregrounding ACB farmer experiences and connecting food production disparities to broader inequities in the food system, as it prioritizes resistance against dominant knowledge forms shaping policies and communication theories, centers local perspectives for culturally relevant solutions, and explores communication erasure within broader ecological contexts. In the section below, I overview CCA's philosophical underpinnings and outline its four conceptual anchors.

The Culture-Centered Approach to Health Communication

The CCA is a methodological and theoretical framework for foregrounding the local experiences, perspectives, and practices of marginalized communities. The CCA has critical foundations in subaltern and postcolonial studies (Fanon, 1963; Spivak, 1988). Conceptualized in opposition to "top-down" health communication approaches agendas that are often controlled by outside "experts" and center post-positivist knowledge as universal in constructing health problems and interventions, CCA prioritizes mutual dialogue with community members to interpret, communicate, and address health issues. Fundamentally, the CCA is a critical endeavor, in that:

> it is expressly concerned with identifying and mitigating asymmetries of power and control within spaces of knowledge production that are related to health inequalities, the loss of health status, and the concomitant erasure of the voices and agendas of marginalized communities across the globe.
>
> *(Sastry et al., 2021)*

The CCA is guided by the dynamic interplay between three central concepts: culture, structure, and agency (C-S-A).[2] In his article outlining CCA's methodological "nuts and bolts," Dutta (2018) built upon the C-S-A triad to introduce a typology of four conceptual anchors.[3] These anchors, including participation, communication infrastructures, partnerships, and reflexivity, serve as methodological tools to interrogate structural forms of communicative erasure and center subaltern voices into mainstream hegemonic spaces. Despite the wide range of interdisciplinary CCA research, this project is one of the first to directly apply its four conceptual anchors in this way. Below, I outline each anchor in more detail.

Participation. CCA builds on community-based participatory research (CBPR) that adopts power-sharing strategies to address health disparities by centering voice, lived experience, and the cultural context of local communities in understanding health problems and articulating solutions (Airhihenbuwa, 1995; Dutta, 2008). While there are widespread debates about what "counts" as authentic participation in community-based research contexts, a defining feature of CCA from other participatory methods is its focus on culture as the primary focus of research. CCA takes culture as an entry point for constructing locally grounded theoretical models of participation that emphasize community assets, resource identification, and partnership cultivation (Yehya & Dutta, 2010). The CCA also incorporates participatory action research principles in that researchers actively engage in participation and activist activities with the community through collaborative and iterative processes (Baum et al., 2006; Dillard et al., 2018).

Partnerships. The CCA underscores the significance of partnerships between marginalized communities and external stakeholders with access to power, aiming to effect change within dominant structures. CCA methodologies prioritize community expertise, initiating problem-solving through community-led identification and theoretical mapping, rather than using community input merely as formative data for future interventions, as many dominant public health models do. Through iterative communication processes and dynamic academic-community and other external partnerships, the CCA methodologically addresses community-specific needs, fosters solidarity-based relationships, and advocates for subaltern voices within dominant power structures.

Communication infrastructures. The CCA empowers marginalized communities to participate in decision-making and knowledge creation processes by creating access to alternative infrastructures that exist outside of dominant communication frameworks. Alternative communication infrastructures can be either discursive (e.g., community-led advocacy campaigns, PhotoVoice, community performances, community podcasts, digital story telling) or material (e.g., physical locations such as temples and churches, community and village spaces, and local health fairs), and work to resist structural inequity and foster community agency by centering subaltern voices into mainstream discourse (see Bradford & Dutta, 2018; Elers et al., 2021; Jenkins, 2014; York & Tang, 2021).

Reflexivity. Reflexivity within the CCA involves critically examining inherent power dynamics that emerge within academic-community collaborations—acknowledging the unequal distribution of power both within communities and between academics and community members (Dutta, 2018). Awareness of these power dynamics is essential for fostering genuine community participation in knowledge generation processes, ensuring that community agendas are not co-opted by expert-driven agendas. By making power dynamics visible, reflexivity enables communities to question and hold accountable the structures of power shaping decision-making processes (Dutta & de Souza, 2008). Academic partners must remain mindful of their own positionalities and the influence of power in shaping what is considered knowledge and best practice, fostering an environment where community voices shape the definition of knowledge. Ongoing reflexive processes work to democratize knowledge production, challenge unequal power structures, and create opportunities for meaningful community participation and shared meaning-making (Dutta, 2008).

Applying CCA's Four Conceptual Anchors to My Critical Research Processes

In this section, I employ CCA's four conceptual anchors as articulated by Dutta (2018) as a guiding heuristic to document my critical research process with NWIAA. The featured case study details examples of how I actively participated with the organization and interrogated my positionality throughout the research process, drawing attention to some of the tensions and power gaps that emerge in academic-community partnerships. Additionally, the conceptual anchors provide a critical framework for centering participant voice in articulating NWIAA's resistance and mobilization strategies, particularly through cultivating partnerships with external stakeholders and developing alternative communication infrastructures.

Participation: Dialogue and Solidarity

Given the activist and applied nature of action research, participation is a vital process for researchers to better understand emic contexts and perspectives of in-group members and foster support in co-constructing local community participation theories. In this section, I document examples of how I participated with NWIAA through the scope of our academic-community partnership.

From a participatory action research context, I engaged with NWIAA since September 2021 in a scholar-activist capacity, serving multiple roles such as political ally (e.g., giving testimony on behalf of the organization at the White House), advisor (e.g., providing feedback on press releases, grant applications), and community partner (e.g., connecting NWIAA with other stakeholders) over the course of our three-year collaboration. In order to foreground NWIAA chapter leader and member voices and lived experiences, I drew from critical data collection methods including ethnography, community-level and stakeholder in-depth interviews, and advisory group discussions (Dutta, 2018).

Dialogue between researchers and the community is a core methodological tool for developing local participation theories (Dutta & Pal, 2010). One theoretical frame that emerged from my community dialogues with NWIAA stakeholders was *internal recognition*, which participants described as an important community asset for navigating race and gender-based challenges resulting from their unique social position. Many participants described this approach as a primary reason for joining NWIAA. As Black women, they often were not taken seriously for their agricultural skill and leadership capacities in dominant agricultural spaces—repeatedly describing instances of being ignored or left out of important USDA funding opportunities, Census of Agriculture reports, and farm conferences and other industry gatherings. Given that dominant communication platforms have largely erased Black women's voice and political agency from the modern agricultural landscape, NWIAA acts as an enclave to navigate hyper-racialized and gendered spaces, build social support and trust networks, and recapture cultural food and farming legacies.

Participant narratives identified how NWIAA fostered *internal recognition* as a way for them to remain encouraged to farm, receive consistent support, instill self-empowerment, and feel seen and valued as leaders. As noted by a U.S. South chapter leader (member three to five years), "… when it comes to NWIAA, they actually sit down with you, understand your value, and maximize your potential by utilizing you for the value that you've presented." Participant narratives reinforced interdisciplinary justice scholars who have underscored the value of recognition as a requisite condition of justice across diverse social and political contexts (Taylor, 1994). MacKinnon and Derickson (2013) define recognition as promoting "a sense of confidence, self-worth and self- and community-affirmation that can be drawn upon to fuel the mobilization of existing resources and argue for and pursue new resources" (p. 265).

CCA also promotes building solidarity with local communities by "walking alongside the margins" and "being there" amid struggles for social change (Dutta et al., 2019, p. 4). One example of how I fostered solidarity with NWIAA was in November 2023, when the leadership team met with White House administration staffers to discuss their proposal to become a congressionally chartered organization and pilot a 4-H program for Black youth in agriculture. I was invited to share my communication expertise as a consultant to help them strategize key talking points, press release content, and presentation materials. The leadership team also asked me to provide testimony about the organization on their behalf during the meeting, where I discussed the extent of our academic-community partnership and shared published scholarship based on this work. The White House meeting led to additional discussions with other offices and Congresspeople to levy political support (e.g., co-sponsoring their "Equity and Inclusion" bill), which is where the deliberations currently stand in 2024.

Communication Infrastructures: Developing Alternatives and Infiltrating the Mainstream

Central to making subaltern communities visible to the mainstream is gaining access to alternative infrastructures for participation in knowledge creation (Estrada et al., 2018). Examples such as community-led media channels, advocacy campaigns, and local performances serve as spaces where historically disenfranchised voices can disrupt marginalizing structures and re-shape cultural narratives (Pavarala & Malik, 2021). In this section, I critically document how NWIAA built community capacity by investing in alternative communication infrastructures.

Scene: National Women in Agriculture Association's 15th Year Anniversary

The NWIAA's 15th year anniversary conference and farm expo took place on February 21–22, 2023. The two-day event was meant to celebrate the organization's quindecennial year and bring together chapter leaders from its 70+ locations in the United States, U.S. Virgin Islands, and Africa. The event included a panel of retired NBA, WNBA, and NFL athletes who started second careers as agricultural entrepreneurs, officers from the USDA Foreign Agriculture Services and U.S. Agency for International Development, and remarks from Oklahoma state legislators, U.S. Congresspeople, and members of the House Committee on Agriculture. Over 200 people attended the conference. During the expo, participants shared updates on their local operations and engaged in networking and fellowship across chapters. For attendees, the 15th anniversary symbolized a form of resistance that centered local knowledge and fostered a dialogic space for contesting existing power relations.

NWIAA created alternative communication infrastructures that were accessible to its members. For example, to combat members' perceptions that they were ignored when reaching out individually to food and agriculture administrators, NWIAA brought resources and support from top-down entities directly to its stakeholders. In 2023, when the National Black Farmers Association wanted to promote workshops highlighting the $2.2 billion Inflation Reduction Act class action discrimination lawsuit, they sought out NWIAA chapter leaders to host, knowing their trusted role in the Black farming community. In 2024, NWIAA chapter leaders hosted virtual "Resource and Equity" summits for local communities where live USDA and NRCS representatives answered questions and provided information.

Other NWIAA alternative communication infrastructures, such as their monthly (virtual) chapter leader meetings, the mobile app (a public platform to provide updates about the organization), the "Women in Ag Wednesdays" talk show (a YouTube show featuring interviews with leading Black women in agriculture), and social media channels fostered community agency, allowing the women's voices to infiltrate dominant discursive spaces. In the excerpt below, a newer Nigerian chapter leader described how NWIAA's alternative infrastructures "opened up" discursive sites for ACB women farmers at the margins:

> That is one of the benefits of [NWIAA] collaboration, it brings women together to collaborate…You talk to women. You're getting to see information, good information on how you can do your thing if it did not work this way, good information. That information, when it comes to me, I pass it down to the grassroot farmer because that's really my aim. I just want the minority farmers to be included in whatever the government is doing, in whatever we are doing, so that it can make money for the farmer and it can be impactful in their community.

Given the activist nature of participatory action research, the researcher-as-interlocutor also plays an important role in helping the community bring collective voice to dominant communication platforms. In this way, I brought our collaborative research to mainstream platforms across diverse disciplines, sectors, and audiences. For example, I gave presentations on this work at leading U.S. academic departments, including Princeton University's Department of Politics, UCLA's Fielding School of Public Health, NYU's Grossman School of Medicine, Stanford

University School of Medicine, and California State University Long Beach's College of Health and Human Services. I also shared my published research with White House administration staffers and with audiences from the Environmental Protection Agency and National Fish and Wildlife Foundation. Publicly, I have written Op-Eds that feature this work in national outlets *Newsweek* and *The Hill*. These efforts represent a first step in infiltrating dominant knowledge platforms by centering the women's stories. For example, many of the spaces where I presented my research were considered Historically White Colleges and Universities (HWCUs) and housed in departments that privileged top-down, positivist assumptions of science (Bonilla-Silva & Peoples, 2022). Often during the Q+A portion of my talks, many attendees expressed shock that Black women were actively doing this work with the potential to meaningfully impact public health interventions.

Partnerships: From Grassroots to Grasstops

Developing partnerships with external stakeholders with access to power is crucial for marginalized groups to drive change and resist oppression. NWIAA incorporated a multi-level approach to partnership development, combining grassroots (bottom-up, collective community-level mobilizing) and grasstops (i.e., top-down outreach via targeted decision makers) advocacy efforts (Grefe, 1997). Below, I critically document some of these strategies as they emerged throughout the research process.

Scene: Research Site Visit to NWIAA's Virgin Islands Chapter

In June 2023, I traveled to St. Croix in the U.S. Virgin Islands to conduct an ethnographic study of the region's food system and collaborate with the NWIAA USVI leadership team. As a U.S. territory with a history of structural discrimination, I aimed to understand how local agricultural practices compared to the broader U.S. food system. I visited 12 farms varying in size and scope, from a family growing vegetables on a porch using pottery and recycled materials to a landowner who had recently purchased 100+ acres rife with different fruit and vegetable varietals. The stark contrasts in farm size and operations mirrored the inequalities within U.S. food production, where abundance and subsistence often fall along race and gender lines.

In addition to learning more about the Crucian food system, a primary goal of my visit was to attend the inaugural meeting of the Virgin Islands Women in Agriculture Association (VIWIAA), a newly created farm advocacy collective. Held at the St. George Botanical Gardens in Frederiksted,

I facilitated a Round Robin discussion to learn more about the members' backgrounds, their lived experiences as agriculturalists, and perceived connections with the U.S. food system.

VIWIAA's inauguration is reflective of the multi-level strategies that lie at the heart of NWIAA's partnership model. Many participants discussed searching in the "proverbial dark" for other ACB women to quell their feelings of isolation and reinforce their resolve to continue farming. NWIAA's key strength in forging external partnerships lay in its ability to form "weak tie" connections with ACB women from diverse communities beyond its direct member network (Granovetter, 1983). Often the mere bringing of women together galvanized the participants to seek out of other partnerships and opportunities, even with a scarcity of power and resources.

Many of the participants mentioned the various collaborations and partnerships they made through informal, casual interconnections outside of their main social networks. The excerpt below demonstrates an example of how participants' involvement with the organization created new opportunities for them to merge weak ties with their own initiatives.

> Just recently, last week, I've been invited to be a keynote speaker at Blue Ridge Women in Ag Association Conference. And they found me through National Women in Ag Facebook—I mean, through their page. And so that right there is huge. So when [NWIAA] put us out there representing the organization, then, I mean, that goes back to making those outreach connections because Blue Ridge—they're in the mountains, Boone, North Carolina. So being able to be seen and heard by your peers that look like you is huge.
> *(US South Chapter leader, member 3–5 years)*

Other participants described partnering their own organizations with NWIAA, either formally or informally, to support shared facilities or services, leverage external resources, and share new knowledge and practices. Below, a U.S. South chapter leader (member for three to five years) provided context into the extent of such partnerships:

> Usually, we do site visits together. I've invited [NWIAA] to different farms for us to harvest different things together. They've invited me to different farms to harvest things together. We initiated the West End Farmers Market, which historically, the West End is a very crime-ridden area. But prior to that, it was a historic area because Martin Luther King and all of his friends would be over there. And so we reinitiated a farmers' market over there.

In addition to grassroots community-level partnerships, NWIAA built grasstops partnerships with political stakeholders, including leadership at the USDA, NRCS, and local, state, and national policymakers. Particularly in the context of their mission to becoming the first chartered Black organization, NWIAA developed important grasstops partnerships with White House and Congressional leaders in support of their "Equity and Inclusion" pilot proposal.

Reflexivity: Positionality, Legitimacy, and Power Tensions

Reflexivity involves continuously engaging in internal dialogue and self-evaluating one's positionality and the extent to which it impacts the research process (Seubert et al., 2023). Reflexivity is a key component for identifying power inequities in academic-community partnerships (Minkler, 2005). In this section, I reflexively interrogate some of the power imbalances and political tensions that emerged during my field experiences.

Entrée: Reflecting on Positionality When Establishing Academic Community-Based Partnerships

As NWIAA and I developed our academic-community partnership, I constantly reflected on power flows in our interactions and the extent to which I was, conscientiously or not, upholding and/or resisting top-down assumptions and cultural logics. As someone trained as a community health scientist who works in an academic department of public health, I was intimately aware of the insidious histories of cultural co-optation, erasure, and violence on local communities under the guise of altruistic, well-intentioned public health participatory campaigns. From this standpoint, I clarified my role with NWIAA as community partner, using my communication training to bring attention to the participants' hidden and erased stories, not co-opt them. Particularly since NWIAA had been engaging in this work since 2008, it was clear that they had the requisite expertise and foundational knowledge to understand and develop their own solutions. What they needed was access to mainstream communication platforms to disseminate and normalize their message. I contributed my journalism training to draft/edit press releases, speech transcripts, correspondence emails, grant proposals, in addition to "power-sharing" by providing access to dominant communication platforms and helping craft *their* rhetorically persuasive messages to external stakeholders. Interventions such as sustainable funding via the "Equity and Inclusion" bill were exclusively grounded in community logics and contexts (e.g., what the intervention should comprise, what types of knowledge "count," how stakeholders should allocate resources).

Navigating "Legitimacy" Discourses

Reflexivity illuminates who has power and how it embeds in the production of knowledge (Alexander et al., 2020; Wallerstein et al., 2019). One inequitable power gap that persisted across our academic-community partnership centered on taken-for-granted assumptions around who was seen (and who saw themselves) as legitimate and an expert. Participants' multiple marginalized positionalities as Black women often led to their expertise being relegated to the margins.[4] For example, a U.S. South chapter leader noted "we just don't think people are really listening to us when we go to talk to them and not taking seriously what we are saying to them about what we're trying to do as National Women in Ag."

I was often asked by the NWIAA leadership team to serve as a power broker to help them foster legitimacy in top-down spaces. For instance, when the team conducted outreach efforts with policymakers in strategizing their protest march and White House meeting, I was asked to reach out to them because, as noted by a team member, "these type of people take men and people with degrees more seriously." During the White House meeting and other stakeholder visits, the executive team referenced the name of academic publishers that housed my work and noted some of the institutions where I had previously given talks as a rhetorical strategy for fostering agency and legitimacy.

For organizational leadership, the process of navigating such discourses presented a quandary of sorts—despite wanting to resist hegemonic assumptions of expertise, their perceived survival required that they work within existing structural figurations. Much of the "legitimacy discourses" referenced above have foundational roots in predominately white institutions (e.g., U.S. agriculture system, elite academic universities and publishers), which have historically de-centered (and erased) the voices and lived experiences of Black communities (Zuberi & Bonilla-Silva, 2008). To combat this hegemony, I reflexively interrogated the communication processes between the organization, its external stakeholders, and myself, often declining opportunities to speak on the organization's behalf and carving out discursive spaces for them to center their voice. For example, when giving a keynote talk at Princeton University, I invited the organization's executive director and several of its members to join virtually and invited them to lead the Q+A section of the presentation. This action simultaneously provided a space for the community to share their stories and build legitimacy toward my work for the audience in attendance.

Tensions between CHC Training and Community Epistemological, Ontological, Ideological Context

As CBPR methods become more popular, recent attention has been given to the tensions and ethical dimensions that emerge from such collaborations (Jamshidi et al., 2014). Rooted assumptions in CBPR include an emphasis on social justice, community collaboration, and an activist orientation to research. CHC practitioners build on these principles to adopt a more explicit focus on power by incorporating critical theory in interrogating how meanings of health are tied to structural power inequities (Zoller & Kline, 2008). To date, most CHC projects document how critical analysis can be used to amplify community voices; though less attention is dedicated to situations when community partners reject or do not align with the values of the research team (see Zoller, 2019).

NWIAA adopted an "any means necessary" approach to advocacy in its willingness to partner with whoever would vouch for and support their cause, regardless of identity or political affiliation. Several instances emerged during our partnership where I had to navigate discordances between my scholarly and ethical CHC orientation and the lived realities and ideological presuppositions of the community.

In one instance, I was approached at an advocacy event to introduce and draft written remarks from a former Congressperson whose political ideologies I recognized as creating harm for marginalized communities. This individual had significant political sway with the USDA and other stakeholders on Capitol Hill. In navigating this tension, I realized that if I agreed to the request, I may have been seen as passively supporting the individual politically. As a junior faculty without tenure and a public advocate for Black farmers, I refused the request as it would have comprised my personal values and was too risky professionally. Micro-level negotiations such as this are often overlooked in CBPR projects that do not consider the multiple power relationships at play in addition to the researcher's own positionality.

Another navigable tension during our partnership emerged from some of the participants' philosophical orientation to advocacy, which often involved supporting top-down, neoliberal policies and rejecting traditional notions of solidarity and Black feminism. For instance, some of the chapter leaders sought alliances with policymakers who were anti-liberation and whose voting records upheld racist and patriarchal platforms in their quest to receive bipartisan support for their pilot proposal. Relatedly, some participants rejected traditional Black feminist ideals, citing ideological discordances and concerns with being viewed as hostile. For example:

> ...Black women that are in leadership positions, as well as Black men and white women. Those are the three primary groups that I have the

most barrier issues with. The ones that I have okay or true partnership help are, again, back to the Caucasian males. They usually accept us, help us understand this, listen to us because, again, they're business people. Their mind is constantly thinking, 'Oh, this is big money. This is a big move. This is going to-- I'm satisfying the government needs of making sure minorities are connected, and I have big numbers'.
 - *(US South Central Chapter Leader, member 9 or more years)*

Because I don't like to think that woman is a minority or something. I don't feel women are. That's not how I really go about my day like, 'Yeah. F the patriarch.' Nah. [laughter] I'm not a feminist or one of those things.
 - *(USVI member, member 0–2 years)*

In managing these tensions, I took a cultural relativist approach to the study context, understanding that it was my job as a critical-qualitative researcher to tell a holistic account across participant experiences by connecting their on-the-ground narratives to broader structural conditions. Specifically, I understood their advocacy approach as a means of survival to foster agency within an oppressive system and took a critical approach when documenting my scholarly findings (e.g., connecting participant white legitimacy logic appeals to broader patriarchal and racist structures in agriculture). Conversely, NWIAA leadership did not identify these tensions and were not discussed during the scope of our partnership.

These above examples demonstrate how reflexive engagement can illuminate hidden tensions and power gaps that persist in academic-community partnerships. By documenting the nuances of when and how power manifests throughout the research process, reflexivity can amend both top-down models that frame the interventionist as "expert" and community as a passive, voiceless, marginalized group, and romanticized emancipatory models that assume full agency to the community that do not account for disagreement or incongruencies between parties. As a note, NWIAA is a deeply liberatory and social justice-oriented organization—the individual-level perspectives and strategies communicated to me and others were important to document the diversity of community member conceptualizations of power and mobilizing strategy, highlighting how collective community voice is rarely monolithic and often contradictory.

Discussion and Conclusion

This chapter documented how I used critical methods at various stages of the research process with NWIAA to demonstrate the utility of such frameworks to community-based research projects. By applying CCA's four conceptual anchors to the methodological case study, I highlighted the organization's multi-level advocacy and communication strategies, and reflexively identified power imbalances and political tensions that emerged in our academic-community partnership. The case study contributes to interdisciplinary scholarship documenting the applicability of the critical paradigm to strengthen community partnerships and develop more effective health communication intervention models.

One of the central contributions of this chapter highlights the complexities and tensions that come with "doing" collaborative, on-the-ground advocacy work with local communities. Much CHC and critical public health scholarship focuses on the activist and "power-sharing" dimensions of participatory action research and emphasizes the grounded theoretical and formative stages of the research process (e.g., listening, problem definition, interpretation). Researcher reflexivity often considers how academics limit their privilege and power in community partnerships, with the assumption that power flows in a linear direction. While useful for centering subaltern voices and theorizing local participatory processes, this research does not always examine the multiple and dynamic power relations that the researcher must juggle across *other* external stakeholders. Throughout my analysis, I referenced several examples of when I had to reflexively negotiate assumptions of community legitimacy and expertise with diverse groups (e.g., White House aides, academic audiences). In each instance, power negotiations were not neutral and shifted depending on the context. For example, during the White House meeting, I was asked to speak on behalf of the organization and provide scholarly evidence of my work to prove *NWIAA's* legitimacy and lend voice to their experiences; conversely, during my Princeton talk, having the executive director and members of the organization present built a legitimacy and authenticity for *my* community-based research agenda among academic colleagues. These examples underscore the multi-directional and fluid nature of power in academic community contexts and the extent to which it may influence the process and outcomes of CHC research.

The findings also highlighted some of the nuanced power gaps and philosophical discordances that emerged between NWIAA and my training and positionality as a CHC scholar. As described above, most CHC research emphasizes social justice principles and critical theory to make power gaps transparent and center marginalized voices. Yet there is limited work exploring these differences as they emerge in academic-community partnerships across epistemological, ontological, and ideological contexts (Jamshidi et al., 2014). For example, many of the participants rejected certain components of Black feminism as they sought legitimacy from external stakeholders within existing hegemonic power structures, interpreting them as a way for external power brokers to mark them as Other and dismiss their knowledge. Specifically, participants described not wanting to be "seen as a troublemaker" or inferior by political leaders. Such perspectives do not align with critically oriented traditions such as Black feminist thought (Collins, 2022), a theoretical framework that centers ACB women's unique standpoint and positionality and critiques politics of assimilation. To navigate these discordances, I took a cultural relativist approach to understand participants' stories on their own terms, with a specific focus on documentation and understanding rather than moral judgment and paradigmatic hierarchy. My "critical" role as an activist came when I connected participants' micro-level, on-the-ground experiences to broader structural inequities outside of their control in my research, and marching and offering testimony in solidarity with their cause. This tension between cultural relativists' obligation to tell the *authentic* story versus critical theorists' obligation to tell the *just* story is part of larger interparadigmatic debate around the capacity of both philosophies to co-exist (Hammer, 2019). Such tensions are even more salient in applied CHC contexts as researchers face real-world impacts in how they decide to interpret and disseminate their work.

Another key takeaway of this chapter—which aligns with the broader scope of this text—highlights the importance of centering critical perspectives in the health communication field more generally. The existing canon of CCA and other CHC research documents the importance of such methods to prevent reductionist narratives of health that reify West-centric expertise and cultural norms (Dutta-Bergman, 2005; Lupton, 1994; Sastry et al., 2021). Paralleling recent disciplinary calls to action, such as the #communicationsowhite movement in 2018 and the increase in number of communication journals dedicating special issues to discussions on equity and justice (particularly in the context of the 2020 social crises) (Chakravartty et al., 2018; Kreiss, 2022), health communication scholars can build on this momentum to think about ways to incorporate critical methods in their work and the field.

In the context of this study, many health communication interventions addressing food access and insecurity draw on top-down logics that privilege positivist assumptions of science and do not interrogate the broader structural factors which often birthed such conditions (see de Souza, 2019; Dutta et al., 2016). Regarding community food security, this means providing surface-level solutions (e.g., food charity, donation programs) that are situated within a food system that simultaneously reproduces on-the-ground oppressive conditions for the consumer (e.g., geographic zoning laws that create food deserts, food policies that privilege which foods are considered "healthy," disproportionate access to unhealthy foods) and farmer (e.g., cultural erasure via seed innovation interventions, land theft, co-optation, diminished representation and leadership in health-promoting initiatives such as the alternative food movement, low political representation) alike (Conrad & Zuckerman, 2020; James et al., 2014). Against this backdrop, the incorporation of critical perspectives centers non-dominant voices and interrogates root causes that reify on-the-ground health outcomes, prevent certain communities from participating in the food system, and uphold existing status quo realities. The participant narratives featured in this study disrupted normative assumptions of ACB women farmer experiences by documenting how they developed alternative communication infrastructures and external partnerships.

Notes

1 Black/African refers to persons with Sub-Saharan African ancestral origins with Brown or Black complexion. The term Black or African American signifies a geographical origin or African descent with attempts to describe a cultural group. Caribbean refers to the people, culture, and communities that are of African descent and reside in the Caribbean.
2 Culture can be understood as the negotiated values, practices, and meanings within a local community. Structure refers to the landscapes and/or systems within which social systems are allocated. Agency is the capacity of local communities to act and make decisions within structures that encompass their daily lives.
3 The CCA entails other ancillary components, such as voice and dialogue, context and space, listening, among others, emphasizing dialogic knowledge co-construction with marginalized communities (see Sastry et al., 2021 for a detailed overview of where CCA has been applied previously in the field)—however most empirical research to date has applied various applications of the C-S-A matrix.
4 Carter et al. (2024) provide a more detailed analysis of these findings.

References

Abrahamowicz, A. A., Ebinger, J., Whelton, S. P., Commodore-Mensah, Y., & Yang, E. (2023). Racial and ethnic disparities in hypertension: Barriers and opportunities to improve blood pressure control. *Current Cardiology Reports*, 25(1), 17–27. https://doi.org/10.1007/s11886-022-01826-x

Airhihenbuwa, C. O. (1995). Culture, health education, and critical consciousness. *Journal of Health Education*, 26(5), 317–319. https://doi.org/10.1080/10556699.1995.10603125

Akamani, K. (2021). An ecosystem-based approach to climate-smart agriculture with some considerations for social equity. *Agronomy*, 11(8), 1564. https://doi.org/10.3390/agronomy11081564

Alexander, S. A., Jones, C. M., Tremblay, M. C., Beaudet, N., Rod, M. H., & Wright, M. T. (2020). Reflexivity in health promotion: A typology for training.

Health Promotion Practice, 21(4), 499–509. https://doi.org/10.1177/15248399 20912407

Alkon, A. H., Bowen, S., Kato, Y., & Young, K. A. (2020). Unequally vulnerable: A food justice approach to racial disparities in COVID-19 cases. *Agriculture and Human Values*, 37, 535–536. https://doi.org/10.1007/s10460-020-10110-z

Baum, F., MacDougall, C., & Smith, D. (2006). Participatory action research. *Journal of Epidemiology and Community Health*, 60(10), 854. https://doi.org/10.1136/jech.2004.028662

Bonilla-Silva, E., & Peoples, C. E. (2022). Historically white colleges and universities: The unbearable whiteness of (most) colleges and universities in America. *American Behavioral Scientist*, 66(11), 1490–1504. https://doi.org/10.1177/00027642211066047

Bradford, S., & Dutta, M. J. (2018). Academic-activist partnerships in struggles of the oppressed. *Palmerston North, NZ: Center for Culture-centered Approach to Research and Evaluation (CARE)*.

Brown, A. F., Ma, G. X., Miranda, J., Eng, E., Castille, D., Brockie, T., Jones, P., Airhihenbuwa, C. O., Farhat, T., Zhu, L., & Trinh-Shevrin, C. (2019). Structural interventions to reduce and eliminate health disparities. *American Journal of Public Health*, 109(S1), S72–S78. https://doi.org/10.2105/AJPH.2018.304844

Canfield, M. (2022). The ideology of innovation: Philanthropy and racial capitalism in global food governance. *The Journal of Peasant Studies*, 50(6), 2381–2405. https://doi.org/10.1080/03066150.2022.2099739

Carter, A. (2023). Sowing seeds of sovereignty: A qualitative exploration of chapter leader experiences who belong to an African, Caribbean, and Black women's agriculture advocacy collective. *Journal of Racial and Ethnic Health Disparities* 11(1), 1–13. https://doi.org/10.1007/s40615-023-01777-1

Carter, A., Broad, G., & Reeves, V. (2024). Recapturing communicative erasure: Black women farmers' lived experience, political voice and cultural knowledge as critical health communication praxis. *Health Communication* 40(1), 1–12. https://doi.org/10.1080/10410236.2024.2328919

Carter, A. L., & Alexander, A. (2020). Soul food: [Re] framing the African-American farming crisis using the culture-centered approach. *Frontiers in Communication*, 5, 5. https://doi.org/10.3389/fcomm.2020.00005

Chakravartty, P., Kuo, R., Grubbs, V., & McIlwain, C. (2018). # communicationsowhite. *Journal of Communication*, 68(2), 254–266. https://doi.org/10.1093/joc/jqy003

Chancel, L. (2020). *Unsustainable inequalities: Social justice and the environment*. Harvard University Press.

Clause, C. J. (2021). Bodies and documents: The material impact of collaborative information- sharing within the seasonal agricultural worker program. *Frontiers in Communication*, 6, 666652. https://doi.org/10.3389/fcomm.2021.666652

Collins, P. H. (2022). *Black feminist thought: Knowledge, consciousness, and the politics of empowerment*. Routledge.

Conrad, A., & Zuckerman, J. (2020). *Identifying and countering White supremacy culture in food systems*. Duke Sanford World Food Policy Center.

Dankwa-Mullan, I., Rhee, K. B., Stoff, D. M., Pohlhaus, J. R., Sy, F. S., Stinson, N., Jr., & Ruffin, J. (2010). Moving toward paradigm-shifting research in health disparities through translational, transformational, and transdisciplinary approaches. *American Journal of Public Health*, *100*(S1), S19–S24. https://doi.org/10.2105/ AJPH.2009.189167

de Souza, R. T. (2019). *Feeding the other: Whiteness, privilege, and neoliberal stigma in food pantries*. MIT Press.

Dillard, S., Anaele, A., Kumar, R., & Jamil, R. (2018). Bridging theory to practice: Utilizing the Culture-Centered Approach (CCA) to address gaps in Community Based Participatory Research (CBPR) processes. *Athens Journal of Health*, *5*(3), 175. https://doi.org/10.30958/ajh.5-3-1

Dutta, M., & Pal, M. (2010). Dialog theory in marginalized settings: A subaltern studies approach. *Communication Theory*, *20*(4), 363–386. https://doi.org/10.1111/j.1468-2885.2010.01367.x

Dutta, M., Pandi, A. R., Zapata, D., Mahtani, R., Falnikar, A., Tan, N., Thaker, J., Pitaloka, D., Dutta, U., Luk, P., & Sun, K. (2019). Critical health communication method as embodied practice of resistance: Culturally centering structural transformation through struggle for voice. *Frontiers in Communication*, *4*, 67. https://doi.org/10.3389/fcomm.2019.00067

Dutta, M. J. (2008). *Communicating health: A culture-centered approach*. Polity Press.

Dutta, M. J. (2018). Culture-centered approach in addressing health disparities: Communication infrastructures for subaltern voices. *Communication Methods and Measures*, *12*(4), 239–259. https://doi.org/10.1080/19312458.2018.1453057

Dutta, M. J., & de Souza, R. (2008). The past, present, and future of health development campaigns: Reflexivity and the critical-cultural approach. *Health Communication*, *23*(4), 326–339. https://doi.org/10.1080/10410230802229704

Dutta, M. J., Hingson, L., Anaele, A., Sen, S., & Jones, K. (2016). Narratives of food insecurity in Tippecanoe County, Indiana: Economic constraints in local meanings of hunger. *Health Communication*, *31*(6), 647–658. https://doi.org/10.1080/10410236.2014.987467

Dutta-Bergman, M. J. (2005). Theory and practice in health communication campaigns: A critical interrogation. *Health Communication*, *18*(2), 103–122. https://doi.org/10.1207/s15327027hc1802_1

Elers, P., Elers, S., Dutta, M. J., & Torres, R. (2021). Applying the culture-centered approach to visual storytelling methods. *Review of Communication*, *21*(1), 33–43. https://doi.org/10.1080/15358593.2021.1895292

Estrada, E., Ramirez, A. S., Gamboa, S., & Amezola de herrera, P. (2018). Development of a participatory health communication intervention: An ecological approach to reducing rural information inequality and health disparities. *Journal of Health Communication*, *23*(8), 773–782. https://doi.org/10.1080/10810730.2018.1527874

Fanon, F. (1963). *The Wretched of the Earth*. Grove Press.

Gist-Mackey, A. N., & Dougherty, D. S. (2023). Unemployment and food (in)security: (Un) just governance in unemployment organizations. In Dempsey, S. (ed.). *Organizing Eating* (pp. 95–113). Routledge.

Gordon, C., Hunt, K. P., & Dutta, M. J. (2022). Food systems communication amid compounding crises: Power, resistance, and change. *Frontiers in Communication*, *7*, 1041474. https://doi.org/10.3389/fcomm.2022.1041474

Gordon, C., Pezzullo, P. C., & Gabrieloff-Parish, M. (2020). Food justice advocacy tours: Remapping rooted, regenerative relationships through Denver's "Planting Just Seeds". In Crick, N. (ed.). *The Rhetoric of Social Movements* (pp. 299–316). Routledge.

Granovetter, M. (1983). The strength of weak ties: A network theory revisited. *Sociological Theory*, 201–233. https://doi.org/10.2307/202051

Grant, G. R., Wood, S. D., & Wright, W. J. (2012). Black farmers united: The struggle against power and principalities. *Journal of Pan African Studies*, 5(1), 3–22.

Grefe, E. A. (1997). Grassroots or grasstops: Your call…your gamble. *Economic Development Review*, 15(2), 15.

Hammer, E. (2019). Critical theory and the challenge of relativism. In Kusch, M. (ed.). *The Routledge Handbook of Philosophy of Relativism* (pp. 247–255). Routledge.

Hinson, W. R., & Robinson, E. (2008). "We didn't get nothing:" The plight of Black Farmers. *Journal of African American Studies*, 12, 283–302. https://doi.org/10.1007/s12111-008-9046-5

Hite, A. H., & Carter, A. (2019). Examining assumptions in science-based policy: Critical health communication, stasis theory, and public health nutrition guidance. *Rhetoric of Health & Medicine*, 2(2), 147–175. https://doi.org/10.5744/rhm.2019.1009

Horst, M., & Marion, A. (2019). Racial, ethnic and gender inequities in farmland ownership and farming in the US. *Agriculture and Human Values*, 36, 1–16. https://doi.org/10.1007/s10460-018-9883-3

Hunt, K. P. (2023). "The rules for the food system we all eat by": How the US Farm Bill (re) structures capitalist food politics. In Dempsey, S. (ed.). *Organizing Eating* (pp. 48–68). Routledge.

James, P., Arcaya, M. C., Parker, D. M., Tucker-Seeley, R. D., & Subramanian, S. V. (2014). Do minority and poor neighborhoods have higher access to fast-food restaurants in the United States?. *Health and Place*, 29, 10–17. https://doi.org/10.1016/j.healthplace.2014.04.011

Jamshidi, E., Morasae, E. K., Shahandeh, K., Majdzadeh, R., Seydali, E., Aramesh, K., & Abknar, N. L. (2014). Ethical considerations of community-based participatory research: Contextual underpinnings for developing countries. *International Journal of Preventive Medicine*, 5(10), 1328.

Jenkins, J. J. (2014). Communicating community: A culture-centered approach to racial/ethnic (in) equality. *Carolinas Communication Annual*, 30(1), 34–51.

Kreiss, D. (2022). Communication theory at a time of racial reckoning. *Communication Theory*, 32, 161–168. https://doi.org/10.1093/ct/qtab020

Layman, E., & Civita, N. (2022). Decolonizing agriculture in the United States: Centering the knowledges of women and people of color to support relational farming practices. *Agriculture and Human Values*, 39(3), 965–978. https://doi.org/10.1007/s10460-022-10297-3

Lunsford, L., Arthur, M. L., & Porter, C. M. (2021). African and Native American foodways and resilience: From 1619 to COVID-19. *Journal of Agriculture, Food Systems, and Community Development*, 10(4), 241. https://doi.org/10.5304/jafscd.2021.104.008

Lupton, D. (1994). Toward the development of critical health communication praxis. *Health Communication*, 6(1), 55–67. https://doi.org/10.1207/s15327027hc0601_4

MacKinnon, D., & Derickson, K. D. (2013). From resilience to resourcefulness: A critique of resilience policy and activism. *Progress in Human Geography*, 37(2), 253–270. https://doi.org/10.1177/0309132512454775

Minkler, M. (2005). Community-based research partnerships: Challenges and opportunities. *Journal of Urban Health*, 82, ii3–ii12. https://doi.org/10.1093/jurban/jti034

Niakouei, A., Tehrani, M., & Fulton, L. (2020). Health disparities and cardiovascular disease. *Healthcare* 8(1), 1–12. https://doi.org/10.3390/healthcare8010065

Odoms-Young, A., & Bruce, M. A. (2018). Examining the impact of structural racism on food insecurity: implications for addressing racial/ethnic disparities. *Family & Community Health*, 41, S3–S6. https://doi.org/10.1097/FCH.0000000000000183

Pavarala, V., & Malik, K. K. (2021). Community radio for social change: Restoring decentralized democratic discursive spaces. In Melkote, S. R. & Singhal, A. (eds.) *Handbook of Communication and Development* (pp. 190–212). Edward Elgar Publishing.

Pilgeram, R., Dentzman, K., & Lewin, P. (2022). Women, race and place in US Agriculture. *Agriculture and Human Values*, 39(4), 1341–1355. https://doi.org/10.1007/s10460-022-10324-3

Sastry, S., Stephenson, M., Dillon, P., & Carter, A. (2021). A meta-theoretical systematic review of the culture-centered approach to health communication: Toward a refined, "nested" model. *Communication Theory*, 31(3), 380–421. https://doi.org/10.1093/ct/qtz024

Schraedley, M. K., Bean, H., Dempsey, S. E., Dutta, M. J., Hunt, K. P., Ivancic, S. R., LeGreco, M., Okamoto, & Sellnow, T. (2020). Food (in) security communication: A Journal of Applied Communication Research forum addressing current challenges and future possibilities. *Journal of Applied Communication Research*, 48(2), 166–185. https://doi.org/10.1080/00909882.2020.1735648

Scollon, R., & Scollon, S. W. (2007). Nexus analysis: Refocusing ethnography on action. *Journal of Sociolinguistics*, 11(5), 608–625. https://doi.org/10.1111/j.1467-9841.2007.00342.x

Seubert, L., McWha-Hermann, I., & Seubert, C. (2023). Critical reflection and critical reflexivity as core processes for critical WOP: Precarious employment as an example. *Applied Psychology*, 72(1), 106–125. https://doi.org/10.1111/apps.12424

Spivak, G. C. (1988). Can the subaltern speak? In C. Nelson & L. Grossberg (Eds.), *Marxism and the Interpretation of Culture* (pp. 271–313). University of Illinois Press.

Taylor, C. (1994). *Multiculturalism: Expanded paperback edition* (Vol. 15). Princeton University Press.

United States Department of Agriculture. (2020). Food environment atlas.

United States Department of Agriculture Natural Agricultural Statistics Service. (2017a). Black producers. Washington, DC: US Department of Agriculture, National Agricultural Statistics Service.

United States Department of Agriculture Natural Agricultural Statistics Service. (2017b). Female producers. Washington, DC: US Department of Agriculture, National Agricultural Statistics Service

Wallerstein, N., Oetzel, J. G., Duran, B., Magarati, M., Pearson, C., Belone, L., ... & Dutta, M. J. (2019). Culture-centeredness in community-based participatory research: Contributions to health education intervention research. *Health Education Research*, 34(4), 372–388. https://doi.org/10.1093/her/cyz021

Yehya, N. A., & Dutta, M. J. (2010). Health, religion, and meaning: A culture-centered study of Druze women. *Qualitative Health Research*, 20(6), 845–858. https://doi.org/10.1177/1049732310362400

York, F. N., & Tang, L. (2021). 'Picture me heart disease free': Understanding African Americans' cardiovascular disease experiences through a culture-centered approach. *Journal of Applied Communication Research*, 49(3), 247–266. https://doi.org/10.1080/00909882.2021.1912377

Zoller, H. M. (2019). Critical health communication methods: Challenges in researching transformative social change. Frontiers in Communication, 4, 41. https://doi.org/10.3389/fcomm.2019.00041

Zoller, H. M. (2024). Addressing health inequalities through worker and consumer cooperatives: Co-op cincy's organizing for food justice. In Dempsey, S. (ed.). *Organizing eating* (pp. 166–189). Routledge.

Zoller, H. M., & Kline, K. N. (2008). Theoretical contributions of interpretive and critical research in health communication. *Annals of the International Communication Association*, 32(1), 89–135. https://doi.org/10.1080/23808985.2008.11679076

Zuberi, T., & Bonilla-Silva, E. (Eds.). (2008). *White logic, white methods: Racism and methodology*. Rowman & Littlefield.

Critical Methods in Health Communication Research and Practice

9
BIOCRITICISM IN A TIME OF PRECARITY

Inventional Resources for Critical Health Communication

Lisa Keränen, Liliane Campos, and Jennifer Malkowski

The study and practice of health communication in the latter part of the twentieth century coincides with the "age of biology," a description that has been applied to both the second half of the twentieth (Toulmin, 1964) and the beginning of the twenty-first centuries (Stavridis, 2014). The "age of biology" denotes a period of intensifying interest in biological, immunological, and genetic domains ushered in by the 1953 publication of the structure of DNA. As terms and ideas from fields like genetics, immunology, neurobiology, and oncology seeped into everyday language, they in turn incorporated digital imagery and key concerns of the culture writ large (Hayles, 2020; Wald, 2008). The promises of genomic mapping, genetic cloning, xenotransplantation, and immunotherapies commingled with the perceived threats of resurging infectious diseases, bioterrorism, and growing antimicrobial resistance to ensure the prominence of biological concerns in public and popular discourses (Campos & Patoine, 2022; Keränen, 2011). These concerns prompted closer attention to how biological and genetic knowledge influenced and was influenced by public and popular discourses and practices.

Just as biologically inflected language increasingly pervaded public and popular discourses and imagery, numerous academic and nonacademic fields—including science studies, literary criticism, composition, technical writing, art, the rhetoric of science and technology, health humanities, and medical anthropology—also attuned to the power of biological discourses and practices. Terms that index the rising prominence of *bios*—a "bio-troping" of the lifeworld—have proliferated in recent decades. *Bio-rhetorics* (Lyne, 1990), *biosemiotics* (Barbieri, 2008; Favareau, 2010; Kull, 1999;

DOI: 10.4324/9781003426530-12
This chapter has been made available under a CC BY-NC-ND license.

Sebeok & Umiker-Sebeok, 1992), *biocapital* (Birch & Tyfield, 2013), *biocriticism* (Campos, 2022; Keränen, 2011), *biocritique* (Séginger, 2015), *biopolitics* (Foucault, 2003; Lemke, 2011; Rose, 2007), *biofictions* (Gill, 2020; Kucukalic, 2022), *biocitizenship* and *biosociality* (Rose & Novas, 2005), *bioimagination* (Kucukalic, 2022), *biovalue* (Waldby, 2000), and *bioidentification* (Johnson, 2023), to name just a few, capture the bridging of the biological and the cultural/political. While the proliferation of such bio-terminologies may seem excessive to some, this terminological effervescence signals a shared drive, across the humanities and social sciences, toward examining and reformulating linguistic tools to account for the profound imprint of the biological in twenty-first-century Western life.

In this chapter, we address one of these terms, *biocriticism,* and consider its utility for scholars and practitioners of critical health communication (CHC). We begin by defining biocriticism as an act of critical invention that seeks to analyze articulations of the relations among biology, culture, representation, and politics. We next outline the theoretical underpinnings and development of two strands of biocriticism, one that emerged from communication and one from literary and performance studies. We then explore several applications of the concept, and we consider how the concept of biocriticism allows CHC scholars to unpack the dynamics and implications of biological discourses, contexts, artifacts, symbols, images, and assemblages with an eye on power relations and subjectivities. In this way, biocriticism allows for extensions of CHC's concepts, theories, audiences, and collaborators. Ultimately, we maintain that biocriticism is necessary in a time of environmental, economic, and political precarity. Through its attention to the semiotic fabric of the age of biology, biocriticism offers inventional resources for forging our individual and collective futures.

Biocriticism as Critical Invention and Intervention

Biocriticism is a neologism combining *bios*—the ancient Greek word for life from which terms like *biology* and *antibiotic* developed—and *criticism,* which also derives from an ancient Greek term, as we explain below. Although some scholars in English and literary studies have occasionally used the term *biocriticism* as shorthand for "biographical criticism," that is, to describe analyses of literary and cultural texts that examine how aspects of the author or creator's life are reflected in the work under investigation, this is not our purview. Our notion of biocriticism focuses on the intersections of biology as discourse and disciplinary practice, and criticism, understood here as the analysis of the symbolic/semiotic workings, consequences, and entailments of text(s), object(s), practice(s) and images(s).

Biocritical investigation extends to artworks, images, practices, objects and sounds as well as textual artifacts, because all these constructions emerge from a discursive context. In this way, criticism is a form of qualitative inquiry that offers, as Zoller and Kline (2008) highlight, "a unique, well-argued and defended interpretation of a discourse [or any symbol] to impart some insight into the multiple ways in which communication fosters particular meanings" (p. 93). Criticism often takes the form of a critical essay that details the context, rhetorical situation, possible meanings, structure, aesthetics, ethics, persuasive operations, power dynamics, and politics of a textual and/or extra-textual artifact(s), but critics also present biocritical work as art, blogs, performance, or literature. We caution against the conflation of biocriticism and rhetorical analysis, although the two can and often do converge (see, e.g., Derkatch, 2022; Krebs, 2021; Sastry & Dutta, 2011, 2012). What makes a work biocritical is a combination of methodological sensibility and substantive focus. More specifically, it involves the use of invention to reinterpret the meanings, power relations, dynamics, and consequences of biologically-attuned objects, discourses, practices, assemblages, and materials.

The complex etymology of the term *critique* in English offers insight about its creative, epistemic, and inventional capacity. In English, the term dates to the seventeenth century, appearing in the works of Shakespeare and Bacon in reference to evaluations of plays (Stypinska, 2020). In French, the term bears an older history with relations not back to *krisis*, as is commonly assumed, but to *krinein*, a verb meaning to "judge" or "decide." In Ancient Greek, the analytic act was performed by a *kritikos* or critic. This etymology reminds us that modern uses of the word "criticism" are inflected by medical roots: in Ancient Greece, doctors of the Hippocratic school defined the *krisis* of an illness as a moment of change, though not necessarily for the worse. In this medical vein of thought, *krinein* designates a discerning examination of a situation (Stypinska, 2020). Crucially, this discernment is based on the interpretation of signs/symbols.

Our definition of biocriticism emphasizes this hermeneutic and symbolic/semiotic dimension, rather than viewing criticism as mere judgment or negative evaluation. As Raymond Williams (1985) reminds us, we should resist equating criticism with fault-finding. Criticism should instead aim to apprehend "the specificity of response, which is often not an abstract 'judgment' but even where including, often necessarily, positive or negative responses a definite practice, in active and complex relations with its whole situation and context" (p. 86). Biocritical practices thus do not need to make value judgments about the artifacts and discourses they examine, although some—particularly in rhetoric and critical/cultural communication studies—often do so. Loosely extending Scott and Gouge's

(2019) explanation of the functions of theory in the rhetoric of health and medicine (RHM) to the realm of biocriticism, we see that biocriticism can be used to:

1. Track how "entangled discourses" about biology and culture/politics mutually shape one another
2. Extend or disrupt an existing biocritical concept or theory (such as biocitizenship, biovalue, and bioeconomies)
3. Propose a new model to understand biological and biopolitical discourses
4. Build upon an existing line of research or artistic example of biopolitics
5. Propose a new metaphor, analogy, or image for viewing the interactions of biology and culture/politics
6. Identify and respond to gaps in current biocritical literature
7. Unpack how a biological or biotechnological text, discourse, or artifact reconfigures identity, subjectivity, or personhood
8. Amplify muted or erased voices and perspectives about biological knowledge, texts, and practices.

As iterative, critical-interpretive work, biocriticism can be assessed by considering how well it encourages others to view its subject in a novel way. Table 8.1 offers a heuristic set of sample research questions a CHC scholar might pose from a biocritical perspective.

In sum, biocriticism aims to analyze the symbolic/semiotic structures and rhetorical strategies that operate in representations of health, medicine, and biology, and to explain how these structures and strategies engage with their epistemological, ethical, and political context. Attention to the specificity of discourse involves analytic moves shared with other forms of CHC. As Zoller and Kline (2008) maintain, "critical theorizing involves deconstructing dominant, taken-for-granted assumptions about health, often with the hope of introducing possibilities for alternative, more inclusive meaning systems" (p. 94). Embodying this spirit, biocriticism can be both dismantling *and* productive, encompassing the unmasking/deconstruction of discourses and practices and their envisioned re-construction.

Theoretical Influences and Two Strains of Biocriticism

Biopolitics, a catch-all phrase for the intersection of biological being and political life, supplies the theoretical scaffolding of biocriticism. Although competing conceptions of biopolitics abound and can be traced to antiquity (Lemke, 2011), the French philosopher Michel Foucault's development

TABLE 9.1 Sample Biocritical Research Questions

Heuristic	Sample Questions
Relationships	How do two sets of "bio" discourses mutually inform one another and with what consequences?
	What do verbal and visual representations of a text, artifact, or practice reveal about how biology and politics intermingle?
	How does a certain practice (medical, journalistic, artistic, or other) engage with a biomedical, bioeconomical, or biopolitical context?
Representations	How does a practice, text, or object intervene in a society's representations of biology, medicine, and health?
	What does this practice, text, or object do if we consider it as a rhetorical intervention in a discursive field? With what discourses or rhetorics does it engage and with what implications?
Conceptual implications	What are the political, ethical, linguistic, and epistemological implications of this object or practice?
	How does a concept, a text, a practice, or an object redefine life, health, and/or the interrelations of the life sciences and politics?
	How does a concept, text, practice, or object redefine other key concepts, such as subjectivity, ethics, agency, or immunity?
Disruption/ resistance	How does this text/artifact/discourse/image/practice disrupt (or resist or challenge) conventional understandings of life, medicine, health, or their interrelations?
	How do certain objects, practices, or vocabularies disrupt, resist, or aid the biomedical management of disease?
Time and culture	How is this artifact, text, or discourse a response to anxieties about biotechnology that emerged during a unique moment in culture/time?
	How do the temporal rhetorics of this artifact, text, or discourse configure identity and agency?
Continuity and Change	How do discourses of this artifact or text extend continuing discourses and themes, and in what ways do they depart from them? That is, what are the major continuities and mutations in the discourse?
Power, agency, and control	How does this text, discourse, artifact, or practice enable or constrain agency and identity? What does it afford or forestall?
	Whose interests are being served by this discourse, artifact, or text?
Identity	How does this text, discourse, or artifact configure identity as biological?
	How does this artwork construct or deconstruct biological belonging?
	What communicative strategies do groups adopt as they co-construct biosocial identities and communities?

of the concepts of *biopolitics* and *biopower* offers considerable analytical capacities for biocriticism. His well-known writings on the intersection of power, institutions, knowledge, discourse, and subjectivities have focused on how power operates in and through bodies and how power, discourse, and knowledge, what he calls "power/knowledge," are inextricably linked (Foucault, 1998). For Foucault, power is omnipresent, relational, and inseparable from discourse that structures thought and action. In his later work, Foucault became concerned with governance, how mechanisms of control guide the conduct of individuals and society.

For Foucault, biopolitics involves the governance of human populations through biological characteristics. In the *History of Sexuality, Volume I*, Foucault proposes that mechanisms of state power began to change in the seventeenth century away from the power of the sovereign (i.e., a king or ruler) to "take life" (i.e., a ruler's pronouncement of a death sentence or the conscription of citizens to war) to a wide set of initiatives a state (and other institutions and groups) took to ensure the health of the population both by disciplining individual bodies and by controlling the broader population. In his words, biopower, which crystallized in the nineteenth century, represents "an explosion of numerous and diverse techniques for achieving the subjugation of bodies and the control of populations," a disruption in the conventional, sovereign exercise of power (Foucault, 1998, p. 140). This move toward biopower represented an enlargement of state power from "the right over life and death" to the oversight, optimization, and ultimately biologification of individual bodies and the population at large. Rather than sentencing people to die, the state and other entities engaged in a host of practices meant to secure and promote life, and these initiatives inescapably involve power and control. Birth control, and statistical analyses of body mass are two examples that reveal the "numerous and diverse techniques" for the "subjugation of bodies and the control of populations" (p. 140).

Foucault's writings on biopolitics and biopower have been adopted, extended, and challenged by numerous scholars including Giorgio Agamben, Judith Butler, Roberto Esposito, Michael Hardt, Achille Mbembe, Antonio Negri, Carl Novas, Paul Rabinow, Nikolas Rose, and Jana Sawicki. While excavation of these ideas exceeds the scope of this essay, the extension of Foucault's ideas has occupied a particularly prominent position in the health humanities. Many of these authors have traced how, in the wealthy Western world, people increasingly understand themselves and others in biological terms, "as beings whose individuality is, in part at least, grounded within our fleshly, corporeal existence, and who experience, articulate, judge and act upon ourselves in part in the language of biomedicine" (Rose, 2007, p. 26).

Reproduction, race, and genomic medicine comprise three valences of biopower in the early twenty-first century. Biocriticism positions these issues within the broader economics and politics of life, which are increasingly shaped by the discourses of health optimization, genetic susceptibility, neurochemical conceptions of the self, and new forms of biosociality arising from shared medical conditions. Often these discourses position people as "responsible" for safeguarding their own health and well-being (Novas & Rose, 2000; Rabinow, 1996; Rose, 2007).

Rhetoric/Communication

To illustrate this approach, we outline two interrelated strains of biocriticism that circle around a common set of concerns at the intersection of *bios* and politics/culture. The first comes from rhetoric/communication studies as practiced in a North American context and the second from a European literary tradition. In the communication/rhetoric strand, the concept of biocriticism grew out of a subfield of rhetoric studies known as the rhetoric of science and technology. Through the 1980s and 1990s, scholars across the humanities and social sciences in general and in rhetoric in particular offered critiques of the discourses and practices of "geneticization," (Condit, 1999; Novas & Rose, 2000; Van Dijck, 1998), raising concerns that individuals were increasingly expected to understand themselves at the molecular level, as, say, collections of genes, in ways imbued with ethical concerns and vexed power relations. In 1990, rhetorician of science John Lyne defined bio-rhetoric as "a strategy for inventing and organizing discourses about biology in such a way that they mesh with the discourses of social, political, or moral life" (p. 38). In his analysis of the traffic between science and popular culture embodied in discourses about "the selfish gene," Lyne demonstrated the appropriation of a scientific vernacular to make social judgments.

Extending Lyne's focus on biological discourses, first author Lisa Keränen (2011) provisionally identified two visions of biocriticism. In a narrow sense, she called for "a sustained and rigorous analysis of the artifacts, texts, discursive formations, visual representations, and material practices positioned at the nexus of disease and culture" (p. 225). In a broader sense, she called for analyses addressing the "administration of life" that "would apply the complement of rhetorical tools (and for those inclined and able, those of allied fields such as anthropology, sociology, and science studies) to more fully engage" biopolitics (p. 238). She explained:

> In this broader inflection, biocriticism would address the range of discursive formations and material practices that comprise "life" by

investigating "vitality," the politics, possibilities, and perils of [Foucault's] "making live."

(p. 238)

In focusing on the "vital" politics of securing and optimizing life, biocriticism would plumb the dynamics of a wide swath of life-focused practices spanning genetic engineering and bioweapons development through transhumanism, neurobiology, and biogovernance. It would also explore how each of these domains "prompts new visions of identity and belonging" (p. 239). Keränen conceived of biocriticism as methodologically flexible so long as it focused on the range of exchanges involved in administering life and ensuring population security. While she hoped this label would unite a disparate group of scholars from English, composition, rhetoric, and health communication around a common project, biocriticism became a methodological footnote (Malkowski et al., 2016; Melonçon & Scott, 2019; Stormer, 2014) until its recent uptake (Derkatch, 2022; Johnson, 2023; Krebs, 2020).

Literary and Performance Studies

In 2022, second author Liliane Campos defined the remit of her "BioCriticism" project as threefold: (a) "critical examinations of contemporary artistic engagement with biological images, discourse and practices;" (b) "critical theory currently engaging with the concepts and discourse of the life sciences;" and (c) "art as a space which engages critically with biological theory, technology and rhetoric." Campos's definition of biocritical practices includes the notion of *"biocritique"* proposed by French Literature scholar Gisèle Séginger (2015), a mode of reading that brings to light literature's dynamic treatment of biological knowledge. Campos's definition of biocriticism, however, extends its scope beyond literature, to other artworks as well as to contemporary theory, and to semiotics beyond the textual. Campos's definition also emphasizes that biocritical practices are carried out by many different actors: not only scholars and theorists but also artists and, potentially, any person who engages critically with medical and biological representations or with the art inspired by such representations.

The BioCriticism online seminar, hosted by Campos at the Sorbonne Nouvelle University in Paris, invites scholars, artists, and art-lovers to discuss artworks and texts that engage with both the discourse and the images of medicine and biology. A prominent strand of these representations is provided by the rising current of bio-art, where artworks tend to be "part critique, part irony, and sometimes part hard science" (Anker, 2015, p. 6). But the current artistic and theoretical interest in the discourse of biology, health, and medicine is a broader trend, where visual artists, performers, and writers who do not identify as bio-artists are increasingly engaging with biological and medical rhetoric. The BioCriticism project examines these artistic and theoretical engagements with our shifting representations of health and biology, and it asks what critical roles they might play in this century's emergent biopolitics.

In both the strand emanating from communication/rhetoric and the one emanating from literary and artistic criticism, biocriticism, as we have defined it here, is an inventive critical practice which is distinct from rhetorical, literary, or artistic criticism, but which can be practiced within those fields, as well as within CHC (and beyond). Literary and artistic criticism are biocritical when they engage with the discursive, semiotic, and political structures that shape our representations of biology, health, and medicine. Biocritical questions tend to arise, in the arts, whenever creative work questions representations of the body and of the body politic (Bernard, 2022), and more generally, whenever art engages with the images and discourses of medicine and biology (Campos & Patoine, 2022). CHC is biocritical when it uses symbolic/semiotic analysis to unpack the dynamics and implications of biological texts, contexts, artifacts, images, and assemblages with an eye on power relations and subjectivities, as we will demonstrate in the forthcoming section.

Examples of Biocriticism

Biocriticism operates at the intersection of several academic and non-academic fields spanning the health humanities and social sciences, including communication and rhetoric, literary and performance studies, and aesthetics. It encompasses a set of practices that may be carried out by scholars as well as by health professionals, artists, and even nonprofessionals. In this section, we offer several examples of biocritical work in communication/rhetoric, CHC, and literary criticism and art.

Communication/Rhetoric/Critical Health Communication

Scholarly borders and boundaries are contested and remade. The relationships between communication/rhetoric, the RHM, the health humanities, and CHC as distinct and interrelated traditions have been discussed elsewhere (see, e.g., Dutta, 2022; Gouge, 2017; Lynch & Zoller, 2015; Sastry et al., 2019). Here, we provide examples of biocriticism from across these areas. Regardless of disciplinary subfield, each example shares concerns about how power operates in and through bodies in ways that rely on biotechnology and biological sciences.

First, Condit (1999) has examined the meanings of the gene in public, popular, and scientific discourses. Condit's longitudinal exploration of textual portrayals and audience understandings of genes identified four major epochs in U.S. public genetics discourses across newspapers, magazines, television broadcasts, and congressional records from 1900 to 1995. In the classical era of genetics from 1900 to 1935, she found that the metaphor of genetics as stockbreeding predominated. This imagistic system was replaced by notions of family genetics from the 1930s–1950s, which included expressions of fear and resurgent concern about eugenics. After the publication announcing the structure of DNA in 1953, a new era of "wild exploration and eager enthusiasm" followed in the era of "experimental genetics" (p. 19). Discourses about ethics and recombinant genes also emerged, and the focus shifted from "normal babies" to genetically "healthy ones," revealing genetics as an emerging mechanism of biopower. At the close of the century, when the Human Genome Project loomed large, the blueprint metaphor dominated discourse, portraying DNA as "instructions for life." For Condit, these major shifts in genetic representations were not neutral but carried problematic assumptions about bodies, heredity, and commercialization. These discourses pivoted around three major themes: genetic determinism, discrimination, and perfectionism, which shifted in focus over time, both enabling and constraining new ways of conceptualizing life.

We selected Condit's work on genetic discourses because it represents an early and sustained example of biocriticism that identifies changes in genetic understandings over time. Condit's work is biocritical because it consistently focuses on how biological ideas interface with social ideas and materials and because her two primary foci—genetics and abortion (Condit, 1989)—sit squarely at the intersection of biotechnology and embodiment. Her analyses expose the interplay among power, culture, and biological discourses, and they invite us to reconsider the implications of emerging genetic and reproductive subjectivities.

Second, Amy Koerber's studies of the discursive construction of women's health across scientific, popular, and lay contexts demonstrate deep attention to the intersections among biology, politics, and embodiment. In her book on infant-feeding controversies, Koerber (2013) blends rhetorical analysis, archival research, and interviews to chronicle shifting debates about the value of breastfeeding from 1940 to 2005. She tracks how the discourses of biomedical articles, policy statements, and pro-breastfeeding materials coalesced into an immunological view of breastfeeding, which promoted the current Western, biomedical "breast is best" paradigm. Placing these discourses in conversation with muted feminist discourses about breastfeeding and interviews conducted with racially and ethnically diverse women, she illuminates how the lived realities of breastfeeding challenge the dominant biomedical paradigm.

Similarly, Koerber (2018) investigates how scientific conceptions of female reproductive health transitioned gradually over centuries from womb/hysteria-based explanations to hormonal explanations in the twentieth century. Drawing from French philosopher Michael Serres's concept of time as topology, that is, as involving blending, stretching, twisting, and folding back in on itself, she traces how key texts related to the science of women's health undermine the "scientific progress" narrative. Instead, evolving scientific and cultural explanations of women's reproductive health coalesced in ways that reify gender stereotypes and limit female autonomy and agency. Koerber carefully untangles how ideas about the "wandering womb" morphed into explanations of hormones as the cause of disparate conditions such as "postpartum depression," "pregnancy brain," or "premenstrual tension" (pp. xvi, 204). Despite the changed discourse, gendered stereotypes about women's supposed "frailty" or "unpredictability" persisted in remixed form.

Koerber's biocritical analysis is evident in her exposure of mutations in biomedical discourses, demonstration of the reassortment of previous ways of configuring women's health, and in the connections she makes between discursive changes and material consequences for women. By calling attention to the entailments of, say, immunological understandings of breastfeeding or to hormonal explanations of women's health, she uncovers how these biologically inflected discourses configure culturally and historically specific ways of being and acting, revealing the mutual influence of biomedical knowledge, cultural ideologies, and identities.

A third example of biocriticism from communication/rhetoric appears across the works of numerous proponents of the culture-centered approach (CCA) to health communication (Basnyat, 2014; Dutta, 2008; Sastry & Basu, 2020). Influenced by postcolonial and subaltern studies (Airhihenbuwa, 1995; Guha & Spivak, 1988) and emerging from Mohan Dutta's fieldwork with the Santali in West Bengal, India (Dutta-Bergman, 2004), CCA asks whose voices and interests are erased from health care discourses and how people who are already vulnerable are left out of health care interventions. CCA seeks to question dominant assumptions of health communication and re-center marginalized voices. As the "most identifiable and formalized critically oriented approach to health communication," (Sastry et al., 2021, p. 380), CCA encourages collaborative, participatory research that makes sense of health in terms of active, thoughtful, and self-reflexive engagement with local and marginalized perspectives (Dutta, 2008; Sastry et al., 2021).

While much CCA work seeks to empower repressed voices through participatory research and is geared toward improving practice, one vein of biocritical CCA work uses postcolonial theory to examine the meanings of infectious diseases in publicly circulating texts (Khan, 2013, 2020; Sastry & Basu, 2020; Sastry & Dutta, 2011, 2012, 2017). We chose the examples below because they employ criticism, in contrast to participatory methods, although a clear demarcation between the two is difficult. In one early example of biocriticism, Sastry and Dutta (2011) conducted a postcolonial analysis of U.S.-media coverage of HIV/AIDS in India and found that mainstream news discourse problematically represented India as primitive, featuring the "third world" as a site needing U.S. intervention, defining U.S. altruism as uplifting, and focusing on AIDS, economics, and security. Sastry and Dutta (2012) then published a postcolonial reading of a Congressional report detailing President George W. Bush's President's Emergency Plan for AIDS Relief (PEPFAR) program that critiqued its focus on the U.S. as a "savior" of the "third world." Later, examining how Ebola was configured in the 2014 outbreaks in Guinea, Liberia, and Sierra Leone, Sastry and Dutta (2017) offered a "theoretical interrogation of the interrelated dynamics of power, culture, and allocation of material resources that accompany large-scale public health crises in the global South" (p. 10). Problematizing the construction of Ebola as a global risk, they found that conversations about indigenous cultural responses to Ebola were forestalled in broader media discourses (p. 14). Extending this line of focus, Sastry and Basu (2020) explored what CCA offers to our understanding of pandemics, whether HIV/AIDS, Ebola, or COVID-19, while Khan (2013, 2020) similarly traced the logics of domination and control in HIV/AIDS public service announcements and public health discourses in India.

Together, these CCA authors call for excavations of who and what are erased from pandemic discourse and how structure, agency, and culture exclude certain communities from needed pandemic responses. Their analyses, like those of other CHC scholars, seek investigations of the power dynamics and inequities inherent in health and medical discourses. Foregrounding the power relations inherent in constructions of people, cultures, and diseases, they show how discourses problematically represent, and often harmfully neglect, the "Other." In so doing, they address the biocritical question of how disease, medicine, power, culture, and identity intersect in problematic, power-soaked ways.

Literature, Art, and Criticism

Biocriticism also foregrounds artistic work as a locus of scholarly and practical reflection. CHC has often taken the form of art-based communication interventions, ranging from installations and graphic fiction to poetry and theater (Baglia et al., 2024; Conaty et al., 2024; Czerwiec et. al., 2015; Harter et al., 2017; Hodges, 2014; Johnson, 2023; Scale Free Network, n. d.; Shi & Wang, 2024). Here, we highlight how biocriticism foregrounds forms of artistic practice that *engage critically with*, but do not *constitute a form of* interventional health communication. Artistic practice, in other words, may itself comprise a form of biocriticism when it engages critically with the visual and verbal rhetoric of contemporary medicine and biology. Adam Dickinson's poetry collection *Anatomic* (2018) offers a striking example. Dickinson's poems were written while the poet underwent extensive biomedical testing, taking samples from his own body to measure the microbiological components of his biological self, including microbes, enzymes, hormones, and various chemical compounds. Dickinson's introduction emphasizes that the project of writing the self must engage with how the self is already "written" by biological terminology:

> How can I read me? How can I write me? I collect my blood, urine, sweat, and feces. I send them to laboratories to determine the levels and types of chemicals and microbes I find. [...] I also tune in to the signal of my microbiome by swabbing various areas of my body for bacteria – hand, genitals, ear, nose, and mouth.
> *(Dickinson, 2018, p. 9)*

Each poem in the collection reacts to the results that Dickinson receives from laboratories. The scientific language of chemical compounds mostly appears in the paratext, before, after, and between the poems, as well as in the epigraphs and notes of each poem. But the discourse of contemporary biology is audible throughout, and Dickinson draws particular attention to the metaphorical drift of popular microbiology: "My gut," he muses, "is a tropical forest of microbes. [...] My body is a spaceship designed to optimize the proliferation and growth of its microbial cosmonauts" (p. 42).

Between these incursions into figurative biological language, the poems engage critically with the discourse of health and hygiene, which Dickinson juxtaposes with the reality of ubiquitous microscopic pollution. The poem "Agents Orange, Yellow and Red," for instance, focuses on one of the molecules found in his fatty tissue: chemical dioxin, which was used as an herbicide, as a weapon during the Vietnam war, and which is a byproduct of chlorine blanching in paper manufacturing:

> Agents Orange, Yellow, and Red
> *2,3,7,8-Tetrachlorodibenzodioxin (serum): 1.304348 pg/g lipid*
> You are either for chlorine

or for the plague.
Right now is the cleanest
we have ever been, and for this
you must love aerial defoliants
or you love communism. [...]
Northern rivers are warmed
by the paper mill's piss, which,
like making the world safe for democracy,
slowly leaked into my childhood, yellowing
the lipophilic paperbacks of my
adipose fat. You are for pulp
or for poverty. (p. 15)

This poem satirizes the binary structure of hygienic discourse, which it overlays with the binary politics of cold war ideology. Not only is the body already written by the environment it sets out to write, it is also constrained by a discursive field where words such as "clean" or "safe" are tainted by their political use. Dickinson's poem functions biocritically because it historicizes such terms, as well as the chemical terminology, whose apparent neutrality is complicated by the history of its industrial and military uses. Elsewhere in the collection, Dickinson similarly describes the ubiquity of polychlorinated biphenyls as a demonstration of how our biologies are written by our industrial histories: "PCBs constitute a form of writing in the Anthropocene, a recursive script where industrial innovations find their way back into the metabolic messaging systems of the biological bodies that have created them" (*Anatomic*, p. 31). Reflecting on these multiple levels of "script," *Anatomic* construes bodies, medical practices, and environments as semiotic structures that are constantly writing one another. For scholars and practitioners of CHC, these poems demonstrate the critical potential of *investigative poetics* (Hartnett, 2007, n. p.).

In a more visual vein, Marie-Sarah Adenis' project *Le Virus Que Donc Je Suis* (*The Virus Which Therefore I Am*) (Adenis, 2024) offers another example of biocritical artistic work. In 2020, Adenis created a series of "virus-masks," which she conceived as an homage to the role that viruses other than SARS-CoV-2 play as "sculptors" of the living world and as "messengers" between species who carry fragments of DNA from one species to another (Adenis, 2021). Without the evolutionary help of viruses, she notes, we would not have the human placenta. To draw attention to their crucial role, Adenis imagines these masks as long lines composed of fragments of DNA and RNA, which she describes as reminiscent of trajectories on oceanographic maps. Designed to be worn by humans, but unlike medical masks, Adenis' masks connect rather than separate. This artwork

Biocriticism in a Time of Precarity   **199**

questions the military terminology of pandemic: instead, the emphasis on messages, travel, and shamanic rites makes viruses communication vectors and emphasizes that viral life cannot be reduced to infectious disease. Adenis' masks have appeared in various exhibitions and have also been worn onstage in *Viral*, a performance co-written by Frédérique Aït-Touati and Bruno Latour (2021). Together, Adenis' creation and Aït-Touati's dramaturgy constitute a biocritical intervention in the rhetoric surrounding the Covid-19 pandemic. Through the paradox of the virus-mask, they foreground that we only perceive viruses through their representation: they are, inevitably, signifiers constructed by a cultural/political discursive field (Figure 8.1).

Artworks such as those of Dickinson and Adenis nourish biocritical thought in artistic and literary criticism. In a study of British writer Ali Smith's "seasonal quartet" novels, Catherine Bernard reads fiction through the lens of Roberto Esposito's philosophy of immunity. Esposito (2002) argues that immunity is a central concept in contemporary politics, because immunity and community are engaged in a relation of reciprocal definition: any political community depends on an "immunitary" apparatus, which includes legal, technological, and rhetorical means of defense. For Esposito, it is crucial to analyze how society speaks of immunity, because this discourse is a locus of political thought, which determines how we think of the "body politic." Bernard uses this framework to read the novels

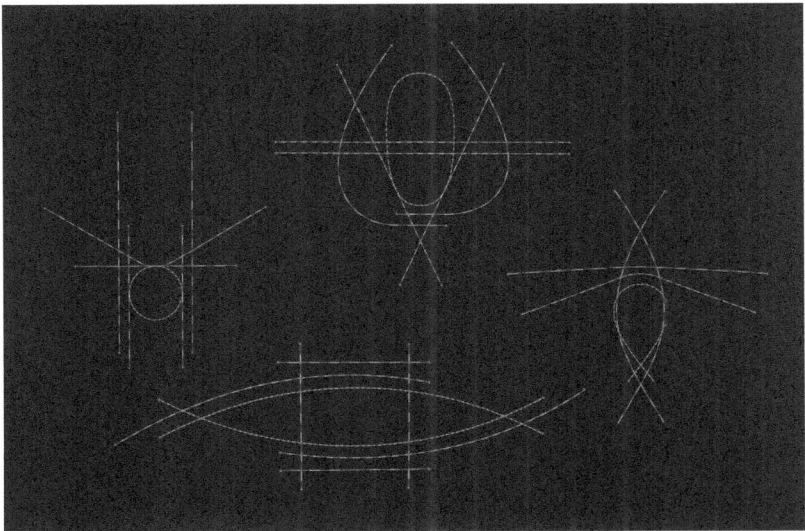

FIGURE 9.1 *Masques virus* © Marie-Sarah Adenis, 2021 (carbon fiber, beads and wire). Courtesy of the artist.

that Smith wrote just before and during the pandemic, arguing that Smith uses the rhetoric of immunity to explore the defensive rhetoric of political isolation and resistance to immigration in post-Brexit Britain. Bernard focuses on key images that function as allegories in Smith's fiction: she reads the fence, for instance, as a trope that spells "the long history of nationalist differentiation, and a literal fencing off of the commons here and now" so that it becomes "one of the vibrant allegories allowing Smith to probe the logic of political immunity" (Bernard, 2022, p. 23). The work of art, in Bernard's reading of Smith, becomes a locus of resistance to a certain rhetoric of immunity.

In parallel to this productive vein of biocriticism, critics may also identify problematic issues within the artwork's relation to biology. Pieter Vermeulen, in his study "Depopulating the Novel: Post-Catastrophe Fiction, Scale, and the Population Unconscious," critiques a strand of contemporary pandemic fiction that indulges in the portrayal of "cosy catastrophe" (Vermeulen, 2022, p. 234). In novels such as Emily St John Mandel's *Station Eleven*, Vermeulen argues, the problems of post-pandemic life are resolved too easily through a focus on a drastically reduced scale of population. This "good life" hinges on demographic reduction, which Vermeulen connects to an implicit Malthusian logic that he refers to as the "population unconscious" (p. 229). Fiction, here, is criticized for not problematizing the discourse of planetary overcrowding that it perpetuates. In this way, biocriticism may use problematic case studies to flag broader political or ethical tensions in our representations of planetary, national, and individual health.

A biocritical approach to artistic work thus draws attention to the wealth of creative and receptive practices that either magnify or resist current representations of health and medicine, and thereby shape our relations to health communication. This engagement is particularly strong in bio-art, which as a genre tends to question the conceptions of self, body, and community emerging in contemporary biotechnological and medical discourse. But as the examples above demonstrate, artistic work does not need to focus explicitly on biological or medical questions to influence our perceptions of health.

Emerging Trajectories for Biocriticism: Expanding Critical Health Communication

Biocriticism supplies a transdisciplinary, multi-methodological, and multi-concept approach to critical invention that promotes reconsideration of the relations among biology, health, medicine, politics, power, culture, and identity. For scholars and practitioners of CHC, biocriticism affords opportunities for theoretical development and for broadening CHC's audiences and collaborators. First, biocriticism provides the theoretical scaffolding for producing analyses of the texts, contexts, audiovisual and material artifacts, assemblages, practices, and infrastructures of contemporary life to demonstrate how these resituate the relations between biology and culture/politics. More specifically, biocriticism offers resources for illuminating how the biological sciences are implicated in systems of power, representation, and resistance in health discourses (Khan, 2013, 2020). By excavating how biomedical knowledge is constructed and mobilized to reinforce or challenge power structures, biocriticism allows us to understand how biomedical knowledge may be used to exacerbate power imbalances and inequities in healthcare systems or how it might be used to create more humane and compassionate systems (Dutta, 2008; Sastry & Dutta, 2011, 2012, 2017). Consistent with the emancipatory aims of CCA, biocriticism can also be used to call into question Western biomedical dominance (Khan, 2013, 2020), opening spaces for indigenous or culturally suppressed voices and perspectives (Dutta, 2008) and for employing a range of methods, including embodied methods (Ellingson, 2019; Kline & Khan, 2019), as well as creative and artistic expression.

Conceptually, biocriticism can be used to reconsider and even revise key concepts in health communication and to examine how particular discursive fields are transformed by contemporary biology and medicine. For instance, in reaction to the developing rhetoric of postgenomic science, neurobiology, and microbiomics, humanities researchers are redefining words such as "identity" and "self" (Malabou, 2007), concepts of "sociality" and "citizenship" (Heath et al., 2007; Novas & Rose, 2000; Rabinow, 1996), and categories such as "legal right-holders," which are currently expanding to include non-humans, and even hypothetically, to microbiomes (Bapteste et al., 2021). Terms like "biosociality," "biocitizenship," "biovalue," or "biocapital" are emergent, debated concepts that require ongoing scrutiny (Birch & Tyfield, 2013; Rose, 2007). A simple way of understanding these terminological transformations would be Hayles's (2020) suggestion that formulations are important because they "can lead to better futures for us and for the more-than-human organisms with which we share the planet" (n.p.). As performative interventions, these neologisms invite reconsideration of key assumptions in the discursive fields of law, ecology, economics, sociology, and political citizenship. By linking to these existing humanities conversations, CHC scholars can build theory and spur conceptual development across discourse domains.

Engaging with these broader humanities authors and frameworks creates opportunities for CHC scholars to expand their transdisciplinary audiences and collaborators. Kline and Khan (2019) recently called for increased

CHC transdisciplinary collaboration, while acknowledging that "the path of collaborative research is not easy" (n.p.). Humanities scholars comprise one such broader set of audiences possessing affinities with CHC, and they present numerous possibilities for collaboration. Especially relevant connection points include projects conducted under the label "biohumanities" (Séginger, n. d.; Stotz & Griffiths, 2008). Philosophy is a prominent actor in contemporary biohumanities, where the rhetoric of immunology, for instance, spurs ongoing reflection on the relations between individuals and communities, and reassessments of our conceptions of the body politic (Esposito, 2002; Neyrat, 2011).

Covid-19 has energized the biohumanities. Hayles (2020) maintains that our philosophical terminology needs to adapt to current biological and medical discourse post-pandemic. "We need a thorough reconceptualization," she argues, "of the concepts and vocabularies with which to describe and analyze these complex interdependencies, as well as the ways in which humans, as a species, are interdependent with one another as well" (n.p.). Similarly, Butler's search for a philosophical terminology appropriate to the pandemic may also be stimulating for CHC, because Butler engages critically with the Covid-19 catch-phrases permeating media reporting and everyday discussions. Butler (2022) reinterprets "the health of the economy" as "life-taking figuration" (p. 53) that masks the sacrifice of human lives under the anthropomorphization of the economy. Butler also criticizes certain forms of pandemic communication for constructing a "metric of grievability" (p. 86), whose normalization of acceptable death rates masks the biopolitical violence of social and racial inequalities. These philosophical interventions may sometimes adopt different aims than CHC work on Covid-19. Nonetheless, CHC scholars might engage productively with Butler's (2022) concept of "differential grievability" (p. 94), for instance, or with Mbembe's (2023, p. 30) critique of ecological metrics or Barnett's (2022) work on the power of naming, archiving, and making visible "ecological grief," to problematize conceptions of acceptable loss.

Biocriticism is also increasingly engaging with three areas of study that transcend disciplines: ecocriticism, cultural studies of synthetic biology and artificial intelligence, and care ethics, creating further possibilities for CHC scholars to extend their work into these domains. Ecocriticism, which grounds critical work in environmental questions, offers valuable frameworks for biocriticism at a time when the biosciences and public discourse are increasingly configured in ecological terms (Campos, 2021). Consider, for instance, what is gained and lost by viewing the human or animal body as an "ecosystem" or a "zoo" (Bapteste, 2018; Enders, 2014; Yong, 2017) or by understanding biological discourses as situated within an escalating ecological crisis. In the environmental humanities, microbiology has stimulated the emergence of new terminology that can be described both as biocritical and as ecocritical, such as Haraway's *sympoiesis*, a practice of "making-with" non-human life forms (Haraway, 2016). In outlining an emergent *symbiopolitics*, other humanities researchers are problematizing the "densely political relations among many entangled things ... coexisting, incorporating, and mixing with one another" (Helmreich, 2014, p. 56). Engaging in ecologically attentive biocriticism is one way that CHC scholars can continue to extend literatures and frameworks in environmental health communication (see, e.g., de Los Santos Upton et al., 2021, de Onís, 2021; Ivancic, 2020; Juanals, 2020; Zoller, 2012) in conversation with ecocriticism and biohumanities.

Additionally, the rapidity with which AI and synthetic biology are stretching the bounds of what is human, blurring distinctions between life forms, and merging with cybernetic intelligence (Bhaskar & Suleyman, 2023) suggests the importance of tracking newly emerging cyber-biological assemblages and subjectivities. These developments also prompt the need for unraveling the implications of cyber-biological beings across domains such as popular scientific entertainments, artistic works, scientific discourses, and vernacular rhetoric. Such focus facilitates conceptual reconsideration of cyborg embodiment (Haraway, 2016). Finally, the recognition that ecological, individual, and collective health are intertwined has increasingly led scholars to embrace care ethics (de Onís, 2021; Dutta, 2008; Pezzullo, 2023; Puig de la Bellacasa, 2017) that stress relational interdependence, attentiveness, and responsibility to other humans and other life forms, and respect in building interconnected systems of care. CHC scholars can use biocriticism to reformulate models and conceptions of care.

Efforts to address these areas can build on an already promising trove of biocritical CHC work (see, for starters, Bennett, 2009; Condit, 1989, 1999; Cooke-Jackson, 2021; de Los Santos Upton et al., 2021; de Souza, 2024; Dutta, 2022; Happe, 2013; Ivancic, 2020; Johnson, 2018, 2023; Juanals, 2020; Kalin & Gruber, 2018; Keränen, 2011; Khan, 2013, 2020; Malkowski, 2014; Mitchell, 2013; Rowland, 2020; Sastry & Basu, 2020; Sastry & Dutta, 2011, 2012, 2017; Scott, 2003; Winderman et al., 2019, 2023; York & Tang, 2021; Zoller, 2012). The wide range of scholarship that falls under the umbrella of biocriticism presents an opportunity to identify and assess the major concepts and findings across work from CHC and various allied fields. This effort would establish a baseline of research topoi, findings, and approaches on which future biocriticism projects could build.

We close this chapter at a time when environmental degradation, mass extinction, global poverty, terrorism and violence, authoritarianism, food insecurity, resource scarcity, and high disease rates punctuate the precarity of human and planetary life. Through its attention to the mutual relations of biology, power, and culture/politics, biocriticism constitutes a necessary and important response to these urgent challenges. By facilitating ongoing sensemaking about power relations as the "age of biology" confronts environmental and human crises, biocriticism encourages CHC scholars to develop resources not only for concern but also for hope, resilience, and shared futurity. Simply put, biocriticism offers an inventional and interventional reservoir for the "arts of living on a damaged planet" (Tsing et al., 2017, i).

References

Adenis, M.-S. (2021). *Masques virus* [carbon fiber, beads and wire]. Artist's collection.
Adenis, M.-S. (2024). *Le virus que donc je suis* [artist's website]. https://mariesarahadenis.com/Le-virus-que-donc-je-suis-1
Airhihenbuwa, C. O. (1995). *Health and culture: Beyond the Western paradigm*. Sage.
Aït-Touati, F., & Latour, B. (2021). *Viral* [performance]. Nanterre-Amandiers Theatre, France.
Anker, S. (2015). Foreword. In W. Myers, (Ed.), *Bio art: Altered realities* (p. 06). Thames & Hudson.
Baglia, J., Defenbaugh, N., & Foster, E. (2024). Healthful, heartful, and hopeful narrative in medicine: An autoethnographic performance text. *Liminalities: A Journal of Performance Studies, 20*(1 & 2). http://liminalities.net/20-1/healthful-heartful-hopeful.html
Bapteste, E. (2018). *Tous entrelacés: Des gènes aux super-organismes: Les réseaux de l'évolution*. Belin.
Bapteste, E., Gérard, P., Larose, C., Blouin, M., Not, F., Campos, L., Aïdan, G., Selosse, M. A., Adénis, M. S., Bouchard, F., Dutreuil, S., Corel, E., Vigliotti, C., Huneman, P., Lapointe, F. J., & Lopez, P. (2021). The epistemic revolution induced by microbiome studies: An interdisciplinary view. *Biology, 10*(7), 651–665.
Barbieri, M. (Ed.). (2008). *The codes of life: Rules of macroevolution*. Springer.
Barnett, J. T. (2022). *Mourning in the anthropocene: Ecological grief and earthly coexistence*. Michigan State University Press.
Basnyat, I. (2014). Lived experiences of street-based female sex workers in Kathmandu: Implications for health intervention strategies. *Culture, Health & Sexuality, 16*(9), 1040–1051.
Bennett, J. A. (2009). *Banning queer blood: Rhetorics of citizenship, contagion, and resistance*. University of Alabama Press.
Bernard, C. (2018). *Matière à réflexion: Du corps politique dans la littérature et les arts visuels britanniques contemporains*. Presses de l'Université Paris-Sorbonne.
Bernard, C. (2022). Vibrant allegories: Questioning immunity with Ali Smith's *Seasonal Quartet* (2016–2020). *Études anglaises, 1*(75), 13–29.

Bhaskar, M., & Suleyman, M. (2023). *The coming wave: AI, power, and the twenty-first century's greatest dilemma*. Bodley Head.

Birch, K. & Tyfield, D. (2013). Theorizing the bioeconomy: Biovalue, biocapital, bioeconomics or … what? *Science, Technology, & Human Values*, 38(3), 299–327.

Butler, J. (2022). *What world is this? A pandemic phenomenology*. Columbia University Press.

Campos, L. (2021). Microbiome poetics: Metaphors and narrative strategies in popular biology [online talk]. https://evol-net.fr/2021/02/19/international-interdisciplinary-colloquium-new-challenges-induced-by-microbiomes/

Campos, L. (2022). *BioCriticism*. https://biocriticism.hypotheses.org/about

Campos, L. & Patoine, P.-L. (Eds.). (2022). *Life, re-scaled: The biological imagination in twenty-first-century literature and performance*. Open Book Publishers. https://www.openbookpublishers.com/books/10.11647/obp.0303

Conaty, S., Ike, J. D., Lane, W., Bayerle, H., Logan, R. A., & Parker, R. M. (2024). Understanding breast cancer images in art history as a form of health communication. *Journal of Health Communication*, 29(5), 340–346.

Condit, C. (1989). *Decoding abortion rhetoric: Communicating social change*. University of Illinois Press.

Condit, C. M. (1999). *Meanings of the gene: Public debates about human heredity*. University of Wisconsin Press.

Cooke-Jackson, A. (2021). Emergent health communication scholarship from and about African American, Latino/a/x, and American Indian/Alaskan Native peoples. *Health Communication*, 37(9), 1057–1060.

Czerwiec, M. K, Williams, I., Squier, S. M., Green, M. J., Myers, K. R., & Smith, S. T. (2015). *Graphic medicine manifesto*. Penn State University Press.

de Los Santos Upton, S., Tarin, C. A., & Hernández, L. H. (2021). Construyendo conexiones para los niños: Environmental justice, reproductive feminicidio, and coalitional possibility in the borderlands. *Health Communication*, 37(9), 1242–1252.

De Onís, C. (2021). "*La justicia ambiental es para ti y para mí*": Translating collective struggles for environmental and energy justice in Puerto Rico's Jobos Bay communities. *Frontiers in Communication*, 6. https://doi.org/10.3389/fcomm.2021.723999

de Souza, R. (2024). Women in the margins: A culture-centered interrogation of hunger and "food apartheid" in the United States. *Health Communication*, 39(9), 1855–1865.

Derkatch, C. (2022). *Why wellness sells: Natural health in a pharmaceutical culture*. Johns Hopkins University Press.

Dickinson, A. (2018). *Anatomic*. Coach House Books.

Dutta-Bergman, M. J. (2004). Poverty, structural barriers, and health: A Santali narrative of health communication. *Qualitative Health Research*, 14(8), 1107–1122.

Dutta, M. (2008). *Communicating health: A culture centered approach*. Polity.

Dutta, M. (2022). The whiteness of the rhetoric of health and medicine (RHM): A culture-centered framework for dismantling. *Departures in Critical Qualitative Research*, 11(1–2), 54–79.

Ellingson, L. L. (2019). Embodied methods in critical health communication. *Frontiers in Communication, 4*. https://doi.org/10.3389/fcomm.2019.00073

Enders, G. (2014). *Gut: The inside story of our body's most under-rated organ.* Faber & Faber.

Esposito, R. (2002). *Immunitas: The protection and negation of life* (Zakiya Hanafi, Trans.). Polity.

Favareau, D. (Ed.) (2010). *Essential readings in biosemiotics: Anthology and commentary.* Biosemiotics 3. Springer.

Foucault, M. (1998). *History of sexuality, Volume I.* Pantheon.

Foucault, M. (2003). *Society must be defended: Lectures at the Collège de France 1975–1976.* Picador.

Gill, J. (2020). *Biofictions: Race, Genetics and the Contemporary Novel.* Bloomsbury.

Gouge, C. (2017). Health humanities baccalaureate programs and the rhetoric of health and medicine. *Technical Communication Quarterly, 27*(1), 21–32.

Guha, R., & Spivak, G. C. (1988). *Selected subaltern studies.* Oxford University Press.

Happe, K. (2013). *The material gene: Gender, race, and heredity after the human genome project.* New York University Press.

Haraway, D. J. (2016). *Staying with the trouble: Making kin in the Chthulucene.* Duke University Press.

Harter, L. M., Pangborn, S.M., Ivancic, S., & Quinlan, M.M. (2017). Storytelling and social activism in health organizing. *Management Communication Quarterly, 31*, 314–320.

Hartnett, S. J. (2007). Investigative poetics. In G. Ritzer (Ed.), *The Blackwell encyclopedia of sociology* (pp. 2420–2424). https://doi.org/10.1002/9781405165518.wbeosi074

Hayles, N. K. (2020). Novel corona: Posthuman virus. *Critical Enquiry, 47*(S2), S68.

Heath, D., Rapp, R., & Taussig, K.-S. (2007). Genetic citizenship. In D. Nugent & J. Vincent (Eds.), *A companion to the anthropology of politics* (pp. 152–167). Blackwell.

Helmreich, S. (2014). Homo microbis: The human microbiome, figural, literal, political. *Thresholds, 42*, 52–59.

Hodges, N. (2014). The American dental dream. *Health Communication, 30*(9), 943–950.

Ivancic, S. R. (2020). "No one's coming to save us": Centering lived experiences in rural food insecurity organizing. *Health Communication 36*(8), 1039–1043. https://doi.org/10.1080/10410236.2020.1724644.

Johnson, J. (2018). (Ed.). *Graphic reproduction.* Pennsylvania State University Press.

Johnson, J. (2023). *Every living thing: The politics of life in common.* Pennsylvania State University Press.

Juanals, B. (2020). Communication and environmental health in critical American approaches. In I. Pailliart (Ed.), *New territories in health* (pp. 49–68). Wiley. https://doi.org/10.1002/9781119706731.ch3

Kalin, J., & Gruber, D. R. (2018). Gut rhetorics: Toward experiments in living with microbiota. *Rhetoric of Health & Medicine, 1*(3), 269–295.

Keränen, L. (2011). Addressing the "epidemic of epidemics": Germs, security, and a call for biocriticism. *Quarterly Journal of Speech*, 97(2), 224–244.
Khan, S. (2013). Manufacturing consent?: Media messages in the mobilization against HIV/AIDS in India and lessons for health communication. *Health Communication*, 29(3), 288–298.
Khan, S. (2020). Examining HIV/AIDS-related stigma at play: Power, structure, and implications for HIV interventions. *Health Communication, 35*, 1509–1519.
Kline, K. N., & Khan, S. (2019). Doing critical health communication: Negotiating the terrain of transdisciplinary collaboration. *Frontiers in Communication, 4*, https://doi.org/10.3389/fcomm.2019.00051.
Koerber, A. (2013). *Breast or bottle? Contemporary controversies in infant-feeding policy and practice*. University of South Carolina Press.
Koerber, A. (2018). *From hysteria to hormones: A rhetorical history*. Penn State University Press.
Krebs, E. (2020). Combating the ills of involuntary intake: A critical rhetorical analysis of Colorado's state psychiatric policies for suicidal patients. *Journal of Applied Communication Research, 48*(3), 310–327.
Kucukalik, L. (2022). *Biofictions: Literary and visual imagination in the age of biotechnology*. Routledge.
Kull, K. (1999). Biosemiotics in the twentieth century: A view from biology. *Semiotica, 127*(1/4), 385–414.
Lemke, T. (2011). *Biopolitics: An advanced introduction*. New York University Press.
Lynch, J. A., & Zoller, H. (2015). Recognizing differences and commonalities: The rhetoric of health and medicine and critical-interpretive health communication. *Communication Quarterly, 63*(5), 498–503.
Lyne, J. (1990). Bio-rhetorics: Moralizing the life sciences. In H. W. Simons (Ed.), *The rhetorical turn: Invention and persuasion in the conduct of inquiry* (pp. 35–57). University of Chicago Press.
Malabou, C, (2007). *Les nouveaux blessés. De Freud à la neurologie, penser les traumatismes contemporains*. Bayard.
Malkowski, J. A. (2014). Beyond prevention: Rhetorics of resistance and containment in social scientific discourse about bug chasing. *Journal of Medical Humanities, 35*, 211–228.
Malkowski, J. A., Scott, J. B., & Keränen, L. B. (2016). Rhetorical approaches to health and medicine. *Oxford Research Encyclopedia of Communication*. https://doi.org/10.1093/acrefore/9780190228613.013.180
Mbembe, A. (2023). *La communauté terrestre*. Editions La découverte.
Mitchell, R. (2013). *Experimental life: Vitalism in romantic science and literature*. Johns Hopkins University Press.
Neyrat, F. (2011). Intact (Roxanne Lapidus, Trans.). *SubStance, 40*(3), 105–114.
Novas, C., & Rose, N. (2000). Genetic risk and the birth of the somatic individual. *Economy and Society, 29*(4), 485–513.
Pezzullo, P. (2023). *Beyond straw men: Plastic pollution and networked cultures of care*. California University Press.
Puig de la Bellacasa, M. (2017). *Matters of care: Speculative ethics in more than human worlds*. University of Minnesota Press.

Rabinow, P. (ed.). (1996). *Artificiality and enlightenment: From sociobiology to biosociality.* In *Essays on the anthropology of reason.* Princeton University Press.
Rose, N. (2007). *The politics of life itself: Biomedicine, power, and subjectivity in the twenty-first century.* Princeton University Press.
Rose, N., & Novas, C. (2005). Biological citizenship. In A. Ong & S. Collier (Eds.), *Global assemblages: Technology, politics and ethics as anthropological problems* (pp. 439–463). Blackwell.
Rowland, A. L. (2020). *Zoetropes and the politics of humanhood.* Ohio State University Press.
Sastry, S., & Basu, A. (2020). How to have (critical) method in a pandemic: Outlining a culture-centered approach to health discourse analysis. *Frontiers in Communication, 5,* 58594.
Sastry, S., & Dutta, M. J. (2011). Postcolonial constructions of HIV/AIDS: Meaning, culture, and structure. *Health Communication, 26*(5): 437–449.
Sastry, S., & Dutta, M. J. (2012). Global health interventions and the 'common sense' of neoliberalism: A dialectical analysis of PEPFAR. *Journal of International and Intercultural Communication, 6*(1), 21–39.
Sastry, S., & Dutta, M. J. (2017). Health communication in the time of Ebola: A culture-centered interrogation. *Journal of Health Communication, 22,* 10–14. https://doi.org/10.1080/10810730.2016.1216205.
Sastry, S., Stephenson, M., Dillon, P., & Carter, A. (2021). A meta-theoretical systematic review of the culture-centered approach to health communication: Toward a refined, "nested" model. *Communication Theory, 31*(3), 380–421.
Sastry, S., Zoller, H. M., & Basu, A. (2019). Editorial: Doing critical health communication: A forum on methods. *Frontiers in Communication, 5,* 637579.
Scale Free Network (n.d.). Small friends books. https://www.smallfriendsbooks.com/
Scott, J. B. (2003). *Risky rhetoric: AIDS and the cultural practices of HIV testing.* Southern. Illinois University Press.
Scott, J. B., & Gouge, C. (2019). Theory building in the rhetoric of health and medicine. In A. Alden et al. (Eds.), *Reinventing (with) theory in rhetoric and writing studies: Essays in honor of Sharon Crowley* (pp. 181–195). Utah State University Press.
Scott, J. B., & Melonçon, L. (2019). RHM's relations and relationships. *Rhetoric of Health & Medicine 2*(4), iii–x.
Sebeok, T. A., & Umiker-Sebeok, J. (Eds.). (1992). *Biosemiotics. The semiotic web 1991.* Mouton de Gruyter.
Séginger, G. (n.d.). Biohumanities webpage. https://www.fmsh.fr/projets/biohumanities.
Séginger, G. (2015). Éléments pour une *biocritique. Flaubert: Revue Critique et Génétique, 13,* 1–13.
Shi, Z., & Wang, Y. (2024). Enhancing health communication through virtual reality-based art therapy: an opinion. *Frontiers in Psychology, 30*(5), 1438172.
Stavridis, J. (2014, January 19). The dawning of the age of biology. *Financial Times,* https://www.ft.com/content/36218738-6355-11e3-a87d-00144feabdc0
Stormer, N. (2014). Biocriticism, or how I learned to love disease. Paper presented at the annual convention of the National Communication Association. https://www.academia.edu/32234490/Biocriticism_or_How_I_Learned_to_Love_Disease

Stotz, K., & Griffiths, P. E. (2008). Biohumanities: Rethinking the relationship between biosciences, philosophy and history of science, and society. *The Quarterly Review of Biology, 83*, 37–45.

Stypinska, D. (2020). *On the genealogy of critique: Or how we have become decadently indignant*. Routledge.

Toulmin, S. (1964, December 31). The age of biology. *New York Review of Books*. https://www.ft.com/content/36218738-6355-11e3-a87d-00144feabdc0

Tsing, A., Swanson, H., Gan, E., & Bubandt, N. (Eds.). (2017). *Arts of living on a damaged planet*. University of Minnesota Press.

Van Dijck, J. (1998). *Imageneation: Popular images of genetics*. New York University Press.

Vermeulen, P. (2022). Depopulating the novel: Post-catastrophe fiction, scale, and the population unconscious. In L. Campos & P. L. Patoine (Eds.), *Life, re-scaled* (pp. 229–258). OpenBook Publishers.

Wald, P. (2008). *Contagious: Cultures, carriers, and the outbreak narrative*. Duke University Press.

Waldby, C. (2000). *The visible human project: Informatic bodies and posthuman medicine*. Routledge.

Williams, R. (1985). *Keywords: A vocabulary of culture and society*. Oxford University Press.

Winderman, E., Mejia, R., & Rogers, B. (2019). "All smell is disease": The sanitary bacteriologic of visceral public health. *Rhetoric of Health and Medicine, 2*, 115–146.

Winderman, E., Rowland, A., & Malkowski, J. L. (2023). *Covid and ... How to do rhetoric in a pandemic*. Michigan State University Press.

Yong, E. (2017). *I contain multitudes: The microbes within us and a grander view of life*. Vintage.

York, F. N., & Tang, L. (2021). "Picture me heart disease free": Understanding African Americans' cardiovascular disease experiences through a culture-centered approach. *Journal of Applied Communication Research, 49*, 247–266.

Zoller, H. M. (2012). Communicating health: Political risk narratives in an environmental health campaign. *Journal of Applied Communication Research, 40*(1), 20–43.

Zoller, H. M., & Kline, K. N. (2008). Interpretive and critical research in health communication. *Communication Yearbook, 32*, 88–135.

10
CULTURE-CENTERED APPROACH AS CRITICAL HEALTH PRACTICE

The Body as Resistance

Mohan Dutta, Satveer Kaur-Gill, Pankaj Baskey, Selina Metuamate, Indranil Mandal, and Venessa Pokaia

The meta-theoretical framework of the culture-centered approach (CCA) dismantles the hegemonic ways of thinking about health by centering the voices of communities in struggle, re-turning the ownership of defining what is health in the hands of communities at the margins. Simultaneously, the CCA engages with postcolonial communication theory, critiquing the Brahminical registers of postcolonial theory controlled by largely upper-caste, upper-class Indian academics descending from families with privilege within the postcolonial context of India (as we write this piece as a collective, we note our differential places of privilege in relationship to the caste-class structure in India and across the global North-South divide, shaping the power inequalities we negotiate in the contexts of caste, settler colonialism, racial capitalism, and imperialism). Based on the argument that epistemic violence—the violent erasure of knowledge systems and ways of knowing at the margins—is intertwined with health disparities, the CCA locates methodological entry points for dismantling the extractive, casteist, settler colonial, racial capitalist, and imperial investments in hegemonic knowledge systems.

Across studies of the CCA, voice infrastructures—systems, mechanisms, and platforms designed to amplify voices of communities that have been historically marginalized and, in extreme forms, erased from discursive registers—serve as sites where communities at the margins describe the structures, name them, and organize to dismantle them (Dutta, 2008, 2011, 2024). Take the example of the Listening 1965 project, co-created with the survivors of the 1965 genocide, where community advisory groups

DOI: 10.4324/9781003426530-13
This chapter has been made available under a CC BY-NC-ND license.

(CAGs) as voice infrastructures co-create songs, poetry, and a storyboard, weaved into a documentary witnessing the U.S.-sponsored genocide carried out in Indonesia that resulted in the destruction of the entire ecosystem of Left party workers, socialist intellectuals, and union organizers and activists (Pitaloka & Dutta, 2021). Voice infrastructures as registers of listening foreground the colonial-imperial violence that shapes the experiences of health and well-being among survivors. Our writing collective here reflects this politics of the ongoing struggle for voice and knowledge within culture-centered scholarship, bringing together two Indigenous community researchers (an Adivasi man and a Maori woman), a Singaporean Sikh woman with caste privileges who is an early career international researcher and an upper-caste, upper-class man who is a full professor. How we negotiate the inequalities in the distribution of power that constitute our relationships while generating knowledge claims is a core concern of the CCA, generating through co-authorships a radical politics that challenge the hegemonic structures that perpetuate injustices.

Drawing upon examples of community-led culture-centered interventions housed under the umbrella of the Center for Culture-centered Approach to Research and Evaluation (CARE), we outline the role of the "body on the line" as critical theory. The CCA, we argue, materializes Gramsci's "philosophy of praxis" (Haug, 1999), articulating the embodied work of theory generation as emergent from within struggles to co-create just material conditions that enable and sustain health. The interplays of community organizing and working-class organizing in the CCA, we argue, is the strongest theoretical contribution as a critical health communication meta-theory, disrupting the neoliberal construction of community as an arm of the market, foregrounding the inequalities and divergences that exist within communities, and turning to the community as the site of radical organizing challenging hegemonic state-market-NGO (non-governmental organization) structures. Our theoretical intervention, therefore, argues that it is through the body placed in values of care and relationality that academic-community-working-class solidarities can start dismantling the racist colonial infrastructures of capital that fundamentally threaten human health and well-being. The theoretical work of dismantling racial colonial capitalism is intertwined with the practical work of agitating in communities and in working-class struggles. Taking some examples of culture-centered interventions, we weave together a narrative account of the history of the CCA that connects contemporary land struggles, resistance to state authoritarianism, anti-racist organizing, worker struggles, and anti-hate organizing to the fundamental struggles for securing health.

Theorizing Health: Culture, Structure, Agency

Drawing upon its roots in the Marxist and postcolonial approaches, the CCA theorizes health at the intersections of culture, structure, and agency (Dutta, 2008, 2011). Because the critical premise of the CCA draws upon the exploration of the health consequences that result from the violent erasure of the cultural context of health, the earliest theoretical interventions within the umbrella of the CCA foregrounded the interplays of health meanings and cultural contexts (Dutta, 2004a, 2004b). In dialogue with the work of Airhihenbuwa (1999) on culture and health, the CCA builds on the theorizing of culture as the ever-changing assemblage of shared values, meanings, and norms to turn to the voices of communities at the global margins in theorizing health. The culture-centered dialogues with Santalis in Eastern India formed the basis for the earliest theoretical interventions into the CCA, foregrounding agency, the capacity of individuals, households, and communities to make sense of their health and co-create land-based struggles around ownership of land, health, and development resources (Dutta, 2004a, 2004b). The expression of agency as voice delineates the structural conditions that shape the everyday experiences of health at the margins, turning to method as listening (Dutta, 2014; Sastry et al., 2021). As the theorizing of the CCA further crystallized, this culture-structure-agency interplay emerged as a key feature of the theory, placing the relationship among meanings, health, communication, and voice at these intersections. CCA studies to date organize how these relationships are reflected in community voices.

Culture

Culture is defined and discussed as the key driver of the CCA with the theoretical perspective emphasizing cultural meanings by listening to the cultural narratives of communities. Cultural narratives in the CCA emphasize grounding insights from community discussions of their health meanings through a culture, structure, and agency fulcra. How participants discuss culture as health from the standpoint of political, social, cultural, and economic struggle and exclusion are central to the CCA's operationalization of culture. Dutta (2004a) explains culture as "both transformative and constitutive, providing an axis for theorizing the discursive processes through which meanings are socially constructed by members" (p. 241). Members in this context are the communities CCA researchers work collectively with to co-constructively challenge and agitate against structural forces that constrain health justice for members in the margins of society.

When guided by the CCA, the goals for centering culture go beyond interpreting culture as surface-level structures. Surface-level structures are cultural elements and characteristics for building health messages tailored to a target audience (Resnicow et al., 2000), what Dutta (2007) describes as cultural sensitivity. The CCA guides health communication scholars toward recognizing cultural meanings in community members' descriptions of culture at the intersections of structure and agency. CCA-guided studies identify cultural meanings and contexts seeking to understand and foreground cultural knowledge in centering health meanings and moving away from stabilizing and essentializing culture as variables classified within brackets and categories for predicting health outcomes. By paying attention to how participants share cultural meanings and how meanings are assigned to health discussions by participants, the structure, culture, and agency nexus pivots to emphasize how participants define culture agentically in the context of health structures (e.g., Basu et al., 2016). To elaborate, this involves identifying how participants negotiate their health meanings in the context of subordination by dominant forms of knowledge production that keep stories of health in the margins.

An example includes the cultures of shame produced around women's bodies and bodily functions across the globe through various forms of constraining structural forms of power (e.g., Pindi, 2020; Rawat et al., 2021). In a study anchored in the CCA, conducted by Rawat et al. (2021) in North India, the authors discuss the intersections of Brahminical patriarchy and casteist structures that perpetuate taboos around menstruation detrimental to women's health outcomes. Here, the intersections of gendered forms of marginalization rooted in patriarchal practices of shaming women for bodily functions have implications for how women sought to address management options for menstruation. Gender policing, surveilling, and shaming operate from and through cultural enactments of harm. The discussion of culture, therefore, is read within the context of structure and agency.

Structure

The interpretation of structures in the CCA structure, culture, and agency nexus locates structures through forms of social organizing that constrain and enable access of individuals, households, communities, and broader societies to health resources (Dutta et al., 2024). Turning to health within a broader constellation of meanings around food, environment, ecosystem, worker rights, cultural rights, etc., shapes how the organizing structures around health are interpreted and approached. Critical health communication theory anchored in the CCA attends to the interplays of settler colonialism, racial capitalism, imperialism, and patriarchy as the driving structures that shape the experiences of health among communities that are disenfranchised (Dutta, 2023a; Elers & Dutta, 2024).

Structures are conceptualized as patterns of social organizing that enable or constrain cultural members' abilities to access health resources and engage in healthful behaviors (Dutta, 2008; Giddens, 2007; Sastry, 2016). The central point of analysis in the approach is how these structures are governed to constrain access to healthful lives of all people in society. How structures are articulated has been outlined in multiple germinal pieces as a key organizing concept of the CCA, which involves recognizing the role of social forces that enact or constrain human agency in achieving good health (see Bates et al., 2019; Carter & Alexander, 2020; Kumar, 2021; Mukherjee & Basu, 2024; Stanley & Basu, 2023). A structural analysis grounded in the CCA unpacks the role structures play in shaping entrenched health inequalities experienced by communities. Community members discuss the context and intersections of power, delineating the roles capitalist-colonial forces play in contributing to health inequities globally from settler colonial violence through the ongoing theft of land from Indigenous communities and occupation of Indigenous land (Elers & Dutta, 2023), food insecurity from stigmatizing neoliberal policy programs (de Souza, 2023), and precarious migration infrastructures aimed at extracting labor for profits (Kaur-Gill & Dutta, 2023; Robb, 2021, 2023). Noting that "the capitalist logic of the colonial project is built upon generating profit through extractive habits that mark the culture of the colonized as needing saving, building the rhetorical basis for the ongoing expansion of whiteness" (Dutta, 2024, p. 407), culture-centered methods explore partnerships that are invested in the dismantling of these structures (Dutta & Pal, 2020). The process of naming the structures, including the naming of the structures occupied by academics, in ways that are legible to communities at the margins, is central to the processes of organizing for structural transformation.

Agency

Building on the work of the Subaltern Studies collective that explores how structures of erasure are scripted into hegemonic sites of knowledge production, the CCA locates voice in the agency of communities at the "margins of the margins." The concept "margins of the margins" attends to the continual erasure of voices built into the organizing of hegemonic structures, the power embedded in sites and processes of knowledge generation, and the ongoing struggles for power over spaces of knowledge generation. The CCA critically engages with Spivak's theorizing of "Can the subaltern speak?" noting that the framing of the question, "Can the subaltern speak?" as a dichotomy is theoretically embedded within the location of caste-class privileged academia in postcolonial India (largely occupied by children of upper-caste upper-class academics, bureaucrats, managers of civil society, and corporate executives), where postcolonial elites with Brahminical privilege pronounce the impossibility of subaltern agency without facilitating the work of social mobilization for structural change (Da Costa, 2023). Worse, the space of alterity is taken over by the Brahminical elite, speaking of the otherness of the Empire while conveniently erasing one's complicity with caste, imperialism, and settler colonialism (Figueira, 2008). Contrast this with the work of the Latin American Subaltern Studies collective and the work of Freire (Beverley, 1999; Freire, 1996; Freire et al., 1997). Similarly, contrast the text-based elitism of postcolonial and Subaltern Studies with the embodied methods of generating knowledge that emerge from Indigenous studies (Xaxa, 2008, 2021). Note that the postcolonial, Subaltern Studies caste elites systematically erase the literature in Indigenous studies while writing about the impossibility of Indigenous agency (Bhukya, 2021; Hokowhitu et al., 2020; Xaxa, 2008, 2021).

The argument posed by Indian postcolonial scholars, and certainly by postcolonial media studies and communication scholars in the mainstream, suggests that an academic by nature of their complicity with structures of power cannot co-construct knowledge with community groups that are marginalized and dispossessed for they suggest that there can never be a recovery of unadulterated knowledge of the subaltern. We refute these rhetorical forms of foreclosure and depart from the premise that co-creation is impossible because of power differentials, approaching subaltern knowledge as a point for social mobilization and structural change. Those of us, Indigenous (and Adivasi) scholars in our collective, note that our struggles for laying claims to postcolonial development are tied to our struggles for asserting our knowledge. Moreover, we note that upper-caste Indian elites precisely use this technique of unseeing Indigenous knowledge to carry out extractive development projects, propped up through police and military violence (Pasternak et al., 2023; Soundadarajan, 2022). Instead, the CCA names the forms of power imbalances (caste, class, gender, settlers of color) as a generative entry point for working through the impossibilities of achieving a space for equal power between communities and academics when academics are employed by the settler colonial, racial capitalist, and imperial university. We argue that the caricature of unadulterated, pure, or transparent knowledge is a violence concocted by caste academics who carry out our critiques without naming our own caste investments.

In the United States, for instance, where most upper-caste, Indian postcolonial scholars write from, such naming of our caste investments and our positions as "settlers of colour" (Patel, 2010) offer critical anchors for connecting with Indigenous struggles against the settler colonial state (Elers & Dutta, 2024; Patel, 2010). Simultaneously, the mobilization to insert the registers of knowledge at the subaltern margins into the hegemonic spaces creates the anchor for social change in anti-capitalist and anti-colonial ways (Elers & Dutta, 2024). For instance, in the Indian context, the organizing of Adivasi Studies, foregrounding Adivasi scholarship and diverse Adivasi subjectivities, is a critical anchor to social change, foregrounding the heterogeneities, complexities, and dynamic cultural spaces across Indigenous contexts (Dutta et al., 2024; Xaxa, 2008).

Postcolonial scholars, a large proportion of whom come from caste elite upper-class families of India, ensconced in the privilege of critique of the text while "writing castelessly" (Da Costa, 2023), fail to account for social justice methods and praxis that read the university as a site for dismantling (academe as a site of political solidarity and reckoning against the neoliberal apparatus) and seek to reimagine the university as an extension of social justice movements, including the development of scholarship that centers pedagogies of radical listening (Freire et al., 1997; Herakova et al., 2024), critical Indigenous pedagogies and methodologies for centering radical care, commitment, and solidarity with subaltern communities at the global margins (Dutta et al., 2023; Dutta, 2023b, Elers & Dutta, 2023). Furthermore, these foreclosures of subaltern forms of knowledge production remove the work of resistance and transformation of the structural conditions within which the subaltern voices are grounded. One of us, Mohan, shares this dialogue with a colleague, Ambar Basu, in an autoethnographic exploration:

> So what I see here, Ambar, is how a certain way of doing postcolonial scholarship, valorizing high theory from afar, it itself a colonizing process. Postcolonial work as high theory rewrites and reworks the colonial enterprise, reiterating the tools of the colonial master in its celebrations of theory as removed from the everyday struggles of/in subaltern communities and detached from the messiness of everyday life. The "theorizing on" instead of "theorizing with" reproduces the colonial relationships of extraction.
> *(Dutta & Basu, 2018, p. 89)*

Resisting Health Communication

The CCA as a critical health practice connects the everyday work of critique to the practices of building community spaces for activism and resistance. Noting that the hegemonic approaches to health communication uphold the agendas of settler colonialism, racial capitalism, and empire, the CCA outlines a framework of health communication as practice organized toward securing health as justice. The framing of health as justice disrupts the individualizing and reductionist logics of hegemonic health communication.

Decentering the Whiteness of Health Communication

The CCA foregrounds the whiteness of health communication, tracing, mapping, and critically interrogating the values of white culture that are upheld and perpetuated as universal (Dutta, 2005). In building registers for theorizing health from the margins, the CCA challenges the hegemonic assumption that Western norms, values, and practices are universally applicable and superior to those of other cultures. Instead, the CCA recognizes the diversity and complexity of cultural contexts, seeking to understand health within its socio-cultural and historical dimensions. By centering the voices and experiences of marginalized communities, the CCA challenges the hegemony of whiteness in health communication and promotes more inclusive, equitable, and culturally relevant approaches to health promotion and intervention.

Additionally, the CCA examines the role of power and representation in shaping health communication discourses and practices. Whiteness is often privileged in mainstream media and advertising, perpetuating stereotypes, and reinforcing inequalities in health outcomes. Through critical analysis and deconstruction of media representations, the CCA seeks to challenge dominant narratives that marginalize and stigmatize racialized communities. This may involve developing counter-narratives that challenge stereotypes, highlight the resilience and agency of marginalized communities, and promote alternative visions of health and wellness. Furthermore, the CCA advocates for structural changes that address the root causes of health inequities, including racism, poverty, and social injustice. Rather than focusing solely on individual behaviors or lifestyle choices, the CCA recognizes the structural determinants of health and advocates for policies and practices that promote equity and social justice (Sastry et al., 2021). This may involve collaborating with community organizations, advocacy groups, and policymakers to address systemic barriers to health, such as lack of access to healthcare, discriminatory practices, and unequal distribution of resources.

Co-Creating Community Spaces

Community spaces of participation take the form of CAGs mobilized in the politics of social change (Dutta, 2014, 2018b). These CAGs serve as voice infrastructures, where community members at the "margins of the margins" articulate their voices, offering interpretive frames through which health is understood. CAGs play a crucial role in the CCA by serving as collaborative partners and catalysts for meaningful community engagement, research, and action. These groups typically consist of representatives from the communities at the margins, including community leaders, activists, advocates, and other stakeholders who bring diverse perspectives, expertise, cultural knowledge, and lived experiences to the research process (Dutta, 2018b). In the CCA, CAGs function as key decision-makers, advisors, and advocates, shaping the direction, design, and implementation of research projects and interventions in ways that are responsive to the needs, priorities, and aspirations of the communities they represent.

CAGs serve as advocates and catalysts for translating research findings into action and driving positive change in their communities. CAGs drive the social change processes directed at transforming the social determinants of health. By actively engaging with researchers, policymakers, and other stakeholders, advisory group members help to disseminate research findings, advocate for policy reforms, and mobilize resources to address pressing social issues and inequities. This collaborative approach ensures that research has real-world impact and contributes to meaningful improvements in the lives of community members. The generation of knowledge within advisory groups and the dissemination of this knowledge through voice infrastructures in the form of white papers, policy briefs, and community-owned media such as community radio and communication campaigns shape the ongoing politics of structural transformation. In summary, CAGs play a multifaceted and integral role in the CCA by guiding research priorities, ensuring cultural relevance and sensitivity, facilitating community engagement and participation, upholding ethical considerations, and translating research into action. By fostering meaningful partnerships between researchers and community stakeholders, advisory groups help ensure that research is conducted collaboratively, ethically, and impactfully, ultimately contributing to positive social change and empowerment within marginalized communities.

Structural Transformation

Whereas on the one hand, the CCA in communication studies emphasizes understanding communication within specific cultural contexts, acknowledging the role of culture in shaping communication practices, meanings, and outcomes, on the other hand, it sees the cultural construction of meanings as a site for structural transformation (Dutta, 2014). In this approach, structural transformation refers to the process of challenging and changing hegemonic power dynamics, social structures, and systems of inequality within and across cultures. Cultures as sites of struggles are dynamic and transformative, placed at the margins of hegemonic forms of organizing. Simultaneously, cultures serve as registers for negotiating power and control within communities (Dutta, 2008). Praxis is intertwined with method in the CCA, working through the research process toward structural transformation, with knowledge claims made by the "margins of the margins" serving as registers for mobilizing against settler colonial, racial capitalist, imperial, and patriarchal structures (Dutta et al., 2019, 2023; Elers & Dutta, 2024). Consider, for instance, the work of the CCA in co-creating voice infrastructures with stateless Rohingya refugees, where mobilizing to lay claims to identity, serves as fundamental sites for resisting the ongoing colonial, authoritarian, and Islamophobic genocidal violence (Rahman & Dutta, 2023).

Across a wide range of contexts, the CCA also engages in policy advocacy and efforts to bring about institutional change through culture-centered communication campaigns co-created by communities at the "margins of the margins." By working to change policies and practices at the macro level, CCA seeks to address the root causes of inequality and create more inclusive communication environments. The work of culture-centered interventions seeking to create spaces for erased conversations in hegemonic registers forms a core element in community-led advocacy, community activism, and mobilization toward broader movements.

Overall, structural transformation in the CCA involves a multifaceted process of challenging power structures, amplifying marginalized voices, promoting cultural anchoring, fostering community participation, advocating for policy change, and facilitating transformative communication practices aimed at creating more equitable and just societies. Consider here some of the key nodes of culture-centered scholarship around Adivasi resistance, worker resistance, anti-racist interventions, and interventions addressing the health rights of gender diverse communities. Across the various spaces, culture-centered interventions often take the form of photovoice exhibits, video-based stories, advertising campaigns, news media kits, songs, poems, performances, protest marches, etc., resisting racism, settler colonialism, capitalism, patriarchy, and imperialism.

CARE as a Transformative Space

CARE created as a space for carrying out culture-centered scholarship, initially in Singapore, and then at Massey University in Aotearoa New Zealand, started experimenting with the work of communication for social change when health meanings emergent from the margins are centered in building voice infrastructures. Within its first three years of inception, CARE offered the space for experimenting with, theorizing, studying, and participating in health activism for health justice, anchored in academic-community partnerships (Dutta et al., 2019). The recognition that the structures that constrain health must be actively challenged through communication turned the praxis of health communication into everyday activism, agitating for an anchor for transformative health communication scholarship that took seriously the work of activism and community engagement within the field of communication studies. An example of CARE's transformative research can be found in its projects focused on health equity and social determinants of health. For instance, CARE has conducted studies examining the impact of structural inequalities, such as poverty, racism, and environmental injustice, on health outcomes in marginalized communities (see the CARE 10th Anniversary Documentary: https://www.youtube.com/watch?v=XKQiccSAqJc). Furthermore, CARE's work extends beyond the academic sphere to encompass advocacy and policy engagement efforts to address systemic injustices and promote human rights. CARE researchers actively collaborate with policymakers, activists, and civil society organizations to translate research findings into actionable policy recommendations, lobby for legislative reforms, and hold institutions accountable for upholding principles of equity and justice (Dutta, 2024).

The Body in Resistance

The criticality of the CCA therefore turns to the body as the site of resistance, recognizing that the work of interrogating power must be intricately tied to the everyday work of dismantling power formations.

Critical Reflexivity in the CCA

Critical reflexivity is pivotal in the CCA, serving as a foundational principle guiding research, practice, and engagement within this framework (Dutta & Basu, 2013, 2018). It encompasses a commitment to self-awareness, introspection, and ongoing examination of one's positionality, familial and network privileges, and ethical considerations in relation to the research process and the communities one seeks to journey alongside (Dutta, 2019). The turn to critical reflexivity in the CCA foregrounds the power tied to the position of the settler colonial academic of color (caste power and settler colonial power are central organizing nodes here, given the engagement of the CCA with Indigenous and Black struggles (see Patel, 2010), noting that the impossibility of listening to subaltern knowledge stems precisely from the power concentrated in the hegemonic positions held by academics (whiteness, caste, settler, patriarchy, cisnormativity, class), then asking, what does it mean to decenter the arrogance of the practices of academic knowledge production by centering habits of listening? At its core, critical reflexivity within the CCA involves a continuous interrogation of the researcher's own assumptions, perspectives, privileges, and situatedness within broader socio-cultural contexts, inviting the researcher to name the sources of privilege and then work through friendships with the subaltern margins to decenter these spaces of privilege. It acknowledges that researchers are not removed observers or textual analysts, but are inevitably shaped by their social location, identities, and experiences. Therefore, embracing critical reflexivity requires researchers to examine how our backgrounds, privileges, and relational investments influence our interpretations, interactions, and ethical decision-making throughout the research process.

One of the key tenets of critical reflexivity is recognizing the inherent power dynamics that exist within the research relationship (Basnyat, 2019). Researchers often hold positions of privilege and authority relative to the communities they study, which can impact the dynamics of knowledge production and dissemination. Critical reflexivity prompts researchers to critically examine how their positions of power may shape their interactions with research participants, the types of knowledge that are valued and prioritized, and the ways in which research findings are communicated and utilized. Moreover, critical reflexivity within the CCA involves a commitment to actively challenging and disrupting dominant narratives and ideologies that perpetuate inequality and marginalization. This requires researchers to critically reflect on our own complicities in perpetuating and/or challenging oppressive structures and systems of power. By engaging in critical reflexivity, researchers can work toward decolonizing knowledge production processes and fostering more equitable and just forms of scholarship and activism. Dutta and Basu, writing about the postcolonial elite capture of social change and social justice rhetoric, note (p. 85):

> We, for the most purposes, perform marginalia in the U.S. academe, muddling the class- and caste-based privileges that have enabled us the entry into the U.S. academe to begin with. This culturalist framework of postcolonial studies, separated from questions of structure, enables a new colonial logic where privileged brown academics become the designated mouthpieces of the postcolonial nation, erasing the voices of the margins that do not conveniently fit into the story of market-driven growth and postcolonial revival.

Practically, critical reflexivity within the CCA is enacted through a variety of methods and strategies. Reflexive journaling, for example, allows researchers to document their thoughts, feelings, and insights throughout the research process, providing a space for self-reflection and introspection (Dutta, 2004a, 2004b; Dutta & Basu, 2013). Reflexive dialogues within the academic team, with civil society partners, with movement leaders and peer debriefings offer opportunities for researchers to engage in critical conversations with colleagues and community members, soliciting feedback and alternative perspectives that can enrich the research process, and simultaneously highlighting the ways in which the specific power positions of academics on the team (Dutta et al., 2018). Writing up, writing in, and writing out these positions of power and privilege invested in the subject positions occupied by the academic team members is a crucial step toward building public registers. For a Savarna male Indian academic, for instance, this call to critical reflexivity is first and foremost about learning to write by including this caste position, then working through strategies of dismantling the privileges that come with the caste position. See for instance Dutta (2004a, 2004b), where the form of writing practice seeks to negotiate the implications of the caste and class position when writing about Adivasi struggles.

Furthermore, critical reflexivity informs the design and implementation of research methodologies within the CCA. Researchers working with the CCA strive to adopt participatory and collaborative approaches that center the voices and experiences of marginalized communities, while also acknowledging the limitations and complexities inherent in their own positionalities. This process of rendering visible the positions of power held by researchers because of our relationships with structures (patriarchy, caste, settler colonialism, racial capitalism, and imperialism) however has to be made accessible to communities we build relationships with, figuring out ways in which these forms of power can be read, challenged, and mobilized toward achieving strategic objectives of social change (Dutta, 2024). Reflexive praxis, therefore, involves actively involving community members in the research process, soliciting their input and feedback, and co-creating knowledge that is grounded in their lived realities and needs (Dutta, 2010; Dutta & de Souza, 2008). Co-creation is itself an invitation to critically interrogate the hyphen in the co and creation, working through carefully the inequalities in the distribution of power, the impossibilities of listening that are tied to these unequal terrains of power, and the hopes that can be carved together through an ethics of friendship (Dutta, 2004a, 2004b). The CCA turns reflexivity into a public and collective exercise, foregrounding the necessity of rendering academic privilege and processes of knowledge generation legible to communities for critical analysis and action (Dutta, 2019). To co-create the capacities for holding academics to account within public spaces is to build public pedagogies within communities for critically unpacking the workings of class, caste, imperialism, patriarchy and cisnormativity (Dutta, 2024). These processes of democratizing knowledge through shared radical commitments to social justice also work simultaneously to reshape authorship practices, inviting in community members, community organizers, and community researchers and activists as co-authors and leaders in writing articles.

In addition to its role in research practice, critical reflexivity within the CCA extends to advocacy and activist efforts aimed at promoting social change and transformation. Researchers recognize that their work has implications beyond academia and seek to leverage their findings and insights to inform policy, mobilize communities, and advocate for structural reforms. By engaging in critical reflexivity, researchers can better navigate the ethical dilemmas and complexities that arise in their efforts to enact meaningful social change. Overall, critical reflexivity is an essential aspect of the CCA, serving as both a guiding principle and a methodological tool for scholars and practitioners engaged in communication research and activism. By embracing critical reflexivity, researchers can work toward more ethical, inclusive, and transformative forms of scholarship and engagement that center the voices and experiences of marginalized communities and challenge systems of power and oppression.

Body on the Line

In the CCA, the concept of "body on the line" begins with an ethic of humility, recognizing that historic casteist, settler colonial, and imperial forms of knowledge production have worked from the arrogance of the text. Resisting this textual hegemony (which itself is a reflection of upper-caste privilege engaged in the service of colonialism and imperialism), "body on the line" politics of method calls for a deep commitment to embodied engagement, activism, and solidarity with marginalized communities, turning toward an ethic of listening that seeks to locate research methods in the hands of communities at the "margins of margins" (Dutta et al., 2019). It emphasizes the importance of resisting the performance of innocent victimhood, opportunism, and careerism that is rampant in the Indian upper-caste academic community in the West, instead of turning toward a community-anchored ethics based on physical presence, emotional investment, and personal risk-taking in challenging oppressive structures of settler colonialism, racial capitalism, and imperialism and advocating for social change through community action (Dutta, 2024; Elers & Dutta, 2024). We build on Dutta's theorizing on "body on the line" within the CCA (Dutta et al., 2019), examining its significance and manifestations, offering some examples of how it is enacted in research, practice, and activism.

At its core, "body on the line" signifies a willingness to put one's physical, emotional, and social well-being at stake in service of a larger social justice agenda defined by communities at the margins. Turning toward communities shifts the accountability of the academic toward community, calling for continual interrogation of the hyphen in academic-community partnerships, exploring the fundamentally unequal power terrains in the academic-community relationship, recognizing the impossibilities in listening to subaltern knowledge claims, and then seeking to unsettle this power terrain through continual interrogation of academic power.

This process of continual interrogation of academic power co-creates a public pedagogy of culture-centered research methods in partnerships with communities, working together through embodied interactions to then build spaces for/with communities, in the form of CAGs, co-creating the research design, collectively making sense of the emergent findings, designing advocacy and activist interventions, and implementing and evaluating the interventions (Dutta, 2014, 2018b). The CCA reflects a recognition that meaningful change often requires that the very concept of intellectual critique or theoretical analysis be decentered, joining here with Indigenous theories such as Kaupapa Maori theory to place theory in struggles for land, food, ecosystems, and justice (Elers & Dutta, 2023; Smith, 1997). The theorizing work of the CCA, by being embedded in struggles, demands tangible action, willingness to sacrifice, and committed solidarity with those who are most affected by injustice and marginalization. Thus, "body on the line" represents a form of embodied activism that is deeply rooted in empathy, compassion, listening, and a sense of moral responsibility toward those at the margins of settler colonialism, extractive neoliberalism, and imperialism.

One of the key manifestations of "body on the line" within the CCA is the active involvement of researchers and practitioners in the communities they study or work with (Elers & Dutta, 2023). Rather than adopting a detached or observational stance, scholars and activists immerse themselves in the everyday realities, struggles, and aspirations of marginalized communities, forging meaningful connections and relationships based on trust, reciprocity, and mutual respect. This embodied engagement allows researchers to gain firsthand insights into the lived experiences of those they seek to empower, thereby enriching their understanding and analysis of communication processes and social change dynamics.

An example of "body on the line" in the CCA can be found, for instance, in how scholars studying healthcare disparities in settler colonial spaces may work closely with community health workers, activists, social movements or grassroots organizations to conduct participatory action research aimed at identifying the theft of land as a barrier to securing health and co-developing land occupations as culture centered interventions (see Elers & Dutta, 2024). Moreover, "body on the line" encompasses a willingness to confront and challenge oppressive structures and systems of power, even at personal risk or cost. This may involve publishing white papers and policy briefs, designing activist campaigns, or co-creating social movements. In other instances, this may involve participating in protests, demonstrations, or direct actions aimed at raising awareness, disrupting injustice, and demanding accountability from those in positions of authority. By physically putting themselves in the line of fire, academics as activists embody their commitment to justice and liberation, serving as visible symbols of resistance and resilience in the face of oppression.

Another example of "body on the line" activism can be seen in the scholarship on migrant worker rights and rights of communities negotiating poverty in Singapore, where researchers at CARE have worked alongside CAGs, built at the "margins of the margins," in risking their livelihoods to challenge the violent erasure of discursive registers around oppression and exploitation (Dutta et al., 2019). Embodied research methods begin with the recognition that no number of risks we negotiate as researchers, embedded in our privileges, compare with the material registers of risks borne by the communities we partner with. Placing the body on the line turns accountability to CAGs co-creating communicative registers for talking about workers' rights and rights of the poor, disrupting the silences reproduced by neoliberalism. The narratives documenting the violence of the hyper capitalist exploitative systems in neoliberal authoritarian spaces serve as registers for the organizing of the poor, the working classes, migrant workers, and civil society organizations (see Dutta et al., 2019). Amidst the backlash carried out by the authoritarian state, this has meant being surveilled, withstanding audits, negotiating planted rumors about financial mismanagement amplified by upper-caste academics, and staying on path amidst threats of being fired (Dutta, 2021). Anti-racist CCA scholarship, often documenting the threats to health and well-being produced by racist disinformation and hate on digital platforms, has negotiated violent attacks and hate campaigns organized by far-right groups (Dutta & Dutta, 2024). In the face of organized hate, researchers are called upon to put their bodies on the line to advance the causes of racial equality and justice emerging from the raced margins (Dutta et al., 2024).

Conclusion

In conclusion, the CCA, as a critical meta-theory of health communication, disrupts the method-theory-praxis division that forms the architectures of whiteness in settler colonial, racial capitalist, and imperial approaches to health communication, instead suggesting that methods for transforming the structures that drive poor health outcomes are intrinsically tied to praxis. The methods of the CCA, from co-creating voice infrastructures to co-creating communication advocacy campaigns, activist interventions, and social movements built on friendships with communities at the margins, challenge the hegemonic approaches to how we do critique and how we do health communication work. Engaging critically with hegemonic approaches to health communication scholarship, the CCA interrogates the interplays of casteism, settler colonialism, patriarchy, and imperialism that shape how knowledge about health, communication, culture, and structure are produced. Ultimately, it builds a practical politics of health communication method as a register for transforming the social determinants of health.

References

Basnyat, I. (2019). Self-reflexivity for social change: The researcher, I, and the researched, female street-based commercial sex workers,' gendered contexts. In D. Zapata & M. J. Dutta (Eds.), *Communicating for social change: Meaning, power, and resistance* (pp. 13–31). Springer Nature. https://doi.org/10.1007/978-981-13-2005-7_2

Beverley, J. (1999). *Subalternity and representation: Arguments in cultural theory*. Duke University Press.

Basu, A., Dillon, P. J., & Romero-Daza, N. (2016). Understanding culture and its influence on HIV/AIDS-related communication among minority men who have sex with men. *Health Communication, 31*(11), 1367–1374. https://doi.org/10.1080/10410236.2015.1072884

Bates, B. R., Marvel, D. L., & Grijalva, M. J. (2019). Painting a community-based definition of health: A culture-centered approach to listening to rural voice in Chaquizhca, Ecuador. *Frontiers in Communication, 4*, 462245. https://doi.org/10.3389/fcomm.2019.00037

Bhukya, B. (2021). Featuring adivasi/indigenous studies. *Economic and Political Weekly, 56*(25), 13–17.

Carter, A. L., & Alexander, A. (2020). Soul food: [Re]framing the African-American farming crisis using the culture-centered approach. *Frontiers in Communication, 5*, 470810. https://doi.org/10.3389/fcomm.2020.00005

Da Costa, D. (2023). Writing castelessly: Brahminical supremacy in education, feminist knowledge, and research. *Meridians, 22*(2), 297–322. https://doi.org/10.1215/15366936-10637690

de Souza, R. (2023). Women in the margins: A culture-centered interrogation of hunger and "food apartheid" in the United States. *Health Communication,*

39(9), 1855–1865. https://doi-org.libproxy.unl.edu/10.1080/10410236.2023.2245206

Dutta, M. J. (2004a), The unheard voices of Santalis: Communicating about health from the margins of India. *Communication Theory, 14*(3), 237–263. https://doi.org/10.1111/j.1468-2885.2004.tb00313.x

Dutta, M. J. (2004b). Poverty, structural barriers, and health: A Santali narrative of health communication. *Qualitative Health Research, 14*(8), 1107–1122. https://doi.org/10.1177/1049732304267763

Dutta, M. J. (2005). Theory and practice in health communication campaigns: A critical interrogation. *Health communication, 18*(2), 103–122. https://doi.org/10.1207/s15327027hc1802_1

Dutta, M. J. (2007). Communicating about culture and health: Theorizing culture-centered and cultural sensitivity approaches. *Communication Theory, 17*(3), 304–328. https://doi.org/10.1111/j.1468-2885.2007.00297.x

Dutta, M. J. (2008). *Communicating health: A culture-centered approach.* Polity.

Dutta, M. J., & de Souza, R. (2008). The past, present, and future of health development campaigns: Reflexivity and the critical-cultural approach. *Health Communication, 23*(4), 326–339. https://doi.org/10.1080/10410230802229704

Dutta, M. J. (2010). The critical cultural turn in health communication: Reflexivity, solidarity, and praxis. *Health Communication, 25*(6–7), 534–539. https://doi.org/10.1080/10410236.2010.497995

Dutta, M. J. (2011). *Communicating social change: Structure, culture, and agency.* Routledge.

Dutta, M. J. (2014). A culture-centered approach to listening: Voices of social change. *International Journal of Listening, 28*(2), 67–81. https://doi.org/10.1080/10904018.2014.876266

Dutta, M. J. (2018). Culture-centered approach in addressing health disparities: Communication infrastructures for subaltern voices. *Communication Methods and Measures, 12*(4), 239–259. https://doi.org/10.1080/19312458.2018.1453057

Dutta, M. J. (2019). Introduction: Theory, method, and praxis of social change. In M. J. Dutta & D. B. Zapata (Eds.), *Communicating for social change.* Palgrave Macmillan. https://doi.org/10.1007/978-981-13-2005-7_1

Dutta, M., Pandi, A. R., Zapata, D., Mahtani, R., Falnikar, A., Tan, N., Thaker, J., Pitaloka, D., Dutta, U., Luk, P., & Sun, K. (2019). Critical health communication method as embodied practice of resistance: Culturally centering structural transformation through struggle for voice. *Frontiers in Communication, 4*, 469040. https://doi.org/10.3389/fcomm.2019.00067

Dutta, M. J. (2021). Universities, civility, and repression in the age of new media: Surveillance capital and resistance. In R. Dutt-Ballerstadt & K. Bhattacharya (Eds.), *Civility, free speech, and academic freedom in higher education* (pp. 41–58). Routledge. https://doi.org/10.4324/9780429282041

Dutta, M. J. (2023a). Culture-centered organizing at the "margins of the margins": Dismantling structures, decolonizing futures. In Pal, M., Cruz, J., & Munshi, D. (eds.). *Organizing at the margins: Theorizing organizations of struggle in the global south* (pp. 157–182). Springer International Publishing.

Dutta, M. J. (2023b). Theorizing southern strategies of anti-racism: Culturally centering social change. In Calafell, B. M. & Eguchi, S. (eds.). *The Routledge handbook of ethnicity and race in communication* (pp. 301–314). Routledge.

Dutta, M. J. (2024). Decolonizing the pedagogy of health communication campaigns: A culture-centered approach. *Communication Education, 73*(4), 405–426. https://doi.org/10.1080/03634523.2024.2403449

Dutta, D., & Dutta, M. J. (2024). *Discursive construction of race and racism in India*. Oxford Research Encyclopedia of Communication.

Dutta, M. J., Baskey, P., Mandi, R., & Mandal, I. (2024). *Indigenous resistance in South Asia*. Oxford Research Encyclopedia of Communication.

Dutta, M. J., & Basu, A. (2013). From the ground to the ivory tower. In Jones, S. H., Adams, T. E.. & Ellis, C. (eds.). *Handbook of autoethnography* (pp. 143–161). Routledge.

Dutta, M. J., & Basu, A. (2018). Subalternity, neoliberal seductions, and freedom: Decolonizing the global market of social change. *Cultural Studies↔ Critical Methodologies, 18*(1), 80–93. https://doi.org/10.1177/1532708617750676

Dutta, M. J., Comer, S., Teo, D., Luk, P., Lee, M., Zapata, D., Krishnaswamy, A., & Kaur, S. (2018). Health meanings among foreign domestic workers in Singapore: A culture-centered approach. *Health Communication, 33*(5), 643–652. https://doi.org/10.1080/10410236.2017.1292576

Dutta, M. J., Collins, W., Sastry, S., Dillard, S., Anaele, A., Kumar, R., Roberson, C., Robinson, T., & Bonu, T. (2018). A culture-centered community-grounded approach to disseminating health information among African Americans. *Health Communication, 34*(10), 1075–1084. https://doi.org/10.1080/10410236.2018.1455626

Dutta, M. J., Kaur-Gill, S., Elers, N. H. C., Mahbubur, M., Rahman, P. J., Mandal, I., Pokaia, V., & Metuamate, S. (2023). Justice-based public pedagogy of care. In J. G., Burchfield & A. A. Kedrowicz (Eds). *Teaching communication across disciplines for professional development, civic engagement, and beyond* (pp. 311–324). Rowan and Littlefield.

Dutta, M. J., Kaur-Gill, S., & Metuamate, S. (2024). Decolonizing impact through the culture-centered approach to health communication: Mobilizing communities to transform the structural determinants of health. *Health Communication, 39*(14), 3581–3589. https://doi.org/10.1080/10410236.2024.2343466

Dutta, M. J., & Pal, M. (2020). Theorizing from the global south: Dismantling, resisting, and transforming communication theory. *Communication Theory, 30*(4), 349–369.

Elers, C., & Dutta, M. (2023). Academic-community solidarities in land occupation as an Indigenous claim to health: Culturally centered solidarity through voice infrastructures. *Frontiers in Communication, 8*, 1009837. https://doi.org/10.3389/fcomm.2023.1009837

Elers, C. H., & Dutta, M. (2024). Local government engagement practices and Indigenous interventions: Learning to listen to Indigenous voices. *Human Communication Research, 50*(1), 39–52. https://doi.org/10.1093/hcr/hqad027

Elers, P., Dutta, M. J., Elers, S., Tau, T. T., & Torres, R. (2024). Subaltern perspectives of developing communication campaigns: Re-examining the culture-centered approach in addressing health disparities. *Journal of International and Intercultural Communication, 17*(1), 39–55. https://doi.org/10.1080/17513057.2023.2274559

Figueira, D. M. (2008). *Otherwise occupied: Pedagogies of alterity and the brahminization of theory*. State University of New York Press.

Freire, P. (1996). *Pedagogy of the oppressed* (revised). Continuum.

Freire, P., J. W. Frazer, D. Macedo, T. McKinnon, & W. T. Stokes (Eds). (1997). *Mentoring the Mentor: A critical dialogue with Paulo Freire*. Peter Lang.

Giddens, A. (2007). *The constitution of society: Outline of the theory of structuration*. University of California Press.

Herakova, L., Newell-Caito, J., McGuire, J., Pelletreau, K., & Maliwal-Bundy, A. (2024). Culture-centered reflexivity as critical assessment. *Communication Teacher*, 39(2), 127–134. https://doi.org/10.1080/17404622.2024.2369719

Haug, W. F. (1999). Rethinking Gramsci's philosophy of praxis from one century to the next. *Boundary*, 26(2), 101–117.

Hokowhitu, B., Moreton-Robinson, A., Tuhiwai-Smith, L., Andersen, C., & Larkin, S. (Eds). (2020). *Routledge handbook of critical Indigenous studies*. Routledge.

Kaur-Gill, S., & Dutta, M. J. (2023). The COVID-19 pandemic and precarious migrants: An outbreak of inequality. In S. Kaur-Gill & M. J. Dutta, *Migrants and the COVID-19 pandemic: Communication, inequality, and transformation* (pp. 1–25). Springer Nature Singapore.

Kumar, R. (2021). Refugee articulations of health: A culture-centered exploration of Burmese refugees' resettlement in the United States. *Health Communication*, 36(6), 682–692. https://doi.org/10.1080/10410236.2020.1712035

Mukherjee, P., & Basu, A. (2024). "Water is life…the problem is there's only one tap": A culture-centered and necrocapitalist inquiry to communicating health and water. *Communication Monographs*, 1–25. https://doi.org/10.1080/03637751.2024.2420962

Pasternak, S., Cowen, D., Clifford, R., Joseph, T., Scott, D. N., Spice, A., & Stark, H. K. (2023). Infrastructure, jurisdiction, extractivism: Keywords for decolonizing geographies. *Political Geography*, 101, 102763.

Patel, S. (2010). Where are the settlers of colour. *Upping the Anti*, 10, 14–16. Retrieved from https://uppingtheanti.org/journal/article/10-where-are-the-settlers-of-colour/

Pindi, G. (2020). "I'm not sick, I'm hairy": Cultural constructions of women's bodies in the OB/Gyn exam. In A. Spieldenner & S. Toyosaki (Eds.), *Intercultural health communication* (pp. 97–124). Peter Lang Verlag.

Pitaloka, D., & Dutta M. J. (2021). Performing songs as healing the trauma of the 1965 anti-Communist killings in Indonesia. In M. S. Micale & H. Pols (Eds.), *Traumatic pasts in Asia: History, psychiatry, and trauma from the 1930s to the present* (pp. 226–244). Berghahn Books

Rahman, M. M., & Dutta, M. J. (2023). The United Nations (UN) card, identity, and negotiations of health among Rohingya refugees. *International Journal of Environmental Research and Public Health*, 20(4), 3385.

Rawat, M., Shields, A. N., Venetis, M. K., & Seth, J. (2021). Women's agentic role in enabling and dismantling menstrual health taboos in Northern India: A culture-centered approach. *Health Communication*, 38(4), 695–704. https://doi.org/10.1080/10410236.2021.1970296

Resnicow, K., Soler, R., Braithwaite, R. L., Ahluwalia, J. S., & Butler, J. (2000). Cultural sensitivity in substance use prevention. *Journal of Community Psychology*, 28(3), 271–290. https://doi.org/10.1002/(SICI)1520-6629(200005)28:3<271::AID-JCOP4>3.0.CO;2-I

Robb, J. (2021). Marginalised health communities: Understanding communities of 'people without papers' as silent networks of survival. *Communication Research and Practice*, 7(4), 311–325. https://doi.org/10.1080/22041451.2021.1978627

Robb, J. S. (2023). A clash of culture and structure: Considering barriers to access for people without papers. *Health Communication, 38*(13), 3003–3011. https://doi.org/10.1080/10410236.2022.2129627

Sastry, S. (2016). Structure and agency in long-distance truck drivers' lived experiences of condom use for HIV prevention. *Culture, Health & Sexuality, 18*(5), 553–566. https://doi.org/10.1080/13691058.2015.1094575

Sastry, S., Stephenson, M., Dillon, P., & Carter, A. (2021). A meta-theoretical systematic review of the culture-centered approach to health communication: Toward a refined, "nested" model. *Communication Theory, 31*(3), 380–421. https://doi.org/10.1093/ct/qtz024

Smith, G. H. (1997). *The development of Kaupapa Maori: Theory and praxis* (Doctoral dissertation, ResearchSpace@ Auckland).

Soundadarajan, T. (2022). *The trauma of caste: A dalit feminist meditation on survivorship, healing, and abolition.* North Atlantic Books.

Stanley, B. L., & Basu, A. (2023). 'Chemical jail': Culture-centered theorizing of carcerality in methadone maintenance treatment and addiction recovery in the United States. *Journal of Applied Communication Research, 51*(5), 463–480. https://doi.org/10.1080/00909882.2023.2180770

Xaxa, V. (2008). *State, society and tribes: Issues in post-colonial India.* Pearson Longman.

Xaxa, V. (2021). Education, assimilation and cultural marginalisation of tribes in India. *Economic and Political Weekly, 56*(36), 10–13.

11
DECOLONIZING HEALTH COMMUNICATION

Reflections on Critical Health Communication Research in Nigeria

C. T. Adebayo, O. O. Olusanya, and O. E. Ambrose

To begin this chapter, it is important to provide details on how we each came into doing critical health communication work in Nigeria. While each of our paths is slightly different, the centrality of dissonance between theory and context is a significant thread across our individual yet similar experiences.

My (Comfort Tosin) entry point to doing critical health communication research in Nigeria began some years ago as a graduate student. In my interpersonal communication theory class, I remember getting excited about doing health communication research that is truly home to me. It was my golden opportunity to publish something "African" in an international health communication journal—and to be clear, my conceptualization of "international" was something published in a U.S. based publisher or outlet. The manuscript in its original form focused on identifying how Nigerians communicated with their healthcare providers. I had just learned about the theory of motivated information management (Afifi & Weiner, 2004) in my theory class. Excited about the underpinnings of the theory and its value for studying health communication, I was intrigued and inspired to apply the theory to my home context of Nigeria. I am glad the paper did not end up the way it had started. It was in that class I recognized my frustration with the Westernization of African healthcare processes and scholarship. I became aware of the lack of communication theories that center the African experience and the day-to-day realities of living in the Global South and in Africa and Nigeria more specifically. After a few failed attempts to use Western theories to explain healthcare practices in Nigeria, my frustration pushed me to start actively exploring theories that explain alternate meanings to health that are embraced in the Global South. These approaches represent a departure from the dominant Western biomedical approach to health.

The reviewers of the manuscript, every one of them, challenged me to interrogate power structures and dominant ideologies that freely paraded the data. Interestingly, dominant assumptions about healthcare processes were so normalized to me that I did not readily acknowledge the power dynamics evident in the data. I tried so hard to "box" the data into a theory that did not acknowledge local factors, structures, and contexts that intrinsically impact how community members experience health. This particular experience served as my launchpad into critical scholarship.

For me (Oluwaseyi), I am still in the very early stage of doing critical health communication research. As a current doctoral student, my introduction to critical health communication work came from my collaborations with Dr. Adebayo, whose work centers on Black women's health in African diaspora. Through our collaborations, I developed a solid interest in maternal and child health, and I am now learning community-based participatory research, particularly focusing on motherhood among women of African descent. Encountering an apparent disconnect between dominant theories and the African contexts that I study has significantly influenced my interest in critical health scholarship. I am particularly interested in highlighting Africa-centered theories in health communication research that focus on Africans.

I (Oyewole) do not remember any specific timeline for my scholarship as a critical scholar. It is an experience that came by default, given the context of my research as a medical sociologist. My research primarily focuses on the sexual and reproductive health of adolescents and young adults. The structural and cultural factors that closely influence health decisions cannot be isolated from this type of research. Thus, centering the uniqueness of the local communities and the cultural beliefs and values have always been necessary considerations when designing my studies. Collaborating with Dr. Adebayo on health communication studies in Nigeria further exposed me to the centrality of communication in critical health research.

A commonality across our journeys is the search for theoretical and methodological frameworks that account for the uniqueness of the context that we studied, which was (still is) visibly absent from much of the critical health communication literature. There is a paucity of health communication research in African contexts (Omenka et al., 2020). To be clear, this is not at all different from the sparseness of African communication research in the discipline in general (Miller et al., 2013). While there have been a lot of groundbreaking critical studies that have examined the experiences of Black people in health communication literature (Adebayo et al., 2020; Pavlish et al., 2010), Africa is still often a missing link in those studies. For studies that examine the experiences of Blacks in the West, Africans are often lumped into the demographic without clear attention to the sociopolitical histories and realities (e.g., colonialism, immigration) that influenced their lived and ongoing experiences.

Additionally, of the few studies that have explored health research in Africa, many have employed West-centric epistemologies, focusing on individual-level changes and health promotion campaigns (see for discussion Sastry & Dutta, 2017), that have limited, sometimes misleading, implications for collectivist African communities. While these approaches, at the very least, have helped gather some knowledge on health practices in these contexts, they often leave behind superficial explanations of health and healthcare processes in Africa. These explanations are often far removed from the tacit meanings that closely influence health behaviors in these communities.

In the following sections, we discuss what critical health communication looks like in our previous and ongoing research in Nigeria. With our experience in the field, our contribution will not only center the voices of Africans in health communication scholarship but also critically highlight the historical and present-day realities of healthcare practice in Africa that can only be understood from a critical, culture-centered approach.

The Outlook of Critical Health Communication Scholarship in Our Work

This section will focus on three fundamental issues that punctuate our critical scholarship in Nigeria. First, we will attend to the issue of context. Second, we will focus on the issue of theoretical frameworks that undergird our work, and lastly we will focus on methodological considerations. We understand other salient issues guide critical work, but for this chapter, we will only highlight these three. Within each of those issues, we give examples of different research projects that we have undertaken that provide practical insights into how each of these factors materialize.

Attention to Context

In critical health communication scholarship, context refers to the material realities of a group of people that shape their understanding of health and interactions with health systems and policies. These include physical, political, sociocultural, and economic factors. The socioecological model of health further categorizes these factors at different layered levels of influence, including the microsystem, mesosystem, and macro system (Adebayo et al., 2024; Kilanowski, 2017). While we have mostly studied health communication in African contexts, we do not at all limit our conceptualization of context to physical or geographical locations only. Beyond physical settings, we position context as a compendium of local systems and experiences, unique to a group, where different factors intersect to shape their health experiences. Given this definition, a context embodies culture, structure, histories, class, and race, to mention but a few, all working together to shape how people experience health in that setting.

Dutta (2008) provides a nuanced argument as to what context means in critical health communication work:

> a locally situated nature of healthcare experiences and is articulated through thick descriptions of the lived experiences of cultural members. Context taps into the dynamics and continuously contested nature of health communication such that health experiences become meaningful only when located in the perimeters of local context.
>
> *(p. 13)*

Health is intrinsically shaped by factors that are local and unique to cultural members. As such, when health is studied and practiced without reference to the factors that shape meanings, beliefs, and attitudes about health, the results are superficial and misleading. This is why doing research from afar, far removed from a context's structural and cultural realities, produces incomplete and often ambiguous conclusions. This is not to say scholars always need to culturally identify with a context in order to engage in research. However, doing critical work should always provide an avenue to dig into the tacit knowledge of the cultural members—practices and activities that are unique, sometimes mundane, but hold important implications for the cultural members. Informed by the culture-centered approach (Dutta, 2008), in our work, three issues punctuate our attention to context: culture, structure, and agency.

To attend to context, critical scholarship in health communication must pay attention to culture. We will not attempt to delve into the much-contested definition of culture. However, for the purpose of this writing, we define culture as "the local contexts within which health meanings are constituted and negotiated" (Dutta, 2008, p. 7). With this, we approach our work by asking important questions like: How is health understood within this cultural context? What are the cultural nuances of a health practice unique to this site or group? These questions are important not just for highlighting the cultural uniqueness of an understudied group. Instead, they provide the necessary basis for providing healthcare interventions both at the local and global levels. For instance, with the Ebola outbreak in Liberia, Guinea, and Sierra Leone in 2014, research shows that cultural beliefs and practices significantly contributed to the spread of the virus in different local communities (Agusto et al., 2015). Until those cultural beliefs were addressed, the virus prevailed in many communities, leading to fatalities. Those cultural influences were not necessarily questions of hygiene or even economic power; they were as simple as cultural and religious practices surrounding caring for the sick or even burying the dead, which further led to the worsening of the Ebola endemic (Manguvo & Mafuvadze, 2015).

In our body of research in Nigeria, prioritizing local and tacit meanings of health is an integral part of our work. This understanding was made possible, first because we are cultural members, but also because we carefully integrate cultural implications into the design and interpretation of our research. These include identifying and understanding cultural practices and how they hold meanings for health experiences. It is a bit incongruous for critical health communication scholars doing fieldwork in places like Nigeria to account for findings without putting those findings into conversations about cultural expectations and beliefs in that context.

Part of our effort to unpack culture within a context is also to interrogate the sociopolitical history of the context of work. Interrogating the discourse of colonialism is at the center of critical health scholarship in Africa. Nigeria, for example, is a previously colonized context, and "Nigeria's health system was built in an ad hoc way, layering traditional community health systems with colonial medicine aimed at maximizing resource extraction" (Abubakar et al., 2022). As such, residues of colonial legacies still intrinsically shape cultural members' engagement with biomedical approaches to health, mainly Western medicine. Such residues further impact the meaning-making process of cultural members as it concerns global health policies. For instance, several studies on COVID-19 in Nigeria highlight the prevalence of vaccine hesitancy due to mistrust of Westerners. Fear of being "swindled by the Whites," an attempt by the Whites to eliminate Africans, among several other political rhetorics, pervades how Nigerians made sense of the vaccine (Ojewale & Mukumbang, 2023, p. 5). The Nigerian sociopolitical context very much shaped how Nigerians made sense of the pandemic, highlighting themes of political mistrust, Western bias, suspicion, and marginalization/otherness, among others.

In addition to cultural context, structural context is also a significant topic in interrogating health. Dutta (2008) presents structure as the human, government, physical, and social infrastructures enabling effective healthcare practice and access, both on the side of providers and healthcare patrons. Many African countries have unique health structures that make it challenging to apply global health policies.

Ranging from different levels of healthcare facilities (federal, state, and local government levels; Adebayo, 2021), to access to technologically driven healthcare (mainly in rural areas), (lack of) health insurance, among others, healthcare in many African countries presents unique challenges that demand an intrinsic knowledge of "how things work here" to be able to interrogate the system.

The role of agency in health outcomes is also significant. Here, we describe agency as the participation and collaboration of cultural members in health care decisions. Dutta (2008) links structure and agency in the culture-centered approach:

> Through the enactment of agency in relationship with structure, individuals, communities, and societies come to experience health. This line of thinking and application development foregrounds the importance of understanding articulations of health by engaging participant voices, particularly in the context of marginalized sectors of the world.
>
> *(p. 56)*

The deliberate use of qualitative research methods has made it possible for us to gain insights into cultural meanings, social structures, and agency. Through interviews, focus group discussions, and ethnographic observations, we are able to engage the voices of community members in Nigeria. The works of scholars like Mohan Dutta and Collins Airhihenbuwa have significantly shaped our approach to interrogating the role of local agents (community members) in this manner. As we will discuss this in greater detail later in this chapter, we want to quickly highlight that attention to the people most impacted by health policies and practices is integral to critical health communication scholarship. The following section provides an example of how we engage local contexts in one of our studies in Nigeria.

Paying Attention to Colonial Context: COVID-19 Study in Nigeria

One of the guiding considerations for us when designing our COVID-19 study in Nigeria was to account for pre- and postcolonial history and realities of the Nigerian society and how that history impacts the meanings of health and health interventions. For example, how can we understand (biomedical) health meanings in Nigeria without addressing questions of Western mistrust?

In this study, the colonial context undergirded tacit meanings of COVID-19 and the willingness of Nigerians to follow international health organizations' recommendations (e.g., World Health Organization

[WHO]). To date, vaccine hesitancy is a significant problem in African countries. This is a major concern for the WHO. However, understanding and tackling that hesitancy requires an analysis of the context and cultural beliefs that so closely shape it. Western mistrust is a major theme in this study. For John, one of the participants, mistrust of the West, led to their mistrust of COVID-19 information as to whether the virus even exists:

> We know that these vaccines are not locally produced, they are actually imported and I'm not sure if when they were doing the test samplings, they actually took a sample of us, how it was actually localized to us, and also apart from that, the government over time, they have failed to earn the trust of the people because of past experiences and how they have tackled certain things... We've heard that some of them are fake vaccines, and we have heard about increasing deaths, some people even still have COVID afterwards. So now, there's no confidence in the vaccine itself.
>
> *(Participant 3- John)*

Blessing reiterated John's perception about the vaccine:

> Like I said, I'm confused about the sincerity of different governments around the world, a lot of politics around this COVID thing. The effectiveness of the vaccine and conspiracy theories – I am not someone that believes in conspiracy theories, most of them are actually stupid. But you can't help but think again.
>
> *(10-Blessing)*

Postcolonial theory, a major influence of the culture-centered approach to health, pushes us to examine and situate the historical contexts of previously colonized nations as a basis for interrogating colonial legacies that still shape the ongoing experiences of citizens. In our data, we honed in on how that sociopolitical history intersects with the meaning-making process of the participants. It would be inadequate to merely highlight how participants felt about the vaccine without situating that perception within the larger cultural discourse of colonialism.

Attention to Theory

Engaging theoretical frameworks that adequately capture the "essence" of our research has been one of the most challenging parts of the scholarship process. Why? Many of the health communication theories were developed in Western contexts, to study Western groups. As such, the theories, mostly post-positivist, do not effectively translate or interrogate the cultural and structural dynamics of healthcare processes in many African contexts. As articulated by Dutta-Bergman (2004), "scholarship and applications in the realm of health communication continue to echo voices of those with power and access" (p. 1107). Often detached from the lived realities of the subaltern context, these approaches often advance the dominant discourse of health as Western and biomedical. Until the mid-nineties to early 2000s, the concept of a culture-centered and critical approach to the study of health was scarce and sparse in health communication scholarship. The works of scholars like Deborah Lupton (1994), Collins Airhihenbuwa (1990), and Mohan Dutta (2008) challenged this. It is on the wings of this critical theorizing of health that our work has found epistemological provisions to interrogate health communication practices in Nigeria and other African contexts.

Thus, in our work, we primarily engage theoretical frameworks that allow us to push boundaries and challenge Western-centric ideologies, which are powerful structures that make it impossible to acknowledge (in meaningful ways) the health experiences of Nigerians. Specifically, we engage frameworks that intrinsically account for the local factors and systems that shape how health is experienced within that cultural context. This approach, thus, includes identifying, examining, and challenging "dominant, taken-for-granted assumptions about health, often with the hope of introducing possibilities for alternative, more inclusive meaning systems." (Zoller & Kline, 2008, p. 94)

Attention to Theory in Sexual Violence Research in Nigeria

Through a National Communication Association (NCA) research cultivation grant for early career scholars, in Summer 2022, Dr. Olusanya (2nd author) and I (Comfort Tosin) began a long-term applied health communication research[1] on the problem of sexual violence in Nigeria. Centered on the critical approach to health communication, we sought to identify institutional barriers within the local healthcare system that influence post-violence support services. Early in the research design process, we were again hit with the reality of the absence of a communication theory that specifically focused on sexual violence in the Global South. However, we have also learned that the advantage of critical theories (in social science) is the *flexibility* to apply and expand a theory in ways that allow for meaningful interpretation of the data in different contexts.

Thus, we adapted and applied the Muted Group Theory (MGT), originally developed by Shirley Ardener in 1975, and then revised by Cheris Kramarae in 1981. MGT is premised on three basic concepts: (1) dominance, (2) acceptability, and (3) subordination (Barkman, 2018; Kramarae, 2005).

However, from our work, applying MGT also gave us an opportunity to identify *how* sexual violence survivors in Nigeria *resist* silencing. The culture-centered approach pushes scholars to highlight how subaltern groups resist power structures. Thus, in this study, we expanded on the theory by focusing on the (communicative) strategies that survivors engage in to resist silencing. Applying MGT to this study was not just an easy way of "using theory." Rather, it was also an opportunity to localize the theory within the Nigerian cultural context.

Thus, we want to emphasize to early career scholars within the field, that the theoretical frameworks that guide our work as critical health communication scholars must not just attend to power dynamics but also provide a framework for its resistance by cultural group members. While critical scholarship helps to critique and challenge dominant structures that usurp power over subaltern groups, it is also important to highlight how subaltern groups resist power structures (Dutta, 2008; Dutta & Kaur-Gill, 2018).

Attention to Methodology

Attention to methodology in our work is first and foremost punctuated by the need to center the voices of cultural members in the process of knowledge production. Centering the voices of cultural members guides us to embrace qualitative research methodology. The context and nature of our research have often required a methodological design that is genuinely culture-centered. Dutta (2008) highlights voice and dialogue as necessary ingredients for doing culture-centered work in health contexts. In their argument, "the very act of engaging subaltern voices is a way of writing health communication from an alternative perspective, demonstrating gaps in the current theory and practice, and showing alternative strategies that might be adopted in health communication" (p. 60). Put differently, engaging alternative meanings of health and illness is hinged on the knowledge production process that provides a space for the voices of Africans to be represented in health communication research. Critical health communication prioritizes voice, dialogue, and, asking questions to engage and center the voices of cultural members. This includes working with cultural members as co-creators of knowledge. To be clear, it is quite easy to do qualitative work without actually engaging the voices of cultural members. Applying qualitative research methodology to health research in Africa does not automatically equate to doing critical work. Qualitative research methodology provides us with the tool to engage, but ultimately engaging the voices of cultural members further includes attention to tacit meanings that help researchers interrogate power structures. Thus, any methodology that does not highlight the role of power and resistance in the meaning-making process of participants ultimately fails the litmus test of critical scholarship in the context of health communication.

Attention to Methodology in Sexual Violence Study: Researcher Identity Versus Site Access and Data Collection

Gender, class, and age are all factors that we consciously attend to as we design and analyze our research in Nigeria. For instance, in our recent sexual violence fieldwork in Nigeria, it became evident that my (Comfort) "Western" scholar identity did come with some power that, in some cases, served as a barrier to accessing research sites. Positionality and reflexivity of the researchers are important considerations in methodological designs for critical health scholarship. In our work, reflexivity goes beyond respecting the participants' culture or awareness of one's strengths and shortcomings as discussed by Tracy (2020). It more centrally embodies critically assessing the methodological choices in the process of knowledge generation. Reflexivity in critical health scholarship includes an "analysis of how, why, and in what ways research is conducted and an understanding of the role of power, privilege, and visibility in the research process" (Jacobson & Mustafa, 2019, p. 2). Being cognizant of the participant-researcher power dynamics and honestly upholding ethical standards, which embodies respect for the participants in the process of data collection and analysis.

When we started recruiting participants for sexual violence research in Nigeria, I (Comfort) visited one of the local higher education institutions to negotiate site access for participant recruitment. My local collaborator (Dr. Olusanya, 2nd author) had warned me not to go by myself. In his argument, I was far removed from the culture. However, driven by the short timeline and the desire to meet my grant completion time requirements, I decided to go. After introducing myself and discussing the research with the gatekeeper, I was hit with the question, "Where are you from?" Although I clearly stated that I am a cultural member of Nigeria, the gatekeeper did not believe me and kept inquiring until I had to disclose that I am also a professor of Communication from a U.S. university.

To be clear, I was not trying to be deceptive; my affiliation information was on the consent form. I wanted my Nigerian identity to be seen and recognized before my "American professor" identity. However, for some reason, I "looked" like an outsider. My accent did not sound "Nigerian." As such, I was seen as an outsider, another American who wanted to do research *on* Nigerians. A Nigerian research assistant who was conginzant of local structures ultimately helped me negotiate with the gatekeeper.

It was in that moment that I materially recognized the intersection of researcher identity and trust in site access.

In another instance, while collecting data, a recruited participant declined to be interviewed by a male member of our team, who happened to be the local collaborator. Their reasoning was, "I would not be interviewed by a man, since I was violated by one." In response to this issue, we respected the participants' valid and important decision and reassigned to them a female team member to interview them. From this experience, we have learned to carefully reflect on our different identities beyond national identities to evaluate and address how our presence in a research context shapes the process and, ultimately, the outcomes.

Conclusion

As we reflect on some of the realities we have had to confront in doing critical health communication research in Nigeria, the three issues (context, theory, and methodology) we highlighted in this chapter are fundamental to this type of scholarship. At the core of doing critical health communication research in Nigeria is the need to *account* for the unique context of our work. Underscoring how colonialism shapes the meanings of health for Nigerians is a history that should parse such work. What makes scholarship critical is not the mere geographical location or the participants involved (these are starting points), but the deliberate and careful accounting of and/for the cultural, structural, and historical (among others) factors that influence meanings and experiences of health. This deliberate evaluation should be reflected in the research design, the fieldwork, the interpretation of the data, and the outlets for the dissemination of the findings.

Additionally, it is important to note that critical scholarship is not critical until it *engages and critiques* the often-hidden, taken-for-granted assumptions that normalize marginalization, suppression, and different forms of silencing, mainly as it concerns Western dominance in understanding health. How can we do critical health communication work in Nigeria and not discuss medical imperialism of the West? How can we not account for the lack of recognition for critical health communication scholarship in the Global South in many communication journals? What are the multiple institutional barriers to access funds for critical health communication research in Nigeria? These are important questions that should guide our work within this field.

Moreover, although Nigeria might be "easily" identified as a ready site (third world, nonwestern) for critical scholarship, we invite early career scholars to see critical health communication as a work that should punctuate everyday health communication scholarship and every context, including the West (e.g., Black maternal mortality in the United States). Critical scholarship focuses on closely examining the often taken-for-granted assumptions as viable sites for interrogating power dynamics (Dutta, 2010; Lupton, 1994; Zoller & Kline, 2008).

We conclude this chapter by calling on early career scholars to take the work further and focus on critical health communication work that leads to tangible and transformative intervention projects—the social justice dimension. Our work should not end with the publications. As Zoller (2024) rightly puts it:

> Embracing praxis as theoretically informed social change means that contextual practice should drive research questions. Additionally, discussion of findings should go beyond brief or general consideration of "practical implications" to identify pathways by which we can share research insights with relevant audiences in order to influence practice.
> *(p. 2)*

We also voice a silent but true bias about our perception of critical work in health contexts. We borrow the words of Nigerian writer Chimamanda Adichie in their book "We Should All Be Feminists." In a similar way, we opine that "we should all be critical health communication scholars." Regardless of our paradigmatic labels, our work as health communication scholars should be united with the goal of improving healthcare access and outcomes for all people. While we may vary in the contexts and approaches that we take, it is important that we are united in the goal of improving healthcare access, particularly for those who are most marginalized.

Note

1 The manuscripts from this study are currently in preparation for journal publication.

References

Abubakar, I., Dalglish, S. L., Angell, B., Sanuade, O., Abimbola, S., Adamu, A. L., Adetifa, I. M. O., Colbourn, T., Ogunlesi, A. O., Onwujekwe, O., Owoaje, E. T., Okeke, I. N., Adeyemo, A., Aliyu, G., Aliyu, M. H., Aliyu, S. H., Ameh, E. A., Archibong, B., Ezeh, A., ... Zanna, F. H. (2022). The Lancet Nigeria commission: Investing in health and the future of the nation. *The Lancet*, *399*(10330), 1155–1200. https://doi.org/10.1016/S0140-6736(21)02488-0

Adebayo, C. T. (2021). Physician-patient interactions in Nigeria: A critical-cultural perspective on the role of power. *Journal of Intercultural Communication Research*, *50*(1), 21–40. https://doi.org/10.1080/17475759.2020.1799845

Adebayo, C. T., Walker, K., Hawkins, M., Olukotun, O., Shaw, L., Sahlstein Parcell, E., Dressel, A., Luft, H., & Mkandawire-Valhmu, L. (2020). Race and blackness: A thematic review of communication challenges confronting the Black community within the U.S. health care system. *Journal of Transcultural Nursing*, *31*(4), 397–405. https://doi.org/10.1177/1043659619889111

Adebayo, C. T., Olukotun, O. V., Olukotun, M., Kirungi, J., Gondwe, K. W., Crooks, N. K., Singer, R. B., Adams, S., Alfaifi, F. Y., Dressel, A., Fahmy, L., Kako, P., Snethen, J., & Mkandawire-Valhmu, L. (2024). Experiences of gender-based violence among Somali refugee women: A socioecological model approach. *Culture, Health & Sexuality*, *26*(5), 654–670. https://doi.org/10.1080/13691058.2023.2236163

Afifi, W. A., & Weiner, J. L. (2004). Toward a theory of motivated information management. *Communication Theory*, *14*(2), 167–190. https://doi.org/10.1111/j.1468-2885.2004.tb00310.x

Agusto, F. B., Teboh-Ewungkem, M. I., & Gumel, A. B. (2015). Mathematical assessment of the effect of traditional beliefs and customs on the transmission dynamics of the 2014 Ebola outbreaks. *BMC Medicine*, *13*(96), 1–17. https://doi.org/10.1186/s12916-015-0318-3

Airhihenbuwa, C. O. (1990). A conceptual model for culturally appropriate health education programs in developing countries. *International Quarterly of Community Health Education*, *11*(1), 53–62. https://doi.org/10.2190/LPKH-PMPJ-DBW9-FP6X

Barkman, L. L. S. (2018). Muted group theory: A tool for hearing marginalized voices. *Priscilla Papers*, *32*(4), 1–5. Retrieved from: https://www.cbeinternational.org/resource/muted-group-theory-tool-hearing-marginalized-voices/

Dutta-Bergman, M. J. (2004). Poverty, structural barriers, and health: A Santali narrative of health communication. *Qualitative Health Research*, *14*, 1107–1122. https://doi.org/10.1177/1049732304267763

Dutta, Mohan J. (2008). *Communicating health: A culture-centered approach*. Polity Press.

Dutta, M. J. (2010). The critical cultural turn in health communication: Reflexivity, solidarity, and praxis. *Health Communication*, *25*(6–7), 534–539. https://doi.org/10.1080/10410236.2010.497995

Dutta, M. J., & Kaur-Gill, S. (2018). Precarities of migrant work in Singapore: precarities of migrant work in Singapore: Migration, (im)mobility, and neoliberal governmentality. *International Journal of Communication*, *12*.

Jacobson, D., & Mustafa, N. (2019). Social identity map: A reflexivity tool for practicing explicit positionality in critical qualitative research. *International Journal of Qualitative Methods*, *18*, 1609406919870075. https://doi.org/10.1177/1609406919870075

Kilanowski, J. F. (2017). Breadth of the socioecological model. *Journal of Agromedicine*, *22*(4), 295–297. https://doi.org/10.1080/1059924X.2017.1358971

Kramarae, C. (2005). Muted group theory and communication: Asking dangerous questions. *Women & Language*, *28*(2), 55–61. https://search.lib.jmu.edu/permalink/01JMU_INST/lvvpvt/cdi_proquest_miscellaneous_60298417

Lupton, D. (1994). Toward the development of critical health communication praxis. *Health Communication*, *6*(1), 55–67. https://doi.org/10.1207/s15327027hc0601_4

Manguvo, A., & Mafuvadze, B. (2015). The impact of traditional and religious practices on the spread of Ebola in West Africa: Time for a strategic shift. *The Pan African Medical Journal, 22*(Suppl 1), 9. doi: 10.11694/pamj.supp.2015.22.1.6190

Miller, A. N., Deeter, C., Trelstad, A., Hawk, M., Ingram, G., & Ramirez, A. (2013). Still the dark continent: A content analysis of research about Africa and by African scholars in 18 major communication-related journals. *Journal of International and Intercultural Communication, 6*(4), 317–333. https://doi.org/10.1080/17513057.2013.787112

Ojewale, L. Y., & Mukumbang, F. C. (2023). COVID-19 vaccine hesitancy among Nigerians living with non-communicable diseases: A qualitative study. *BMJ Open, 13*(2), e065901. https://doi.org/10.1136/bmjopen-2022-065901

Omenka, O. I., Watson, D. P., & Hendrie, H. C. (2020). Understanding the healthcare experiences and needs of African immigrants in the United States: A scoping review. *BMC Public Health, 20*(1), 27. https://doi.org/10.1186/s12889-019-8127-9

Pavlish, C. L., Noor, S., & Brandt, J. (2010). Somali immigrant women and the American health care system: Discordant beliefs, divergent expectations, and silent worries. *Social Science & Medicine (1982), 71*(2), 353–361. https://doi.org/10.1016/j.socscimed.2010.04.010

Sastry, S., & Dutta, M. J. (2017). Health communication in the time of Ebola: A culture-centered interrogation. *Journal of Health Communication, 22*(sup1), 10–14. https://doi.org/10.1080/10810730.2016.1216205

Tracy, S. J. (2020). *Qualitative research methods: Collecting evidence, crafting analysis, communicating impact.* John Wiley & Sons.

Zoller, H. M., & Kline, K. N. (2008). Theoretical contributions of interpretive and critical research in health communication. *Annals of the International Communication Association, 32*(1), 89–135. https://doi.org/10.1080/23808985.2008.11679076

Zoller, H. M. (2024). Applied communication research as a discipline of crisis and care: Meeting the moment. *Journal of Applied Communication Research, 52*(1), 1–4. https://www.tandfonline.com/doi/full/10.1080/00909882.2023.2275038

12
JOURNEYS IN CRITICAL HEALTH COMMUNICATION

Meditations on Being/Becoming CCA Scholars

Balkisa M. Sissy, Usman Bah, Yixuan Qi, and Shaunak Sastry

In 2021, Sastry and colleagues published an article in *Communication Theory*, one of the leading journals of our field, that used a meta-analytical systematic review to define and refine how the culture-centered approach (CCA) was being used in the field of health communication (Sastry et al., 2021). We proposed a refined, "nested" model of CCA as a critical health communication (CHC) theory. We offered a detailed explanation of this tiered view of CCA, and why it makes sense to refine the theory in this way. Rather than repeat that discussion here, our goal in writing this chapter, in this form, is to introduce the journey of doing CCA to junior scholars, graduate and undergraduate students, and perhaps even advanced scholars and practitioners of health communication.

Few can accuse CHC scholars of parsimony. We tend to mistake the profundity of the writing of those that inspire us—Karl Marx, Theodor Adorno, Jürgen Habermas, Michel Foucault, Raymond Williams, Gayatri Spivak, Wangari Maathai, David Arnold, Paul Farmer, or Judith Butler (in no alluded order of verbosity)—as license to construct impenetrable prose. The body of work in the CCA to health communication, with its grounding in Marxist political economy, postcolonial and subaltern studies, and Giddensian structuration, is no exception to this. It tends to adopt a form of jargon-laden academese that betrays the very purpose of the scholarship: to explore how a community's health is a dance between political struggle, cultural identity, and individual autonomy.

Instead, in this chapter, we hope to do away with the theoretical finesse and lexical charms and show (not tell) what it means to do work in the CCA tradition. Or at least, what it means to us. The point is to "look under the hood" of the CCA as one might do to a complex machine assembly: to invite you, our reader, to walk with us as we offer our own perspectives on CHC. Since the point of this edited collection is to bring CHC to the mainstream of health communication, we felt it was important to share what we know, based on our perspectives, our backgrounds, and our positions. We do this in the form of a performed conversational essay. We ask each other questions, speak from our own positionality, pathways, and privilege, and crystallize important differences in how we view the work of CHC. In other words, we invite readers to take a glance into our academic journeys, and our definitions and understanding of CCA at various points in our journeys. "We" here, importantly, refers to a collective of scholars that are at different stages in our academic careers, as well as different degrees of familiarity with the field of health communication—and consequently, the CCA. Here's who "we" are at the time of co-writing this chapter:

Sissy Balkisa (SB): I am a 2nd-year M.A. student at the University of Cincinnati. I am currently writing my M.A. thesis titled: "Voices rising: The untold narratives of maternal mental health in Ghana's Zango communities." This project aims to uncover the experiences and perceptions of Zango women as I delve into how cultural, religious, and biomedical beliefs, as well as societal structures, shape their understanding of perinatal depression. These perceptions influence women's approach to communication and support seeking. Growing up, maternal health had never been my interest, not to mention it being a priority. Giving birth to my first child, whom I refer to as my "Lucky Charm," in Ghana brought up so many questions about the ordeals mothers had to go through before and even after childbirth. These questions continued to linger after I gave birth to my second child, "My Door Opener" in the United States, meaning "the key that opened worlds and opportunities I hadn't imagined." Given how these two childbirth experiences (in Ghana and the United States) were different, I kept asking myself what I could do to assist or make a difference in marginalized communities in Ghana. I may not be as marginalized as the communities I grew up in, but if I could go through these turbulences after childbirth, what about those who did not have the means or any confidence to share their feelings? Was it the pressure from extended family members, finances, and decisions I had to make concerning my birth process, change in physical figure, or taking care of my baby that surfaced all those emotions? My interest revolves around women's health, maternal and infant health, particularly within marginalized and culturally unique communities. My lived experiences made me focus on how our social, cultural, and religious factors influence women's perception of maternal health and mental health issues.

Yixuan Qi (YQ): I am a 1st-year PhD student at the University of Cincinnati. I did my M.A. at Minzu University of China. "Minzu" is a Chinese word to name ethnic groups that share the same culture, language, history, and often the same ancestry. China officially recognizes 56 Minzu, including the Han majority and 55 minority ethnic groups. My research interests lie in health communication, particularly focused on mental health and cancer-related communication. I see health as socially constructed, shaped by cultural standpoints and power relations that influence how people understand and practice health. Currently, I am exploring the mental health needs of young professionals in China and their experiences with mental health services. Given that CCA values individual experiences, especially those of marginalized, normalized, or underrepresented groups, this framework aligns perfectly with my focus. CCA emphasizes cultural diversity, acknowledging that interpretations of even scientific issues vary significantly across cultural contexts. For example, in China, mental health issues like depression and anxiety are often downplayed even though some people recognize their importance and the significant impact on their lives. Even individuals interested in improving their mental health face numerous barriers to taking action. Cultural stigma, inadequate mental health services, structural barriers, and, most importantly, the diverse challenges faced by different individuals all need to be considered when addressing this issue.

From my master's training, my initial research interest was in intercultural communication. I learned about Edward Said's Orientalism and how colonization shapes global cultural narratives. My M.A. research on Tibetan films allowed to work through issues related to minority groups, cultural representation, and the importance of marginalized voices. I began thinking deeply about these issues during the COVID-19 pandemic, which also led to my shift in research interests toward health communication. During the pandemic, two members of my family were diagnosed with cancer. Being quarantined at home brought me physically and emotionally closer to them. I witnessed their experiences and suffering throughout their treatment, as well as the complexities of communication between patients, families, and doctors. I also saw how China's COVID policies affected the treatment plans. I realized that understanding health solely from a scientific or medical perspective is far too limited. Health is deeply human—it is emotional, social, and cultural. We can't simply blame patients for being afraid of cancer, for lacking health knowledge, or for holding on to outdated beliefs. People's views on health are shaped by broader social forces—culture, history, politics, economics, and even geography. Instead, we should reflect on how to bring about change and empower patients. At that point, I realized that from a communication perspective, truly understanding health requires listening to the needs of both patients and their families. Ensuring their voices are heard and incorporated into treatment plans is vital. Furthermore, amplifying their voices in broader social conversations allows them to be seen, gain more understanding and support, and finally challenge the stigma and stereotypes associated with illness. My research starts from a simple wish to promote social equity and equality. That goal pushes me to think critically and focus on people who are silenced or oppressed. I believe that everyone has the right to express themselves freely, to be heard and understood, and to fight for what they need and deserve.

Usman Bah (UB): I am a 1st-year PhD student at the University of Cincinnati. I did my M.A. at Ohio University. My research interests are in health and environmental (climate change) issues. Previously (before my master's and now my PhD program), my research interests were in media, freedom of expression, and community engagement. This was influenced by my work with the Media Reform Coordinating Group (MRCG) in Sierra Leone, a coordinating Secretariat for ten media organizations/institutions in Sierra Leone. At the latter stage of my career with the MRCG, I became more interested in environmental sustainability (climate change). I worked with six coastal communities in Sierra Leone on a climate change awareness campaign for three years before I left home for my master's degree in 2022. Nevertheless, I have always had an interest in health research due to my unforgettable experience with the Ebola crisis in Sierra Leone that claimed the lives of members of my family, friends, neighbors, and fellow Sierra Leoneans. At that time, I was not satisfied with the response of the government and international partners in managing the Ebola outbreak. The country did not have health communication experts to account for factors such as cultural and religious beliefs, distrust of public officials, and ethnic diversity in their response to the epidemic. The country had to rely on external experts who arrived later and were not as informed about the local intricacies and often developed insufficient recommendations. At that moment, I knew culture was an especially important element that the experts ignored and there were power dynamics such that the voices of locals and traditional leaders were discounted.

Shaunak Sastry (SS): I am a Professor of Communication at the University of Cincinnati and advise/mentor the other authors of this chapter. As a "senior scholar," I have worked on applying, refining, and extending the CCA through my academic career. In this conversation, I take the role of the moderator and push the discussion around to explore how our ideas of the theory and its application evolve and crystallize. You would have observed that in introducing their research interests above, my co-authors started talking about their unique lived experiences, cultural contexts, and health. This, in many ways, is the first stop in the journey to becoming a CCA scholar: to develop an academic curiosity about some aspect of a health problem, a cultural process related to health, or an issue of personal relevance to them. For SB, their interest was clearly rooted in very personal, embodied experiences of childbirth. For YQ, it was an observed interest in the changing cultural landscape around mental health of young professionals in China. For UB, it was both the professional experience of working in community organizing for climate change preparedness and the felt experience of climate change in coastal Sierra Leone. This approach is typical for CCA scholars who are entering the field. We tend to learn the theory at the same time as we learn about the health context that we are interested in exploring. In other words, our familiarity with the theoretical concepts of CCA is crystallized at the same time as we learn more about the health context of interest. For some of us, this means applying our personal, cultural, or discovered experiences to the conceptual components of the theory, and for others it means refashioning and re-labeling these experiences with the terminology of the theory. Either way, the "first step" for a CCA scholar is to be socialized into a critical (related to the distribution of power in society) understanding of health.

SB: But if you come from the Global South, then you grow up with a critical understanding of health anyway.

SS: Aha! Say more!

SB: You grow up seeing that health isn't just about access to a clinic or doctors; it's about everyday realities of life spanning through cultural beliefs, family pressures, and ways communities make do without support. You get to understand that maternal health struggles like PND are woven into silence, survival, and resilience about things we've always known and felt but rarely get to say out loud.

UB: Even before being introduced to the CCA in my Communication and Development Studies master's program at Ohio University, I had also held this belief that the culture and beliefs of communities and individuals should be at the center of any planned communication intervention. For instance, during the Ebola crisis in Sierra Leone, when I was in my freshman year in college, I woke up to daily news of how we had lost a relative, a neighbor, friends, or fellow Sierra Leoneans to the virus. Ignoring people's cultural and religious beliefs like touching and caring for the sick and washing and burying the dead in a dignified manner at the start of the crisis contributed to the initial failure of planned health interventions. The frustrating part was that communication experts did not take account of these factors in their response to the epidemic and for the most part, the external experts were not as informed about the local intricacies and often developed insufficient recommendations to respond to the epidemic. This prompted me to pursue a career in health communication that centers culture in health interventions. As such, when I was first introduced to CCA, I was like, "Yes, this is it…"

YQ: I feel like it's a yes and no about the "critical understanding of health." Growing up in China, sure, people deal with all kinds of pressures and confusion around health. It's not like everyone obeys the system without reflection. But it's hard to frame those feelings as a critical understanding of health. It's more like a messy, complicated experience you just live through. When I was in China, I never heard a clear expression that health could be something to think critically.

SS: Those are all excellent points—we see that CCA draws so many scholars from the global South into the discipline of Communication, and this is part of it—that the theoretical impulse of the approach taps into experiences of marginalization that we have witnessed in our cultural contexts—whether that is due to the historical colonial processes that have shaped global health disparities in the global South (Arnold, 1993; Dutta & Basu, 2008; Farmer et al., 2013; Hickel et al., 2022), or the unfair global burden of disease or environmental degradation that we experience in the global South (Coates et al., 2021; Jones et al., 2023; Roberts & Parks, 2007). So, I think this is a very profound point about who is drawn to the CCA and what it means to be CHC scholar—that a lot of the source material is already built in for those of us who have personal or secondary knowledge of marginalization and health. In very distinct ways, the critical edge of CCA is in that it provides an avenue for us to theorize from "where we came from." In that sense, CCA socializes those of us from the global South, and provides an invitation for our lived experiences, our geopolitical and cultural knowledge to be counted as veritable, credible, important knowledge in a field where the norm has often been to universalize the experiences of WEIRD samples (White, Educated, Industrialized, Rich, Democratic). There is also a running thread through so many CCA scholars, young and established, that many of us need to be extricated out of our "home culture" context to speak with authority about it. That perspectival distance—that experience of migration and distance—seems to be critical. The larger question, here, of course, is China's position as a member of the "global South." That political question, while very much a part of current geopolitical trends, is outside of the scope of what we can discuss here. But both Mignolo (2011) and Liu (2022) offer good discussions of the complex politics of locating China within the world order system.

YQ: I think this is exactly the point. My orientation to the field and to exploring my research interest is through the CCA and that prompted me to think about my own cultural context in more detail. I was introduced to CCA while researching Ph.D. programs that aligned with my passion for social justice and health communication. During my master's studies, I often noticed the unreasonable or problematic aspects of social phenomena. When discussing these issues with others, the response was usually dismissive: "What can you do about it?" or "This should not be your concern." Even when selecting a research topic, I'd often hear doubts, such as, "Does your research have an audience?" I would wonder, doesn't anyone else have similar thoughts? Even if there isn't a clear audience, does that mean the research lacks value? And who exactly are these audiences anyway?

When I encountered Dr. Sastry's work on CCA, it was a turning point. CCA seemed to bring a social justice lens into health communication, critically exposing normalized injustices and empowering marginalized voices. I felt it was a framework to articulate the issues I had always noticed yet struggled to express. As I joined the CCA group and studied the theory through various cases—like Nepal's radio program, AIDS communication, and cancer awareness—I realized that CCA isn't limited to marginalized communities alone; it also brings sidelined issues into mainstream discussions. For instance, China's mental health topic may not seem marginalized in terms of the numbers affected or the scope of the audience, yet I feel CCA is still applicable in this context because of the systematic silencing of ideas about mental health, therapeutic interventions, and support in that context. It can clearly highlight ambiguous norms, empower awareness, and enable a new understanding of the issue.

SS: That's a great point. CCA clearly operates as a place for "non-Western" scholars to come to speak authoritatively about human communication processes because it is fundamentally an approach to theory that valorizes alternatives to the "dominant understanding" of health—or what we would call in social sciences a "received view." In that sense, CCA, by its very theoretical stance, seeks to broaden, move, and de-center the "where" of Communication studies—that human communication can have multiple, co-existing, and non-authoritative "centers" instead of "center-periphery" models where existing theory must be adjusted, elaborated, refined, and tailored for different audiences. This "tailoring view" is what Dutta calls the "cultural sensitivity" mode of theorizing (Dutta, 2007).

UB: I was introduced to the CCA in my master's program as one of the powerful methods we can use to co-define and co-create solutions with communities whose voices have mostly been ignored. With my experience with the Ebola crisis and my distaste for top-bottom approach which I saw as "banking system" of spoon-feeding people with information and solutions instead of having them take part in the process of deciding on issues that affected their lives, I knew immediately that this was the perfect approach for me. Realizing that this was the link I was missing to make my arguments on why the communication chains were ineffective and misinformation had its way to greatly fuel the spread of the Ebola virus in Sierra Leone, I opted to learn more about this approach to better situate myself in making a better and an informed argument on why culture should be at the center of the communication process in nations like Sierra Leone, Liberia, and Guinea that are highly cultural, religious, and traditional. I also realized that the voices of most of the communities I had worked in in Sierra Leone were hardly valued by NGOs who had this Eurocentric way of framing and seeing things. They mostly imported ideas and solutions to problems that were specifically unique to these communities, ignoring structural and cultural barriers. At the end, most of these projects failed or faded away when the donors left. It was painstaking for me to see thousands of dollars just wasted like that without creating the desired long-time impact.

SS: Well sure, the critique of Eurocentric thought is at the heart of CCA. But there is also a warning in here against parochialism on the other end of the spectrum. As CCA becomes more popular in the field, there is also a tendency to use "cultural" explanations to elide any critiques of power or any analytical leaps that a "native" takes. For me, this has always been the fine line that CCA has to walk, to avoid the fate where challenging a totalizing system like Eurocentrism produces a homegrown form of totalitarianism. While in graduate school, I read this quote from the Marxist economist Samir Amin that has stayed with me: "There is something highly Eurocentric in assuming that all Eurocentrism comes from Europe (Amin, 1989, p. 264)."

Notice that we are firmly in the first tier of the "nested model" here—defining the problem through a deep engagement with the CCA components of culture, structure, and agency. These sensemaking devices enable us to delimit and empirically establish what health means to the community, cultural group, or population of our interest. This is where a lot of us enter the field of CCA—in doing the definitional work through the concepts of culture-structure-agency. Using these concepts also serve as a guardrail against overdetermining "culture" as an explanatory mechanism for health processes. For instance, regarding your example, Usman, about burial rituals and safety in the context of Ebola, a CCA approach would not, in my understanding, argue for the idea that the cultural practices around burials (touching, hugging goodbye, cleaning and bathing the dead) are sacrosanct and cannot be altered given the very lethal risk of infection. Rather, the point is to have local voices, local cultural practices incorporated within the necessary medical interventions required. The challenge of CCA is to have those decision chains start locally, be led by community voices, and be ready to respond to real-time challenges of speed and efficacy in the context of an infectious disease epidemic like Ebola. The point is not to conduct some sort of "disease exceptionalism," which is a term coined by the ethnographer Adia Benton (2015), but to situate the cultural practice within the constraints of structural pressures.

Could we perhaps move the discussion to the next "tier" or the next stage—we say that the next logical step for CCA interventions is to think about "problem interpretation." In other words, not just defining a health problem but focusing on "how" we know what we claim to know. In the model, we talk about these "ladders" between the tiers. For a CCA project to go from the Tier 1: Problem definition to Tier 2: Problem Interpretation, we use the ladder of methodological reflexivity. What do you understand by this?

SB: A couple of points here. CCA guides my perspectives and engagements with co-participants in my research study by reminding me that this is not just my research but rather our story constructed together. This taught me to see myself as a collaborator, not an expert, and my co-participants feel heard and valued. CCA emphasizes listening deeply not only to words but to silences, and gestures that shape how people express themselves. With this in mind, I prioritized creating environments where my co-participants feel safe and comfortable to share their truths. I ask questions that invite their stories to unfold naturally, and I also acknowledge and respect the ways they choose to communicate whether through metaphors or storytelling the details they choose to share, and what they prefer not to share. I do not see the CCA as only a transformative communicative theory but also a human way of analyzing phenomena or, better yet, real-life occurrences. This involves listening, sharing, and co-creating meanings in spaces where voices are often silenced. It's not about imposing solutions from the outside but about fostering conversations that allow communities to articulate their realities and needs, shifting the focus from the "expert" to the "community." CCA recognizes that communication isn't just about transmitting information but about the relationships and power dynamics that shape how people engage with one another and the systems around them. It challenges us to rethink who gets to speak, who gets heard, and how structures of power influence those processes. What sets CCA apart from other theories is its commitment to centering margins. Most theories I've come across try to explain phenomena in broad strokes or situations, often overlooking the peculiarity of lived experiences in specific contexts. CCA insists that these occurrences are rich spaces of knowledge and people's evidence of resilience against these structural barriers, be it power dynamics or silence from people. CCA grounds itself in the unique realities of the marginalized it seeks to understand or co-create knowledge with rather than seek generalization.

UB: The CCA concepts have helped me as a researcher to try to "disempower" myself during my interaction with participants to overcome the power dynamics that may ensue. Instead of seeing myself as the expert (which I might be in some ways), the CCA has guided me to consider myself as a collaborator and a partner with community members to co-identify, co-define, and co-address the issue (s) that a community may be faced with. I have always had this belief that those who experience a problem or challenge firsthand are experts and are in a better position to tell their lived experiences. As a collaborator or partner, my role would be to collaborate with these people who have these lived experiences to co-create sustainable solutions that take into consideration their cultural values and existing structural constraints like poverty, power dynamics, and identities and minority representations, among others. Additionally, the CCA concepts have taught me to be more of a listener than the main voice. Since there is usually this (un)conscious power dynamics and difference between the researcher or scholar with community members in which the researcher is considered as the authority, I am learning to create a safe and level playing field for my collaborators to partake in the communicative space.

SS: Lot of similar things to discuss in these responses. I really am taken by this notion of "disempowerment"—is that something that is possible to do? The critical edge of CCA will ask what it means to disempower oneself as a researcher. One may argue that as a graduate student, or an early career scholar, trying to build rapport and trust in the community is already relatively disempowering in general. So, what does that process look like, to actively work to disempower one's own interpretations in favor of a more co-constructed viewpoint? Usman, can you talk about an example where this takes place? I am thinking about your insistence of using the term "extinction" to describe how the local community in Conakry Dee, Sierra Leone, describes their situation with relationship to coastal loss and climate change. That discussion and our back-and-forth with the term "extinction" seem relevant.

UB: That is true, and the notion of disempowerment is complicated. For instance, during my thesis research, I realized that most of the participants in our interaction addressed me as "Sir" or would respond saying "Yes sir" even though most of them were way older than me. I then realized that this respect accorded me was due to their assumption of me being an expert and empowered since I had led climate awareness campaign in their community before. This pragmatic emergence of power dynamics made me reconsider my questioning and interaction approach with participants. I then deliberately asked some of them leading questions to test their responses against my notion of them considering me as an expert. Their answers were affirmative to my leading questions. I realized they may think that was what I wanted to hear and as such they were framing their responses toward that end. I then had to reframe my questions that prompted them to focus on what they had experienced or seen. I took my time to allow them to struggle and stutter with their responses. One key term that they brought up with me was the issue of their physical community going extinct. In my expert knowledge, I knew the term "extinct" has usually been scientifically used to refer to species extinction. It was interesting how their use of this term focused on extinction of the "environment" rather than themselves or other species. I saw this as a local knowledge and view, which I had to value and rely on than the predominant expert or science view of the term. Acknowledging that and using it in my thesis and a research paper that is about to be published seemed to me I disempowered my knowledge of such concept and put forward my participants' local knowledge. One reviewer asked me to rephrase the word extinction as being used in the paper. I stood my ground and explained that that was how my participants described their situation in terms of the climate crises they are faced with.

SS: This idea of co-construction is an important one to reflect on—what does co-construction look like? Of course, one way to discuss it is to ensure that the researcher is very aware of their power in the interaction, like Usman mentions above. It is also inherent in recognizing that our "community partners" or co-participants are under no obligation to share with us and may choose at times to actively not share information. How does co-construction work in that context? Sissy, you seem to suggest, in your response above, that in listening to the stories of the women you interviewed in Ghana for your M.A. thesis, there were some things that your participants chose not to share. How did you arrive at this, and how does one work through this contradiction? How does one even sense that something is missing?

SB: For me, co-construction means entering spaces with an understanding that the co-participants are the holders of the knowledge, and I'm not there to listen and to make them feel like I'm extracting. During my field work in Zango communities in Ghana, my co-participants' hesitation to share some experiences was not always obvious. Sometimes it was a long pause, a tight smile or smirk on the face, a shift in tone, or a glance away from me. It was in those subtle moments that I realized those silences were boundaries they were setting to protect certain parts of their stories. This just reminded me of my conversation with SS about my thesis analysis. I told him that no matter how I want to share my postpartum experiences, there are some parts of it that I cannot share.

This personal reflection made me understand that co-construction is about recognizing that my co-participants owe me nothing, and their choice to withhold is as meaningful as their choice to share. I learned to honor gaps as part of the story. My development of that mutual process of trust and care, while building a narrative together, and allowing space for what remains unspoken, defines the basis of co-construction for me. One will say, "how do we get to know the full story if co-participants choose what to withhold & what to share?" I say this feels deeply human because real narratives, especially about experiences of pain or resilience, are never complete or easy. It is layered, and it belongs ultimately to those living it.

SS: The one question that I receive when I speak to students and scholars interested in CCA is the question of timing, effort, and the professional goals of graduate school. In some way, from the tenor of the questions I receive, I suspect that a younger generation of scholars in health communication tends to look at CCA and the fieldwork-heavy nature of CCA as anachronistic to how graduate school and doctoral training are done today. In the age of data mining and data scraping, AI-powered sentiment analysis, and the broader "Tiktok-ization" of culture, I feel that there is this sense that this is an outmoded way of understanding health processes. I guess these are two questions in one. First, what are the pragmatic considerations of doing CCA work as doctoral (and even M.A.) scholars? What do you expect to be the challenges and opportunities along the way? And second, and related but not the same question, what does CHC look like in this political moment? What methods/approaches/gestures must be incorporated? Choose any one to address…

SB: The most significant challenge to me is the inherent complexity of working within culturally diverse contexts. Collecting data that is reflective of community experiences requires establishing trust, which can be difficult, especially when dealing with vulnerable groups. Sometimes people may be wary of outside researchers or have had negative experiences with academic projects in the past. Another challenge is ensuring that the research process is not perceived as an investigation, but rather as an equal conversation between myself and the community. As a 2nd year M.A. student about to enter a PhD program, one of the significant challenges in doing CCA work is the limited access to the field. Unlike established researchers or those with institutional backing, we often lack the authority or resources to enter certain communities for research. Access to the field typically requires trust and sometimes permission from community leaders or gatekeepers, which can be difficult to establish as a novice scholar. Additionally, CCA often calls for a long-term, relationship-building approach that can be time-consuming.

YQ: For me, the greatest challenge lies in explaining the cultural context. The cultural landscape is vast and intricate, and the rapid pace of social change in China further complicates this task. Many influences that seem natural or self-evident are, in fact, deeply embedded in daily life, making them difficult to recognize and even harder to articulate clearly. Moreover, I believe that developing such awareness requires a certain level of detachment, such as a positionality that allows for critical distance. However, because the social context is constantly evolving, the distance risks losing the richness and nuance that come from close, immersive understanding. Additionally, I find that CCA has significantly shaped the way I perceive social issues, offering valuable insights into underlying problems. However, I still experience some uncertainty regarding methodological application, particularly in operationalizing CCA in my research. I realize that within the entanglement of multiple forces, such as political and economic structures, it is challenging to find practical strategies that improve agency, such as strategies that empower marginalized communities, amplify their voices, and enable them to push back against dominant systems. Moreover, how to sustain these efforts remains a challenge. Seeing such strategies truly put into practice and lead to real change would be even more encouraging and inspiring.

UB: In terms of challenges, CCA tends to be theoretically complex for an upcoming scholar especially trying to understand the intersection of culture, structure (power), and agency in the communication and intervention processes. At times, I would feel like I have grasped the concepts but suddenly, when I intend to apply them to certain issues or instances, I find myself struggling between which element challenges or influences the other. There is also the challenge of writing and asking questions that are CCA grounded. However, one thing I have learned in all of these is that it takes time for one to get all these concepts right. Furthermore, I have always had this personal conflict of balancing power dynamics between me as the researcher and community members I collaborate with or research with. Since I know the importance of participants feeling empowered (agency) to tell their own stories, I always have this fear not to unconsciously take away that power (agency) from them. I have been reflecting on how to provide my participants with a platform where they can share their knowledge and how all of us can equally share the benefit of that knowledge. I know that there are many instances in which researchers (consciously or unconsciously) end up exploiting underserved communities for their own personal academic growth when they conduct research about marginalized communities, leave, publish, and never go back to those communities. I do not want to be a party to that. I am sure, with more training and guidance from my mentors, I will find that solution that works for me to avoid this.

SS: I think that is so powerful, Usman. What you talk about here is the idea of conceptual slippage, that is so common to critical work, where at one point you feel like you understand what is happening, and then, suddenly, you slip into uncertainty. I think we are all in that boat—the power of a good theory is that it allows us to experience these movements but provides conceptual anchors for us to reframe and re-establish our bearings. In the CCA model, we talk about these ladders called "methodological reflexivity" and "philosophical reflexivity" and I find those concepts are orienting anchors (Sastry et al., 2021). However, in the end, a lot of this is the practice, the doing, and the engagement with the field that helps us become more dexterous with the concepts.

But I also think there is a broader point about the pressures of graduate school, of developing credibility as a scholar, and identifying how one becomes a CHC scholar. As Heather Zoller reminds us (in her chapter in this book) but also in our interactions with her in the classroom and elsewhere, being "critical" refers to an orientation to how to study and change social processes, and not really in the choice of what specific thing one is interesting in. As graduate scholars, it can seem unnerving to say "I am going to do CCA" if the endpoint of CCA, as described in the model, is to work toward a self-sustaining, community-owned movement around health. That's an idealization of what CCA looks like outside of the tremendous contradictions and paradoxes that go along with the work. Which is to say, the label of being a "CCA scholar" is relevant to our field, and is relevant to discussions in academic spaces, but outside of that, being a CCA scholar is to adopt a certain kind of posture toward social movements, it is a commitment to challenging social injustice (at the personal, institutional, community, and professional) levels, and acting in "pragmatic solidarity" with movements for social change. That is the north star—that's what we call "Philosophical Reflexivity" in the tiered model. That is a recognition that the commitment to social transformation is an orientation, and not just a commitment to expertise in a particular health context. Which is why, as one develops a critical voice in the field, one tends to self-identify as a "critical scholar" rather than a scholar of epidemic disease, or HIV/AIDS communication, or of climate change communication. It is the orientation that is central. And this is where I acknowledge the profound influence of Mohan Dutta's public activism and commitment to critical causes—not only do I feel compelled to pay forward his incredible intellectual generosity but also recognize the need to put what he calls "the body on the line" (see his chapter in this book).

Toward a Conclusion

It was a real challenge to find an organic closure to this rather freewheeling conversation, but page length requirements suggest this is as good a place as any. Working in CHC spaces means embracing the chaotic nature of applied scholarship and balancing the neatness of academic constructs versus the fundamentally contradictory nature of social change. As scholars at different stages of the journeys into (and perhaps out of?) CCA-driven projects, we hope to have reflected on how this approach to doing health communication work changes and evolves through one's contextual, experiential, professional, and activist frameworks. In the end, a critical approach also means a reflexive orientation to the untied end of knots—and we hope that this chapter, in its cyclical, conversational tempo, alludes to the ongoing nature of CHC work. As a collective of scholars on different legs of this journey, we thank you, reader, for staying the course and journeying with us.

References

Amin, S. (1989). *Eurocentrism*. Monthly Review Press.

Arnold, D. (1993). *Colonizing the body: State medicine and epidemic disease in nineteenth-century India*. University of California Press.

Benton, A. (2015). *HIV exceptionalism: Development through disease in Sierra Leone*. University of Minnesota Press.

Coates, M. M., Ezzati, M., Robles Aguilar, G., Kwan, G. F., Vigo, D., Mocumbi, A. O., Becker, A. E., Makani, J., Hyder, A. A., Jain, Y., Stefan, D. C., Gupta, N., Marx, A., & Bukhman, G. (2021). Burden of disease among the world's poorest billion people: An expert-informed secondary analysis of Global Burden of Disease estimates. *PLoS One, 16*(8), e0253073. https://doi.org/10.1371/journal.pone.0253073

Dutta, M. J. (2007). Communicating about culture and health: Theorizing culture-centered and cultural-sensitivity approaches. *Communication Theory, 17*, 304–328. https://doi.org/10.1111/j.1468-2885.2007.00297.x

Dutta, M. J., & Basu, A. (2008). Meanings of health: Interrogating structure and culture. *Health Communication, 23*(6), 560–572.

Farmer, P., Kleinman, A., Kim, J., & Basilico, M. (Eds.). (2013). *Reimagining global health: An introduction*. University of California Press.

Hickel, J., Dorninger, C., Wieland, H., & Suwandi, I. (2022). Imperialist appropriation in the world economy: Drain from the global South through unequal exchange, 1990–2015. *Global Environmental Change, 73*. https://doi.org/10.1016/j.gloenvcha.2022.102467

Jones, M. W., Peters, G. P., Gasser, T., Andrew, R. M., Schwingshackl, C., Gütschow, J., Houghton, R. A., Friedlingstein, P., Pongratz, J., & Le Quéré, C. (2023). National contributions to climate change due to historical emissions of carbon dioxide, methane, and nitrous oxide since 1850. *Scientific Data, 10*(1), 155. https://doi.org/10.1038/s41597-023-02041-1

Liu, H. (2022). China engages the global south: From Bandung to the belt and road initiative. *Global Policy*, *13*(S1), 11–22. https://doi.org/10.1111/1758-5899.13034

Mignolo, W. D. (2011). The global south and world dis/order. *Journal of Anthropological Research*, *67*(2), 165–188. https://doi.org/10.3998/jar.0521004.0067.202

Roberts, J. T., & Parks, B. C. (2007). *A climate of injustice: Global inequality, North-South politics, and climate policy*. MIT Press.

Sastry, S., Stephenson, M., Dillon, P., & Carter, A. (2021). A meta-theoretical systematic review of the culture-centered approach to health communication: Toward a refined, "nested" model. *Communication Theory*, *31*(3), 380–421. https://doi.org/10.1093/ct/qtz024

13
NEW LIGHT

Critical Health Communication and Connections to Experiences from the Field

Urmi Basu, Ambar Basu, Mavis Freeman Essel, and Roopam Mishra

New Light is a not-for profit charitable organization that works with a community of poor women in sex work in Kalighat, Kolkata, India (New Light, 2025). The sex worker community in Kalighat is the oldest in Kolkata. Founded in 2000, New Light provides numerous services to the sex worker community in Kalighat, namely shelter, educational opportunities, healthcare, and legal aid to the children, girls, and women in the Kalighat community. This includes a crèche and night shelter, and three residential homes for young and teenaged children of sex workers working in Kalighat. According to the organization's website, New Light also "operates a Community Clinic to address the medical needs of the sex worker community. The clinic treats gynecological, pediatric, STD, HIV-AIDS, and general medicine cases" (New Light, 2025). Further, the New Light website states that "for those exposed to or infected by HIV, provisions are in place to provide assistance with hospital visits, testing, and treatment, along with additional care and support in the form of food aid."

The history of the Kalighat sex worker community is not readily available and it is likely that the Kalighat sex worker community developed around the Kali temple when a number of dharmashalas (rest houses) were set up to house pilgrims, traders, and travelers to the nearby Kali temple (Basu, 2010). The community now houses more than 2,000 sex workers from Kolkata, suburban areas around the city, and countries such as Nepal and Bangladesh. Most sex workers live and work in the seven bylanes that skirt the northern fringes of the Kali temple, all of which lead to the Adi Ganga waterway that, during the East India Company rule, served as a trade and transit route in the city.

The New Light office and night shelter (for younger children of sex workers in the community) is housed in one of these bylanes and on the second floor of a local temple. Urmi Basu is the founder and leader of New Light. A sociologist by academic training, Urmi Basu has received the Nari Shakti Puraskar (literally translated to mean Woman Power Award), India's highest civilian award that recognizes the achievements and contributions of women. In 2009, she was honored by the Dalai Lama as one of the "Unsung Heroes of Compassion." The story of New Light and Urmi Basu's journey with the Kalighat sex worker community has been featured in the documentary series led by Nicholas Kristof and Sheryl WuDunn, called "Half the Sky: Turning Oppression into Opportunity for Women Worldwide."

This chapter documents excerpts from conversations between Urmi Basu (Urmi henceforth) and Ambar Basu (Ambar), the two first authors, over a two-phase zoom meeting lasting approximately two hours. Ambar has known Urmi for close to 20 years now, having conducted several research studies with members of the Kalighat sex worker community and other stakeholders of New Light (Basu, 2011, 2017; Basu & Dutta, 2008, 2009, 2011). The other co-authors collaborated on writing this chapter, transcribing the conversation between Urmi and Ambar, and in processing the data/conversations.

In this chapter, the conversations between Urmi and Ambar are synthesized and presented in a sequence that will help the reader understand, among other things, how critical health communication (CHC) might play out as a practice on the ground in a setting of utter dispossession and away from the glare and scope of strict theories and accompanying methodologies/best practices of public health interventions. As such, this chapter aims to present to the reader connections (and disjunctures) between CHC theorizing and interventions (such as those of New Light) that intend to make a difference in the lives of the displaced and dispossessed and take shape on the ground—in the communities.

In these conversations, readers might witness Urmi as an interlocutor (Beverley, 1999) who works with organic intellectuals (Gramsci, 1971) in the subaltern Kalighat sex worker community to implement initiatives and organize resources that transform lives of dispossession. The interlocutor can also be understood as a facilitator who creates communicative and material pathways that allow the narratives of the dispossessed to disrupt the linear, mainstream understandings of health and marginality. In *Toward the Development of Critical Health Communication Praxis*, Lupton (1994) called for health communication advocacy that centers CHC praxis. Such a praxis interrogates and actively seeks to transform prevailing discourses in health communication. These prevailing discourses reinforce the primacy of the biomedical model of health while ignoring for the social, cultural, historical, and hence political dimensions of how individuals, communities, and institutions make sense of/communicate about health.

One of the aims of this book is to foreground relationships among local cultural and communicative systems, power, politics, and health inequities and show how such inequities play out on the ground in the lives of those who bear the brunt of these inequities. In another chapter of this book (by Leandra Hernandez), for example, we see a call for a practice of journalism that highlights CHC praxis through ethical witnessing to improve news coverage and public health responses to gender-based violence. This chapter, similarly, seeks to foreground a CHC praxis that explores how local and global knowledge and communicative systems come into play in a marginalized community as an individual or an organization facilitates pathways for the transformation of the health and lives of members of the community. Lessons learned from New Light's and Urmi Basu's journey are illustrative and instructive in this context. Hopefully, the readers will see how this critical health initiative that aimed to transform the lives of the marginalized came to fruition.

This chapter is organized into three sequential themes that collate the conversations between Urmi and Ambar. Each theme speaks to a particular (non-linear) phase of CHC praxis with a marginalized community (with New Light as an exemplar): The Beginning, Sustaining and Expanding, and Into the Future.

Script

The Beginning

Ambar: Urmi di,[1] as I think about your work over the past few decades in public health, I see you as an advocate for the health and well-being of communities that are at the margins. Is this an appropriate way of understanding or framing your work?

Urmi: I'm not sure if there is any appropriate way to frame my efforts. What I can say is I've always known that people from the fringes have very little access to the public healthcare system. And it is becoming increasingly difficult for them to access healthcare even though a lot of new (government) schemes are being instituted.

New Light, which has been in operation for the last 24 years, began on the strength of, you know, an aspiration of a mother, you could say. As a young mother, when I walked into the red-light district of Kalighat, which has been New Light's primary area of operation, 24 years ago, the situation that I saw there was almost abysmal in terms of people's safety, in terms of children's healthcare or a minimum nutritional level. And education. So, for me too, as a young mother, to watch a small child, say a toddler sleeping under the bed of a mother who was with a different client, say every hour, was an extremely traumatic experience. And I don't know where it came from, but I was, I began to wonder if my life had been that way.

So, the answer that I found within my heart was I would try to do the best that I could.

And I think that has been the genesis of the idea of New Light that every child deserves a safe and secure place to grow up in. And to dream about things that they see around themselves, but which were always just beyond their reach. That's what New Light has been trying to do for the communities, you know, that we have worked with over all these years.

Ambar: When you started off...

Urmi: Starting off, and I got a lot of input from people who are my colleagues now, those who have grown up in the area. We identified that we would work toward not having any young girl work as a sex worker in the area, and that we would try to make sure that not a single girl child who's been through the New Light program would ever be employed as a sex worker. The thing is, 24 years ago, there were very, very few young people in the sex worker community here who had finished high school. But today, at least, the community takes that like it's a guaranteed thing that every child growing up in the Kalighat sex worker community will definitely finish their secondary and higher secondary level of education.

Ambar: Let us talk more about the beginnings of New Light. What did you and your team do to get started?

Urmi: You know, reminiscing or recollecting or thinking about what all has actually happened, and this stuff that you have been able to do, there are so many more things that I think about. Like I told you, I was not alone. There were inputs I got from my colleagues who themselves have grown up in that area, Krishna, for example. And I think it was a really, you know, heartfelt observation and very, very inspiring for people from the community to recognize that I could work with them and help to bring about meaningful change.

	New Light has been an audacious project—this enterprise in making these changes, these substantial changes in the community over the past two decades or more—and we did not have any blueprint. There was nothing that the team at that time, primarily me and two other young people from the community, nothing that we could adopt, there was no ready playbook. You know, there was nothing. No set guidelines that we could base our work on. So, everything that New Light has done has kind of grown very organically, and the services that we were able to put together were kind of those that needs of this community dictated, not the other way around. Like I didn't, at the very beginning, begin by saying they needed education, or they needed healthcare, or vaccination, or that they needed other economic opportunities, adult education, no.
Ambar:	What about funding?
Urmi:	New Light is a project that started with only ₹10,000 In the year 2000, so ₹10,000, if you convert that today, it would be like $100 and maybe $120.00. So that's what was the seed money. And with that seed money, what we bought the first day we started New Light was a water filter, a couple of plastic mats, and a small bed where a child could be kept safe and could sleep in comfort. And maybe a couple of plastic plates and a few spoons. That was all. So that's how our journey began.
	And when you begin that way, when you don't have any track record, you can't go to people and ask for money. Nobody believes you. People are not going to open their purses when they see you have nothing. So, I kind of used my common sense. I reached out to friends and family and told them whatever you're discarding please give it to us. If you are throwing out the toys of your kids who have outgrown those, if you are discarding clothes, if you're changing the curtains in your house, and if you give those to us, we can probably use the curtains to have children sit on them on the ground. So, most of the things that we had at the beginning were repurposed, including the clay tiles in the New Light office—those came from a movie set of a friend of mine who was a producer. The windows that you see in the New Light, which in retrospect really look like those that have been there forever, came at the cost of ₹400. I started to tell people if your kids are not using their old exercise books and crayon boxes which are used, you could give those to us. If you have medicines left over and those have not reached the date of expiry, please give them to us. That's how the initial

phase of New Light started. We were open only between 5 pm until 10 pm because that is the peak hour when the sex worker women are working with their clients. And the idea was to keep the kids of these women off the streets, right? At New Light, the kids could come to a safe space, and they were kept in the care of other women from the community who had already exited from sex work.

At the beginning, there was no other face of a stranger other than my face. Everybody else in New Light was from the community.

Ambar: So, why do you think people in the community believed you enough to join hands with you?

Urmi: I have no idea why they believed (in) me or why they thought it would be possible to do what I was proposing, that is, to open a shelter for the kids and the women of this sex worker community. And when you're going to work with a marginalized community, they will not trust you even one bit unless they know that you understand them, like you've sensed them under your skin, you understand their language.

Time is crucial as you continue to work with them. It is important to realize that these women do not quite trust you or me. There is reason to not trust. Some have been trafficked when they were very young. But, being with them, reaching out, and creating spaces where they can talk about their problems, and listening to those problems is important. Listening to the community has been an important characteristic of New Light's work in this community.

Sustaining and Expanding

Ambar: In my research with this community, I have heard from people here that 'New Light listens to us.' This idea of listening, listening to people in the community, can you talk a little bit about this idea and process of listening? How did you bring it to play in your work in the community?

Urmi: The first 'listening' happened, I remember, pretty early on, in a year or so since New Light began work here. I called a few of the mothers who had small kids and toddlers and just asked them: 'If you had a place where you could leave your child, and with a certain degree of safety and care, would you be willing to do that?' And they said, 'yes, of course.' There were other NGOs running programs in this community; none of those were actually running an evening program because it was not considered safe to stay and work in this sex worker community after sundown.

I think New Light became a success because we just addressed that need. Yeah, so, I realized many of these kids were running around completely without adult supervision. You know, running around actually just sensing what was going on around them, absorbing everything. And sometimes, kids were being sent out to buy alcohol, to buy cigarettes, and none of the mothers were cooking because that was their peak earning time. So, we decided we needed to provide a meal for the kids and a safe space where they could rest and be safe.

But, you know, during that initial period, I could not get people to come and work at New Light because the NGO had nothing to show; we were very young. So, I called some of the young people from within the community and they were taking care of the kids and just giving them, you know, alphabet recognition and shapes and sizes and colors and things like that. And also making sure that some of these kids, young people, they had the opportunity to go out and get, you know, the basic computer training like to just sit in front of a PC and start operating. They then started to transfer this knowledge, and once people begin learning automatically their self-esteem goes up, right, and they begin to be treated differently within their community.

So, watching people from within the community getting more skills and getting more knowledge and exposure, all of those things actually mattered, and it took us almost say close to five years before we had the first set of teachers with graduate degrees, and you know a counselor or a therapist or things like that. But what we did right from the beginning was to have a doctor.

Ambar: Why? Can you please talk more about how New Light initiated and grew its healthcare initiative?

Urmi: Because New Light began to deal with so many kids, and every now and then, the kids would fall sick and coming from a doctor's family, I thought it was essential to attend to issues of health of these kids and their mothers. So, we set up a clinic in a small makeshift room in our office and had a doctor volunteer for us. [New Light also later hired a trained nurse.] At New Light, we began to distribute condoms and talk about HIV and AIDS, and our clinic became the first point of entry for a number of people who had already been, you know been exposed to the virus and they were too shy to go to a government clinic, even though antiretroviral therapy was available for free, but they didn't have the documents and you could not access ART without having your documents of identification.

So, at one point in time, I can't remember exactly the year, we also invited the Election Commission to come and set up a temporary office at New Light and we managed to get government ID for people in this community. The Election Commissioner's Office asked me if I knew all of these people here. Because I was underwriting, I was kind of the recommending person that yes, I know there is so and so person and this is where this woman lives and yeah without those documents, the kids could not be brought within the fold of services that they later on went to access from the government. Yeah, and honestly, I have no idea where I got these ideas from or how it happened. But as I mentioned earlier, there was a need and we said okay, fine, what is it going to be?

So all of those things, you know, the fact that we had a doctor coming there, a child specialist and a HIV expert, general physician and a lady doctor all of those things mattered, and in the present scenario, if I see there are no patients coming to our clinic, I am happy because our job has been, you know, our objective has been served. So, my younger colleagues are telling me, 'Oh, there are no patients;' I tell them, 'That is because New Light has helped create for them and their kids the ability to access health care from the government.' The kids here, they have all been given vaccines, so they are not falling sick anymore; their nutritional level, is way higher. So, they're able to fight illnesses that are caused because of compromised health situations.

Ambar: It's fascinating how New Light, a community-propelled system, has been put into place. New Light is not perfect, but there are tangible results that you're able to deliver.

Urmi: Then, there was a point when from being a 5 pm to 10 pm operation, New Light became a 24-hour operation.

How did that happen? One day a child was brought to the New Light clinic. He was six weeks old. He weighed 1.6 kg. His mother was very sick, was an addict, and HIV positive. Dr. Chatterjee, our attending pediatrician, called me, and he said this child needs immediate attention and he pinched the skin of this baby to show me how extremely dehydrated he was. And the doctor said the child needs immediate attention otherwise, we would not be able to save this child. So, we told the mother to come with us; so, it was four or five of us. We got into a taxi and took the child to a pediatric hospital.

The doctor took him inside, did whatever needed to be done and then he came back, and he told us, 'I'm sorry we have six neonatal facilities, but all are full.' I said then, 'Well, tell me, what do I need to do?' They tried to look to give him transfusion but couldn't find his veins. And he said, 'all you have to do is to try and do it manually. Just give it [hydration] to him, spoon by spoon, by spoon.'

So, Krishna (founder trustee of New Light and a member of the community), myself, the boy's mother, the grandmother, and we brought him back, and I called a few mothers from the community and told them that for this child to survive, we all would have to pull our weight and I asked who could volunteer at nighttime. We had one mother, a former sex worker, who herself was raising four kids, volunteer. We asked our clinic nurse to step in as well. We fed the child, one drop at a time. And that was 18 years ago. That point, we decided overnight that we were going to run for 24 hours every day, that no child within Kalighat should lose his or her life because they do not have the required healthcare. That is how we switched to the 24-hour mode. Today, this child goes to boarding school. He is 18 years old and is in 12th grade.

Ambar: What are your ongoing projects and commitments?

Urmi: The New Light shelter for kids in Kalighat, and the health initiatives, continue to be the heart of the project. We have added a toddlers' Montessori training place to make sure that children of sex workers as young as two years old have the chance to have an early start to school bringing them on par with kids from mainstream society. Then, we have three residential homes. One residential home is for girls between the ages of 8 and 18. The other residential home is for boys between the ages of 8 and 18, and the third residential shelter is for young women who are above 18 and are continuing to have either university education or professional training as a nurse or as a teacher or as a beautician.

The older girls in this residential home come from the Kalighat community and other extremely at-risk vulnerable situations. A number of them are survivors either of domestic violence, early marriage, or trafficking. So, these are kids, young women who would not otherwise have the opportunity to go

	and get higher education or degree or professional training. So, this has been a unique experiment, and it has been very successful so far. We have more than 100 graduates from this program.
Ambar:	How did you come upon this idea of operating shelters?
Urmi:	See, within say seven years of New Light being in operation, a number of kids in the program began to be pre-teens and I got a sense that they were already being seen by customers or being prepared to join sex work. I was witness to a couple of instances where the mothers had taken the girls away from New Light and were in the process of selling the kids. So, we began to house the young girls from the community away from the sex worker community.
Ambar:	When you did this, what was the reaction from the mothers of these young girls?
Urmi:	Again, you know, having multiple meetings, convincing the mothers that if your girl stays here, it will become increasingly difficult for you to keep her safe and if she has an opportunity to have a good education, she'd be able to transform your life. In these sorts of surrogate homes, the children have a chance to be formally educated, are exposed to career-skills training skills, social and cultural skills, and are, of course, provided with food, shelter, clothing, and healthcare. So, I told the mothers, 'It's just not you're sending the girl away. You are investing in a future that's going to be secure for her, and it's going to be secure for you as well.'

Into the Future

Ambar:	Now, say you have a student/scholar/public health expert who is very inspired by your work and would want to do similar work. What knowledge would you transfer to this person?
Urmi:	See, when you are dealing with human beings there is no guarantee for success. You just have to do what you do day after day and you're lucky if you find results that you expect. So, two things, your effort has to be 100% and your expectation has to be zero. That's one way I approach this work; otherwise, I know I'd be disappointed every single day and before you can even open your books, it's 'OK. I'm done with this.'
	For instance, there is no guarantee that all the kids you're working with are going to be with you for those many years and finish their education. The mother can decide to leave Kalighat tomorrow.

Also, I am 100% sure I could not have done this same project in another geopolitical and cultural context, say in another city, Mumbai. You need to know the finer cultural nuances and political forces that work in the community. I have gone to communities in Jharkhand, worked with women who are survivors of witch hunting[2]; I have worked with women in prisons, and on multiple occasions I have just sat with them and told them, 'I get you.' And I think it also comes from the training to listen and when we listen, the person that we are listening to must get the sense that you are actually listening. It's something else; it is how you fold your physical body, your mind, and your heart, and you say, 'here I am.'

Ambar: We are often told and taught that what you learn in the classroom is very different from what is out there or what actually works on the ground, and I don't think there is a better person than you to ask how true this is. You've been in the classroom; you've earned educational degrees in social work. How is this work in New Light different from what you learned in the classroom?

Urmi: During our academic training, we had to do our internships at different locations. My supervisor set me up to work with undertrial prisoners in Mumbai. So, I learned a lot from her but there was also a lot of unlearning that I had to do when I came to this work [in New Light]. One of the principles we were taught in the classroom is to control emotional involvement so that we don't burn out. So instead of that, I mean now, at this age and after, you know my work life is coming to an end, I can very easily say that this principle needs to be reworded. Instead of saying 'control emotional involvement with your clients' it should be worded as 'equip yourself to deal with whatever is brought to you.' The moment I seek to control emotion and involvement; I am setting a boundary. And with boundaries you will not be able to gain whatever little trust you can in a community that lives in poverty and stigma. Unless I bring my own vulnerability to the table, and I am willing to stand completely naked to be seen, to be examined, to be, to be understood and seen in and listen in every possible way.

We talk about empathy. Another very important aspect of work with underprivileged people. But empathy is not something that you can teach or learn. I cannot teach somebody how to be empathetic, and I cannot learn to be empathetic by watching someone. Yes, I can bring some of the actions that can be

	termed as actions of great empathy. But unless it is there within me, something that I have nurtured all my life, it will not get translated into your action.
Ambar:	But you know, given the geopolitical changes that are happening around us across the world, empathy is hard to come by. What do you envision will be different for a person who is interested in working with underprivileged communities like you do, in the future?
Urmi:	What public health and human rights advocates need to do now is to remain more in contact with each other, to try and form coalitions, and to be of support to each other. Like a major concern right now is, of course, the climate. And tampering with our seeds and our forests and our water.

How did this happen? This happened on our watch.

I have a friend who's an engineer and he gave up his career to go and work with the tribal people in Madhya Pradesh. His spouse is a tribal woman from there and is a scholar/activist. I have heard that for them, it's an everyday struggle. Just to go out and gather the seeds that they want to keep alive and give to their people to till the land.

Postscript

There are indeed several pathways to interpret this conversation between Urmi and Ambar in ways that might help to connect discourses and materialities of CHC theory and praxis. One of these interpretations could be about how the advocacy work of organizations such as New Light and interlocutors (Beverley, 2004) such as Urmi Basu might lead us to understand the value of pragmatic solidarity in CHC praxis.

Solidarity, according to Mattaini (2006), "is a willingness to make respectful common cause with the vulnerable" (p. 2). In *Subalternity and Representation*, John Beverley speaks about solidarity in terms of aligning scholarship and praxis with social justice, being committed to subaltern histories, and working toward the transformation of dominant power relations (Beverley, 1999). For Farmer (2003), solidarity is how one's scholarly work and praxis are relevant to the suffering of the vulnerable and how such work contributes to the removal of such suffering. Crucial to Farmer's conceptualization of solidarity is the commitment to interrogating and upending material violence that marks lives at the margins. In other words, solidarity needs to be pragmatic in the sense that those in control of power, resources and language, must, at the very least, engage in "ensuring that the rights of the vulnerable are honored, actively focusing one's work on relief of suffering in ways that are consonant with the vision of the vulnerable themselves" (Mattaini, 2006, p. 2). In *Pathologies of Power*, Farmer (2003) writes:

> If solidarity is among the most noble of human sentiments, then surely its more tangible forms are better still. Adding the material dimension to the equation—pragmatic solidarity—responds to the needs expressed by the people and communities who are living, and often dying, on the edge.
>
> *(p. 230)*

New Light has grown from an organization with meager means and limited goals of providing food, shelter, and health for the young children of sex workers in Kalighat, to a multi-faceted charitable organization that

> today serves more than 250 children of various age groups. The services offered by New Light includes education, healthcare, nutritional support, recreational facility, HIV/AIDS care, income generation opportunities for the women and residential care for many of the young children from the community. Legal aid and advocacy against gender based violence are other thrust areas of New Light's operation.
>
> *(New Light)*

New Light's program is, in essence, a health and social intervention with a modest beginning, and without a blueprint for goals and sustainability. It was not planned like funded health campaigns are generally done. While the unplanned nature is not always the case in health campaigns that work toward transformation at the margins (see for example the blueprint of a culture-centered campaign to address health and land rights of indigenous peoples (Dutta et al., 2020), it is critical to note that transformative work with the margins does not quite have a start and end point. Or a blueprint. An inspiration can well serve as a precursor to putting one's body on the line, as is the case with Urmi. Remember that Urmi comes from middle-class Bengali privilege, and this privilege harbors stigma toward people (and not just women) working with or associated with severely stigmatized sex workers. Add to this the fact that Urmi began this work with sex workers in Kalighat without any financial support, a blueprint for success, and without the trust of the most vulnerable women and children she prepared to work with. Taking risks to life, livelihood, and one's position in society points to putting one's body on the line as an act of solidarity. This idea aligns with the idea of accompaniment (Farmer, 2013), where solidarity involves being physically and emotionally present in places of suffering, or the idea that standing with the subaltern also implies a willingness to take risks by challenging structures—discursive and material—that marginalize (Beverley, 1999).

Solidarity—in its discourses and enactments—serves as a praxis for doing CHC work. In Urmi's life, solidarity was how she came in with nothing, had the courage to stake her life and the moral judgment that her middle-class community would subject her to, learn from the community, listen, and work together, often with not much theoretical guidance or an intervention blueprint—to collaboratively make meaningful change in the lives and health of women in sex work and their children. Solidarity actually plants the seeds for transformative work within systems of modernity that, while onerous to dismantle, must always be subject to dismantling. It is often arduous to visualize and enact a change in the system deep entrenched in necrocapital—an advanced capitalist system that punishes, kills, displaces, and dispossesses. Solidarity and advocacy in such times/contexts might mean working in whatever way possible to positively impact the lives of the dispossessed even if that means not being perfect in the execution of an intervention.

This idea of pragmatic solidarity finds resonance in a chapter by Heather Zoller in this book. Zoller situates the idea of critical pragmatism as a central orientation in her CHC praxis. She notes:

> the pragmatic orientation can prevent us from spiraling into arguments based in orthodoxies about the best way to achieve change (e.g., only socialism, government intervention, cultural change, etc.). By embracing more-than and both-and logics over binaries, we investigate how a multitude of experimental efforts (e.g., private, governmental, union, grassroots, corporate) can synergize to promote emancipatory changes.

And then, as a note to conclude and perhaps as a call for further thought, another aspect of such pragmatic advocacy/solidarity is a better understanding of what Urmi calls a strident need for synergy, a need to connect the advocacy dots. To repeat what she says:

> What public health and human rights advocates need to do now is to remain more in contact with each other, to try and form coalitions, and to be of support to each other. Like a major concern right now is, of course, the climate. And tampering with our seeds and our forests and our water.

As forces of necrocapital stifle advocacy, as "battering, child abuse, bullying, human trafficking, detention in contravention of international law and standards, torture and life-threatening poverty among other violations" (Mattaini, 2006) proliferate, all aided by global media and access to weapons, coalition building across struggles becomes critical. As resources available to the margins become increasingly sparse, and as climate, land, seeds, food, health, water, education, medicine, employment, human rights, dispossession, death, and displacement become threaded, so too should advocacy and solidarity synergistically keep up the struggle to distribute such resources equitably among human beings.

Notes

1 Di, short form for 'Didi,' refers to elder sister.
2 In India, witch-hunting is prevalent in several states, including Bihar, Jharkhand, and Odisha.

References

Basu, A. (2010). Communicating health as an impossibility: Sex work, HIV/AIDS, and the dance of hope and hopelessness. *The Southern Communication Journal*, *75*(4), 413–432. https://doi.org/10.1080/1041794x.2010.504452

Basu, A. (2011). HIV/AIDS and subaltern autonomous rationality: A call to recenter health communication in marginalized sex worker spaces. *Communication Monographs*, *78*(3), 391–408. https://doi.org/10.1080/03637751.2011.589457

Basu, A. (2017). Reba and her insurgent prose: Sex work, HIV/AIDS, and subaltern narratives. *Qualitative Health Research*, *27*(10), 1507–1517. https://doi.org/10.1177/1049732316675589

Basu, A., & Dutta, M. J. (2008). Participatory change in a campaign led by sex workers: connecting resistance to action-oriented agency. *Qualitative Health Research*, *18*(1), 106–119. https://doi.org/10.1177/1049732307309373

Basu, A., & Dutta, M. J. (2009). Sex workers and HIV/AIDS: Analyzing participatory culture-centered health communication strategies. *Human Communication Research*, *35*(1), 86–114. https://doi.org/10.1111/j.1468-2958.2008.01339.x

Basu, A., & Dutta, M. J. (2011). 'We are mothers first': Localocentric articulation of sex worker identity as a key in HIV/AIDS communication. *Women Health*, *51*(2), 106–123. https://doi.org/10.1080/03630242.2010.550992

Beverley, J. (1999). *Subalternity and representation: Arguments in cultural theory*. Duke University Press.

Beverley, J. (2004). *Testimonio: On the politics of truth*. University of Minnesota Press.

Dutta, M. J., Elers, C., & Jayan, P. (2020). Culture-centered processes of community organizing in COVID-19 response: Notes from Kerala and aotearoa New Zealand [Original Research]. *Frontiers in Communication*, *5*. https://doi.org/10.3389/fcomm.2020.00062

Farmer, P. (2013). *To repair the world: Paul farmer speaks to the next generation*. University of California Press.

Gramsci, A. (1971). *Prison notebooks: Volume 1*. Columbia University Press.
Lupton, D. (1994). Toward the development of critical health communication praxis. *Health Communication*, 6(1), 55–67.
Mattaini, M. A. (Ed.). (2006). *Editorial: Human rights, pragmatic solidarity, and behavior science* (1 ed., Vol. 5). https://doi.org/10.5210/bsi.v15i1.382
New Light. https://www.newlightindia.org/about_us.php

INDEX

Note: **Bold** page numbers refer to tables and page numbers followed by 'n' refer to notes.

1worker1vote.org 35
1worker1vote union cooperative movement 122, 125–127, 129
4-H program 166

abortion in Latine Community: and abortion laws in Argentina 85–87; decriminalization of 83–85, 88, 89; lack of care 82, 85, 88, 92; in Mexico 83–85, 88–91; misinformation and disinformation 80–83; procedures as public health risk 80, 81, 87; reducing maternal mortality rates 86; Spanish-language coverage of 83–91; stigmatization 80–83, 88; women's access 81–82, 85, 88, 92
academic-community partnership 16, 159, 164, 166, 170, 224
activism 13, 15–17, 41, 59, 64, 68, 149–152; collective reform through Equitable Food Initiative (EFI) 122–125; collective transformation through 1worker1vote union cooperative movement 122, 125–127
Adebayo, C. T. 9
Adénis, Marie-Sarah 198–199
Adichie, Chimamanda 242; "We Should All Be Feminists" 242
Adivasi scholarship 215, 216, 219
Adult Entertainment Sector (AES) 97
advocacy 7, 122, 125, 127–129, 160, 163, 166, 168, 172–174, 224, 274
African American farming crisis 45
African healthcare processes/system 235–236, 238; Westernization of 231
agriculture: farmers' resistance against corporatization 43–45; monopoly 124; subsidies 42–43
Airhihenbuwa, Collins 7, 212, 236, 238
Ait-Touati, Frédérique 199
The American College of Obstetricians and Gynecologists (ACOG) 84
anti-choice abortion discourse 80–84, 89, 92
anti-feminicidal activism 68
anti-violence activism 64, 68
Appalachian identity 41
Appalachian Nutrition Advisory Council (ANAC) 39
Ardener, Shirley 238
#ArgentinaDesdeLaConcepcion 85
Arizona Nutrition Standards (AZNS) 42

artificial intelligence (AI) 203
Asante, G. 12
Ashodaya Academy 139
Ashodaya Samithi 138–154; citizenship and activism 139–141, 149–152; critical ethnography 142; data collection and analysis 143–144; formation of 141–142; identity consciousness 144–147; interactions with police and health care systems 147–149; member participant profile 144
autoethnography 216
autoimmune deficiency syndrome (AIDS) 99, 140, 196, 258, 267; related deaths 138
Avahan, Bill & Melinda Gates Foundation Initiative 141, 144

Babu, S. 12
Baer, H. A. 5
Bah, Usman 248, 249, 251, 252, 254, 255, 258
Baldwin, James 117
Balkisa, Sissy 246, 249, 251, 253, 255
Barnett, J. T. 202
Basnyat, I. 99
Basu, Ambar 140, 196, 216, 221, 262–272
Basu, Urmi 262–274
bearing witness 66
Bejarano, C. 58
Bennett, J. A. 13
Benton, Adia 253
Bernard, Catherine 199–200
Beverley, John: *Subalternity and Representation* 272
Bill and Melinda Gates Foundation 161
bio-art 192
biocapital 186, 201
biocitizenship 186, 201
biocritical practices 192
biocriticism 185–204, 186; biofictions 186; biohumanities 202; bioidentification 186; bioimagination 186; biosemiotics 185; communication/rhetoric/critical health communication 191–196; as critical invention and intervention 186–188; emerging trajectories and critical health communication 200–204; examples 193–200; literature, performance, art, and criticism 196–200; sample research questions 189; theoretical influences and strains of 188, 190–193
biopolitics 186, 188, 190, 191
biopower 190, 191, 194
bio-rhetorics 185, 191
biosociality 186, 191, 201
biovalue 186, 201
Black farming/farmers 159–160; disparities 159–160; tradition 159
Black feminism 172, 174–175
Black Lives Matter movement 98
Black sovereignty 160
Black women: discrimination 49; farmers 158, 160
Bourdieu, P. 34
Bovee, W. G. 65
Brotherhood of Sleeping Car Porters (BSCP) 126
Brüggemann, M. 59
Bush, George W. 196
Butler, Judith 65, 202; work on grievability 65

Campos, Liliane 192
Cano, Brianda Padrón 56
cartel violence 63
caste/casteism 140, 210, 211, 213, 215, 216, 220–223, 225, 226
Center for Culture-Centered Approach to Research and Evaluation (CARE) 211, 219–220
charitable food distribution/programs 35, 38, 39, 41, 42
Child Nutrition Act policy 42
Chilton, M. 37
citizenship 139–141, 149–152
class discrimination 39
co-construction 255–256
coercive communication 101–104
cognitive-behavioral approaches 32
collective consciousness 150
collectivization 139, 148, 153
communication infrastructures 16, 45, 166–168
communication sovereignty 45
communicative disenfranchisement 12
communities: capacity building 139, 142, 152, 166; of color 31, 42, 160

community advisory groups (CAGs) 210–211, 217–218, 224, 225
community-based organization (CBO) 142
community-based participatory research (CBPR) 163, 172
community-engaged 41, 139, 141, 165, 199, 223
community-led structural intervention (CLSI) program 139, 152
Condit, C. M. 194
conscientious objection 85
Conservative Political Action Convention (CPAC) 91
Cooks, L. 37
Co-op Cincy 35, 125, 126
Co-op Dayton 126
Corona, I. 62
corporate agriculture 43–45
corporate irresponsibility 37
counter-hegemony 36, 49, 50, 116–119
COVID-19 pandemic 11–12, 59, 76, 196, 202, 247; affecting marginalized groups 79; antivaccination discourses 76; misinformation and disinformation during 76, 79; study in Nigeria 235–237
Crenshaw, K. 49
criminal justice 49, 61; interventions 57
critical-cultural theory 5
critical ethnography 142; methods 34
critical health communication (CHC): conceptual developments in 11–13; conceptualization 3–4; current state of critical research 8–10; origins and traditions 4–8; scholarship 32, 43, 57, 233–242; *see also individual entries*
Critically Holistic Framework of workplace health promotion 122–125, 128; health activism 122; promoting through transformative change 127–129
critical modernism 32, 49; approach to hunger 32–35; and health communication 33–34
critical pragmatism 129, 274; linking counter-hegemony and social change to 116–119
critical race theory 9

critical reflexivity 220–223
critical theory 3, 4, 33, 34
culture-centered approach (CCA) 6–7, 32, 43–45, 159, 162–164, 176n2–3, 195–196, 210–226, 245–258; agency 8, 44, 214–216, 236; body in resistance 220–225; "body on the line" concept 211, 223–225; CARE as transformative space 211, 219–220; communication infrastructures 163–164, 166–168; community spaces co-creation 217–218; critical reflexivity 220–223; culture 8, 43–44, 212–213; health communication resistance 216–220; methodological reflexivity 258; participation 163–166; partnerships 163, 168–170; philosophical reflexivity 258; reflexivity 164, 170–173; structural transformation 218–219; structure 8, 44, 213–214, 236; theorizing health 212–216; whiteness of health communication 217
culture(s): relativist approach 175; sensitivity 213, 251; of shame 213; stigma 247
cyber-biological beings 203; cybernetic intelligence 203; cyborg embodiment 203

Davis, C. S. 11
dehumanization 37, 63
De Los Santos Upton, S. 58
Dempsey, S. E. 12, 40, 41; *Organizing Eating: Communicating for Equity Across US Food Systems* 40
Derickson, K. D. 165
desconocidas (public women) 62, 63, 66
Dewey, John 117
diagnostic discourses **120**, 120–122
diagnostic reductionism 119–120
Dickinson, Adam 197–199; *Anatomic* 197–198
differential grievability 202
digital activism 13
disease exceptionalism 253
Dooling, D. 39
double-binding risks 79, 81
Dougherty, D. 37
Douglas, N.: *Everybody Eats: Communication and the Paths to Food Justice* 41

Dove, S. A. 11
DuBois, W. E. 126
Dutta, Mohan 2, 5, 12, 32, 40, 43, 45, 99, 140, 161, 163, 164, 195, 196, 212, 216, 221, 222, 224, 234–236, 238, 239, 258
Dutta-Bergman, M. J. 238

East India Company 261
Ebola 196, 234–235, 248, 249, 251–253
ecocriticism 202, 203
ecological crisis 202
ecological metrics 202
economic insecurity 37
embodied activism 224
entangled shame, concept of 39
entertainment establishments 96–99, 101
Entman, R. M. 59
environmental humanities 202–203
environmental justice/injustice 48, 220
Environmental Protection Agency 168
environmental sustainability 121, 126–129
Equitable Food Initiative (EFI) 122–124, 126, 129
"Equity and Inclusion": bill 170; protest march 158
Esposito, Roberto 199
ethical witnessing 64–66
Eurocentric middle-class ideologies 32
Eurocentrism 252
extractive capitalism 35, 124, 126, 127, 214, 224

Facebook 82, 83
Farmer, Paul 6, 7, 32, 98, 99, 272; *Pathologies of Power* 273
farming inequities 162; ACB 176n1; African American 45, 176n1
Farm Labor Organizing Committee 122–123
Farmworker Justice 123
fat/fatness/fat bodies 37
female sex workers (FSWs) 138, 143–145, 149, 152–153
femicides 57–58, 62, 67
feminicidal violence 56, 57, 61, 67
feminicides in Latin America 58; as global public health 57–59; in Mexico 56, 59, 62, 63, 68; news coverage 62, 63, 65, 67, 69; resisting 65–68; structural causes of 61
feminicidios 62–63, 66; definitions and trends 57–71; ethical witnessing and news coverage of 64–66, 68, 69; testimonios 68; violent visual imagery 66–67
feminist: activism 59; Latin American movements 82
Field-Springer, K. 77
Finnegan, N. 68
first-order risks 76–77, 79, 84–87, 91
food: assistance programs 39, 47; banks/banking 39, 40; commodification of 43; community organizing 39–41; corporate 31, 35, 124; corporatization 44; discourses 37–38; disparities 35; free 39; for health and social well-being 41; industry 37; injustices 35, 46; insecurity 31, 37, 38, 44, 46, 49, 161; justice 34, 43, 46, 48; pantries 39–40, 48, 121; place-based organizing in Appalachia 40–41; profit-driven capitalist 35; safety 39; security 34, 37, 41, 45, 160; shortages 34, 37; sovereignty 44, 45; system 46, 159; transformation 33, 121
Foucault, Michel 33, 49, 188, 190; biopolitical theory 42; biopower 115–116; *History of Sexuality, Volume I* 190
free market policies 80
Fregoso, R. 58, 63
Furgerson, J. 80

Gabriela, Jessica 56
Galtung, J. 6, 98
Galvez, Xóchitl 88–89
Geist-Martin, Patricia 12
gender: inequalities 9, 57, 97, 103, 107; labor 45, 105–107, 105–108; power imbalances 101, 107, 108, 147, 152; vulnerabilities 103, 104, 109
gender violence 56–68, 82; journalists' role and practices 59, 64, 66, 67; news discourses and coverage about 61, 64, 263; as public health concern 56, 59, 64, 65, 69; structures of 63; against women 59–64, 67

General Agreement on Trade and Tariffs (GATT) 43
genes 194
genetics 194
George, A. 152
Giddens, A. 42
Glaude, Eddie, Jr. 117
Global Day of Action 88
Godoy, M. 82
Gouge, C. 187
Gramsci, A. 33, 115, 116, 211; hegemony theorizing 115, 116; philosophy of praxis 211

Handbook of Health Communication 8
Haraway, D. J. 203
Harmes, R. H. 58
Harris, Kamala 83
Hawkins, D. S. 9
Hayles, N. K. 202
health activism 7, 116, 122
health communication 5, 32; hegemonic approaches to 216–217, 226; scholarship 8, 31, 39
Health Communication 5, 9
health disparities 11, 31, 39, 40, 41, 44, 46, 47, 108, 127, 250; approaches to managing 120–121; collectively reforming sociopolitical contexts 121; collectively transforming sociopolitical contexts 121; diagnostic discourses and **120**, 120–122; individually adapting to sociopolitical contexts approach 121; ignoring sociopolitical contexts approach 120
health inequities 109, 159, 214, 217; Black 159–160; role of power in 32, 33
Healthy Cities/Healthy Communities 119
hegemony 116; ideologies 34, 36; knowledge systems 210; structures 211, 214; theorizing 115
Hernández, L. H. 58
Hill, The 168
HIV 97, 138, 139, 141–143, 145, 148, 149, 152, 153, 154, 196, 258, 267; anti-retroviral therapy 32; *see also* autoimmune deficiency syndrome (AIDS)
Holling, M. A. 68

House Committee on Agriculture 166
Human Genome Project 194
human rights 19, 35, 50, 57, 58, 69, 98, 122, 274
hunger 31; among Black and Brown communities 35; charity in solving 35; counter-hegemonic assessments of 36; critical communication approach to 36–45; critical modernist approach to 32–35; industrial complex 35; power dynamics in discourses, practices, and policies 33; problem 33; root causes of 32, 37, 38, 46, 48; sustainable solutions to 41; women experiencing 38; *see also* critical communication approach to hunger
Hunt, K. P. 42

identity consciousness 144–147
identity risks 78–79, 89–90
ideological domination 115–119
illness attributions 117–119
Immokalee Workers' Fair Food Fight 125
imperialism 35, 210, 214, 215, 219, 222, 223, 224
Indigenous knowledge 215
Inflation Reduction Act 167
infodemics 76, 127
Institutional Review Board 100
Inter-American Commission on Human Rights (IACHR) 85, 86
International Women's Day 90
intersectional identity 10
intersubjectivity 4
Ivancic, S. 9, 39–42

Jana, S. 153
Joint United Nations Programme on HIV/AIDS (UNAIDS) 138, 152
journalism ethics 63
Journal of Applied Communication Research 161
Journal of the American Medical Association (JAMA) 6

Kalighat sex worker community 261, 262, 264, 266, 269, 273; *see also* New Light
Karnataka Health Promotion Trust (KHPT) 141, 143
Kaupapa Maori theory 224

Keränen, Lisa 191, 192
Khan, S. 201
Kline, K. N. 5, 187, 188, 201
knowledge: co-creation 222–223, 239; construction 9, 34; generation 164, 214, 215, 218, 222–223, 240; production 13, 161, 162, 164, 213, 214, 216, 221, 223, 239
Koerber, Amy 194–195
Kramarae, Cheris 238
Kristof, Nicholas 66; "*Half the Sky: Turning Oppression into Opportunity for Women Worldwide*" 262
Kumudini 100

LaPoe, B. R. 13
Latour, Bruno 199
LeGreco, M. 41, 42; *Everybody Eats: Communication and the Paths to Food Justice* 41
Le Virus Que Donc Je Suis (*The Virus Which Therefore I Am*) project 198–199
LGBTQ+/LGBTS 10, 12
Listening 1965 project 210–211
lived experiences 4, 10, 37, 44, 66, 97, 99–101, 108, 142, 144, 159, 163, 165, 169, 171, 218, 224, 234, 246, 248, 250, 253, 254
lunch: debt 46–47; shaming 46–47, 49
Lupton, Deborah 5, 9, 37, 238; *Toward the Development of Critical Health Communication Praxis* 5, 262
Lyne, John 191

MacKinnon, D. 165
male sex workers (MSWs) 143–145, 149
Mandel, Emily St John 200; *Station Eleven* 200
"Many Helping Hands" 44
#MarchaPorLaVida movement 85
marginalization 34, 35, 39, 40, 43, 47, 79, 97, 99, 101, 106, 139, 140, 152, 153, 250
marginalized communities 7, 8, 47, 138, 140, 141, 151–153, 152, 153, 162, 163, 172, 217, 218, 220, 222–224, 246, 251, 257, 263, 266
Martin, Z. C. 63

Marxist political economy 33, 245
materiality 32, 34, 39, 50; of food 36, 37
Mattaini, M. A. 272
Mbembe, A. 190, 202
McKnight, John 5
media ethics 65
Media Reform Coordinating Group (MRCG) 248
medical communication 5
Menem, Carlos 86
Menon, V. 69
mental health 9, 49, 81, 88, 96, 101, 104, 105, 119, 120, 125, 128, 246, 247, 249, 251
mental stress 99, 105
#MeToo movement 98
Meyers, M. 60
microbiology 202–203
Mindich, David 64
misogyny 57, 58
modernism 33
Mondragon cooperative values 126
Montgomery Bus Boycott 126
Montiel Valle, D. A. 63
moral agency 85
moral risks 77–78, 81; constructions 77; golden rule 87–88
Movimiento Viva Mexico campaign 83, 88
Muted Group Theory (MGT) 238–239

National Black Farmers Association 167
National Communication Association (NCA) 238
National Fish and Wildlife Foundation 168
National Institutes of Health 161
National School Lunch Program (NSLP) 46, 47
National Science Foundation 161
National Women in Agriculture Association (NWIAA) 158–160, 164–174
necrocapitalism 116
necropolitics 9, 12, 63, 65, 116
neoliberalism 13, 35, 39, 40, 45, 75, 129, 224, 225; agrarian reform 44, 45; logics 44, 45; policies 44, 172, 214; privatization 124; and stigma 40–42

Nepal Health Research Council (NHRC) 100
New Light 261–275
news frames/framing: of feminicidios 65; of reproductive feminicides 57; of violence against women 57, 59–64, 69
news production 59, 60
news reception 60, 64
Nigeria, decolonizing health communication in 231–242; context 233–237; COVID-19 study 236–237; critical health communication scholarship 233–242; methodology 239–241; researcher identity *vs.* site access and data collection 240–241; sexual violence research and study 238–241; theory 237–239
Ni Una Más movement 68
Ni Una Menos 59
nutritional needs/subsidies 39, 42–43

obesity 36–37
objectification 37, 97, 107, 108
objectivity 4, 62, 64, 69
occupational safety and health (OSH) 118
Okamoto, K. E. 39, 40
Op-Eds 168
oppression 39, 151; gender 107; neoliberal systems of 44; political-economic 32
Orientalism 247
Our Harvest 126
Oxfam 122

Pal, M. 45
Papa, W. 38
participatory action research 163, 167, 196, 225
patriarchy 57, 58, 221–223, 226; practices 213, 214; structures 44–45, 219
Patterson, Kent 67
PEN-3 model 7
Pesticide Action Network 123
Peters, J. D. 65, 66
Pew Research Center 76
philosophy of immunity 199
place based narrative labor 41
Planned Parenthood v. Casey 80–81
political violence 32

postcolonial elites in India 215, 221
postcolonial scholars/scholarship 215, 216
postcolonial theory 196, 237; postcolonial communication theory 210
postmodernity/postmodernism 33, 75
poststructuralism 49
poverty 31, 38, 217, 220; root causes of 32, 46
power 34; dynamics in public health discourse 76; inequities 116, 152, 159, 170, 172, 210; role in health inequities 32, 33
pragmatic utopianism 35
pregnant women, violence against 56; *see also* abortion
President's Emergency Plan for AIDS Relief (PEPFAR) program 196
pro-abortion 88, 89
pro-choice 88, 89
psychological distress 96, 103, 109
psychological harm 106, 107, 109

qualitative research methods 236, 239
queer theorizing 10
Quinlan, M. M. 11

racial biopolitics 42
racial capitalism 210, 211, 214, 217, 223
racial discrimination 39
racial inequalities 9, 202
racial neoliberalism 48
racial sovereignty 48
racism 217, 220; colorblind 42; environmental 13
Radford, J. 58
Ratzinger, J. 36
Rawat, M. 213
reflexivity 164, 170–173, 240; reflexive dialogues 22; reflexive journaling 222; reflexive modernity 75
reproductive feminicides 58, 63–64; in Mexico 56
reproductive health 82, 195
reproductive justice 81, 92
rhetoric of health and medicine (RHM) 7, 188, 193
risk orders theory approach 75–80, 83; combating medically inaccurate misinformation and disinformation

92; as critical method of examining reproductive health 92; first-order risks 76–77, 84–87; second-order risks 77–79, 87–90; third-order risks 79–81, 91; *see also* abortion in Latine Community
risk society 75
Rodriguez, C. 67
Roe v. Wade (1973) 82, 89, 91
Rohingya refugees 219
Rose, D. 37
Russell, Diana 58

Said, Edward 247
Sastry, Shaunak 8, 196, 245, 248–250, 251, 252, 254, 256
Schmid, A. T. 80
Schuwerk, K. 39
Scott, J. B. 187
Séginger, Gisele 192
self-harm 96
Serres, Michael 195
settler colonialism 214–216, 217, 223, 224
sexual harassment 97, 101, 103, 107, 108
sexual violence 63; research/study in Nigeria 238–241
Sharf, Barbara 12
Smith, Ali 199, 200
social change 116–119, 223, 224, 257–259
social change and CHC 45–49; lunch shaming and lunch debt in public schools 46–47
social class 37, 38
social determinants of health (SDH) 32, 79
social-ecological model (SEM) 6
social inequities 140
social justice/injustices 35, 46, 49, 68, 98, 109, 140, 216, 217, 221, 258
social risks 78, 81, 88–89
social stigma 35, 37, 38, 96, 138, 139, 141, 142, 146, 147, 152
social transformation 35, 43, 223, 258
solidarity 35, 85, 116, 125, 126, 140, 153, 154, 163–166, 172, 175, 216, 223, 224, 272–274, 272–275
de Souza, R. 11, 39; *Feeding the Other: Whiteness, Privilege, and Neoliberal Stigma in Food Pantries* 39, 46
Spieldenner, A. 10
Spivak, G. C. 214
state-sanctioned violence 58, 64
stereotypes 38, 41, 47, 49
STI 97, 139, 141–143, 149, 152
stigmatization 80–83, 88, 96, 97, 141, 151
Striley, K. 77
structural discrimination 138, 139, 141, 146, 150–152
structural racism 42
structural transformation 32, 45, 218–219
structural violence 10, 150, 151
structural violence within entertainment establishments 32, 96–109; coercive communication as 101–104, 108; concept of 98; description 98–99; deteriorating physical health as 104–105, 108; gendered labor as 105–108; lived experiences of women workers and health communication 99–101, 108; semi-structured in-depth interviews 100–101; social exclusion 106; unhealthy behavior normalization 101–105, 107, 108; women workers in Kathmandu, Nepal 100–107
structuration theory 42
subaltern knowledge 215, 220–221
Subaltern Studies collective 214–215
Supreme Court of Mexico 83, 88, 91
Susan B. Anthony Foundation 83
sustainability 2, 35, 48, 121, 126, 248, 273
symbiopolitics 203
symbolic annihilation 60
sympoiesis 203
synthetic biology 203
systemic discrimination 35, 144
systemic inequalities 14, 32, 97, 101, 107–109

Tait, S. 65, 66, 68
targeted regulations of abortion providers (TRAP) laws 81
Taylor, R. 60
Thaker, J. 45
TikTok 82

Total Worker Health initiative 123
Tracy, S. J. 240
trade liberalization 43
transgender people 138
Transgender Persons (Protection of Rights) Bill (2019) 140
transgender sex workers 139, 143–145, 149, 150
trauma-informed journalism 67–69
Truman, Harry 47
Trump, Donald 91
Tucker, R. V. 13

unhealthy foods 35, 44, 175
United Nations 59
United States Department of Agriculture (USDA) 48, 167, 170, 172; Food Environment Atlas 159
U.S. Agency for International Development 166
U.S. Centers for Disease Control (CDC) 123
USDA Foreign Agriculture Services 166
USDA Natural Agricultural Statistics Service (NASS) 160
U.S. Farm Bill 42, 43
U.S. hunger policy 42
U.S. immigration policy 48, 49
U.S.-Mexico border 58, 61
U.S. Supreme Court 91
U.S. Surgeon General 82

Vardeman-Winter, J. 9
Verástegui, Eduardo 83–92; *see also* abortion in Latine Community
verbal abuse 97, 103, 109
Vermeulen, Pieter 200; "Depopulating the Novel: Post-Catastrophe Fiction, Scale, and the Population Unconscious" 200
victim-blaming language 60–61
violence journalism 61–62, 63, 66, 67
Viral 199
Virgin Islands Women in Agriculture Association (VIWIAA) 168–169
virus-masks 198–199, *199*
voice infrastructures 210, 211, 218–220, 226

Voices of Hunger project 44
volunteer labor 38, 39

Waitzkin, Howard 6, 12
Walker, Connie 67
Wallace, L. R. 64
Watson, K. 80, 81
Weick's sensemaking theory 117
Western-centric ideologies 238
Western lifestyle attributions 118–119
Western medicine 235
Western public health 118
white saviorism 41
Whole Foods 123
Williams, Raymond 187
women: of color 34; experiences of working in entertainment establishments 97–99, 101; exploitative practices 97, 101–103, 108; identity and ability to procreate 90; marginalization 34; representations in mass media 60; reproductive health risk discourse 80; rights 68; shaming for bodies and bodily functions 213; smoking and alcohol consumption among 101–105, 109
worker ownership 35, 125, 126
Worker Owner Workbook 126
Working Well 123
workplace health promotion (WHP) 118; *see also* Critically Holistic framework of workplace health promotion
World Health Organization (WHO) 58, 76, 119, 237
Wright 63
WuDunn, Sheryl: "*Half the Sky: Turning Oppression into Opportunity for Women Worldwide*" 262

Yep, G. A. 10
Yixuan Qi 247–250, 257

Zango communities in Ghana 246, 255
Zhao, X. 99
Zoller, Heather 2, 5, 9, 35, 187, 188, 242, 258, 274